THE PSYCHOLOGY OF PAIN

The Psychology of Pain

Edited by

Richard A. Sternbach, Ph.D.

Director, Pain Treatment Center
Scripps Clinic Medical Group, Inc.
La Jolla, California

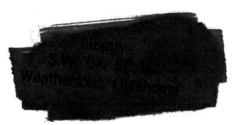

Raven Press ■ New York

Raven Press, 1140 Avenue of the Americas, New York, New York 10036

Made in the United States of America

Library of Congress Cataloging in Publication Data

The Psychology of Pain.

    Includes bibliographical references and index.
    1. Pain–Psychological aspects–Addresses,
essays, lectures. I. Sternbach, Richard A.
[DNLM: 1. Pain–Psychology. WL704 P974]
BF515.P79   152.4   77-84554
ISBN 0-89004-278-0

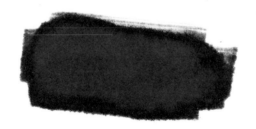

Preface

This text provides a systematic review of the literature on the psychology of pain, gathering in one convenient volume references previously scattered in wide and diversified publications.

The psychological aspects of pain include neurological, behavioral, perceptual, cognitive, and clinical research studies, and the authors of the chapters included in this volume view the phenomenon from these varied points of view. All have contributed extensively to the research literature on pain, both experimental and clinical, and it is this burgeoning literature that makes this survey desirable.

This work will be of interest to psychologists who wish to know what contributions have been (and can be) made to a difficult physiological and medical problem by the unique approaches available to psychology. This book will also be of interest to those in the many other disciplines and professions whose work involves the area of pain and who wish a convenient review of the psychology of pain.

In order to expedite publication, this volume is being produced by photocopying the original manuscripts. Thus the reader will have an up-to-date review, which may serve as a benchmark for later evaluations of the field.

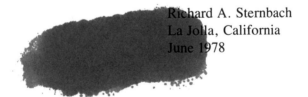

Richard A. Sternbach
La Jolla, California
June 1978

Contents

Contributors

J. Timothy Cannon, Ph.D.: *Postdoctoral Fellow, Department of Psychology, University of California, Los Angeles, Los Angeles, California 90024*

C. Richard Chapman, Ph.D.: *Associate Professor, Departments of Anesthesiology, Psychiatry and Behavioral Sciences, and Psychology RN-10, University of Washington, Seattle, Washington 98195*

Kenneth D. Craig, Ph.D.: *Associate Professor, Department of Psychology, University of British Columbia, Vancouver, B.C., Canada V6T 1W5*

Stephen G. Dennis, Ph.D.: *Postdoctoral Fellow, Department of Psychology, McGill University, 1205 McGregor Avenue, Montreal, Quebec, Canada H3A 1B1*

Wilbert E. Fordyce, Ph.D.: *Professor (Psychology), Department of Rehabilitation Medicine RJ-30, University Hospital, University of Washington, Seattle, Washington 98195*

Hanan Frenk, Ph.D.: *Assistant Professor, Department of Psychology, Tel Aviv University, Ramat Aviv, Israel*

Ernest R. Hilgard, Ph.D.: *Professor Emeritus, Department of Psychology, Stanford University, Stanford, California 94305*

John C. Liebeskind, Ph.D.: *Professor, Department of Psychology, University of California, Los Angeles, Los Angeles, California 90024*

Ronald Melzack, Ph.D.: *Professor, Department of Psychology, McGill University, Montreal, Quebec, Canada H3A 1B1*

Harold Merskey, D.M, M.R.C.P., F.R.C.P. (C), F.R.C. Psych.: *Professor of Psychiatry, The University of Western Ontario, and Director of Education and Research, London Psychiatric Hospital, 850 Highbury Avenue, London, Ontario, Canada, N6A 4H1*

Issy Pilowsky, M.D., F.R.C. Psych., F.R.A.N.Z.C.P., F.R.A.C.P.: *Professor of Psychiatry, The University of Adelaide, Royal Adelaide Hospital, Adelaide, South Australia, 5000*

Richard A. Sternbach, Ph.D.: *Director, Pain Treatment Center, Scripps Clinic Medical Group, Inc., 10666 North Torrey Pines Road, La Jolla, California 92037*

B. Berthold Wolff, Ph.D.: *Research Professor of Psychology, Chief, Pain Study Group, New York University Medical Center, 550 First Avenue, New York, New York 10016*

The Psychology of Pain, edited by R. A. Sternbach.
Raven Press, New York © 1978.

Neurophysiological Foundations of Pain

R. Melzack and S.G. Dennis

Department of Psychology, McGill University, Montreal, Quebec, Canada, H3A 1B1

INTRODUCTION

The problem of pain was long thought to be primarily the concern of the physiologist and anatomist, and the management of pain was almost exclusively the task of the neurosurgeon and neurologist. All this has changed in recent years. It is now recognized that every physiological explanation of pain contains an implicit psychological concept that has a profound impact on both the study and treatment of pain. The problem of pain, therefore, has been investigated increasingly by psychologists, and psychological methods are, accordingly, often used in the treatment of chronic pain problems.

The psychological and clinical phenomena of pain provide the framework for the physiological problems we will consider in this chapter. Pain, we now know (30), is a highly personal, variable experience which is influenced by cultural learning, the meaning of the situation, attention, and other cognitive activities. How does the central nervous system function to permit such powerful cognitive control over the somatic sensory input? Pain, it is generally acknowledged, is primarily a signal that body tissues are being or have been injured; yet pain may persist for years after tissues have healed and damaged nerves have regenerated. How can we account for neurophysiological processes that go on for such long durations? Similarly, pain and trigger zones sometimes spread to distant, unrelated parts of the body. Can we understand such phenomena in terms of the known connections among neurons in the nervous system? While present-day physiology has answers to some of these problems, it is not even close to explaining others.

It is customary to describe the somatosensory system by proceeding from the peripheral receptors to the transmission routes that carry nerve impulses to areas in the brain. However, it is essential to remember that stimulation of receptors does not mark the beginning of the pain process. Rather, stimulation produces neural signals that enter an active nervous system that (in the adult organism) is already the substrate of past experience, culture, anxiety and so forth. These brain processes actively

1

participate in the selection, abstraction and synthesis of information from the total sensory input. Pain, then, is not simply
the end product of a linear sensory transmission system. Rather,
it is a dynamic process which involves continuous interactions
among complex ascending and descending systems.

Because every aspect of pain is the subject of vigorous
debate, it is impossible to discuss pain without taking a theoretical point of view. As we shall see, a seemingly innocuous
phrase such as "pain fibres" presupposes a specific theoretical
position. This chapter, therefore, examines the various facets
of pain from a well-defined theoretical framework.

PAIN MODULATION

The traditional specificity theory of pain, which is still
taught in most medical and graduate schools, proposes that pain
is a specific sensation and that the intensity of pain is proportional to the extent of tissue damage. The theory implies a
fixed, straight-through transmission system from somatic pain
receptors to a pain center in the brain. Recent evidence, however, shows that pain is not simply a function of the amount of
bodily damage alone,but is influenced by attention, anxiety,
suggestion, prior conditioning, and other psychological variables
(30). Moreover, the natural outcome of the specificity concept
of pain has been the development of neurosurgical techniques to
cut the so-called pain pathway. When failures occur, they are
attributed to an escape of "pain fibres", so that operations are
carried out at successively higher levels of the nervous system.
Generally, the results have been disappointing, particularly for
low back pain, the neuralgias, and other chronic pain syndromes.
Not only does the pain tend to return in a substantial proportion
of patients, but new pains may be "unmasked" and other iatrogenic
complications, such as dysesthesias, "girdle pains", and various
sensory-motor losses, may occur (40). The psychological and
neurological data, then, refute the concept of a single straight-
through sensory transmission system.

In recent years the evidence on pain has moved in the direction of recognizing the plasticity and modifiability of events in
the central nervous system. The psychological evidence lends
strong support to the consideration of pain as a complex perceptual and affective experience determined by the unique past history of the individual, by the meaning of the stimulus to him, by
his "state of mind" at the moment, as well as by the sensory
nerve patterns evoked by physical stimulation.

The Gate Control Theory of Pain

It was in the light of this understanding of pain processes
that Melzack and Wall (37) proposed the gate control theory of
pain. Basically, the theory proposes that neural mechanisms in
the dorsal horns of the spinal cord act like a gate which can
increase or decrease the flow of nerve impulses from peripheral

fibres to the spinal cord cells that project to the brain.
Somatic input is therefore subjected to the modulating influence
of the gate before it evokes pain perception and response. The
theory suggests that large-fibre inputs tend to close the gate
while small-fibre inputs generally open it, and that the gate is
also profoundly influenced by descending influences from the
brain. It further proposes that the sensory input is modulated
at successive synapses throughout its projection from the spinal
cord to the brain areas responsible for pain experience and response. Pain occurs when the number of nerve impulses that
arrives at these areas exceeds a critical level.

Wall (62) has recently assessed the present-day status of the
gate-control theory in the light of new physiological research.
It is apparent that the theory is alive and well despite considerable controversy and conflicting evidence. Although some of
the physiological details may need revision, the concept of
gating (or input modulation) is stronger than ever.

Spinal Cord Mechanisms

The dorsal horns, which receive fibres from the body and project impulses towards the brain, provide valuable clues about
information processing at the spinal cord level. The dorsal
horns comprise several layers or laminae, each of which is now
known to have specialized functions. The inputs and outputs of
each lamina are not entirely understood. But the picture which
emerges, based largely on the work by Wall and his colleagues
(see 23), reveals that the input is modulated in the dorsal horns
before it is transmitted to the brain.

Lamina 1 cells are known (43) to receive information from the
small-diameter peripheral nerve fibres (the A-delta and C fibres)
when the skin is crushed or burned, and a portion of them project
directly to higher levels of the spinal cord. It is reasonable,
therefore, to assume that they play a role in pain processes.
However, the picture is far more complex than this. Just below
lamina 1 are the cells that comprise the substantia gelatinosa
(laminae 2 and 3). This region is of particular interest because
it represents a unique system on each side of the spinal cord
which appears to have a modulating effect on the input (60).
Many afferent fibres from the skin terminate in the substantia
gelatinosa, and the dendrites of many cells in lower laminae,
whose axons project to the brain, lie within the substantia
gelatinosa. This region, then, is situated between a major portion of the peripheral nerve fibre terminals and the spinal cord
cells that project to the brain. There is convincing physiological evidence (37) that the substantia gelatinosa has a modulating
effect on transmission from peripheral fibres to spinal cells.

Below the substantia gelatinosa, the cells in lamina 4 have
small cutaneous receptive fields and project to the dorsolateral
pathway ipsilaterally and probably to the lamina 5 cells (23).
Lamina 4 cells tend to respond when gentle pressure is applied to
the skin, and to electrical stimulation of the large A-beta

myelinated fibres. However, their response rate usually fails to
increase when the skin is pinched or crushed or when the A-delta
and C fibres are activated. These cells, then, are selectively
tuned to gentle pressure applied within their receptive fields.

In contrast, lamina 5 cells usually have a wide dynamic range
and are particularly responsive when noxious stimuli are applied
within their receptive fields (23). Their fields have a remarkably complex organization, and they respond with characteristic
firing patterns to stimulation over a wide range of intensities.
Moreover, lamina 5 cells receive multiple inputs. There is reason to believe that they receive inputs from the lamina 4 cells.
In addition, they receive inputs from the small myelinated and
unmyelinated fibres from the skin, from deeper tissues such as
blood vessels and muscles, and from the viscera (44).

It is now known that virtually all dorsal horn cells are under
the control of fibres that descend from the brain. These cells,
moreover, with the exception of the substantia gelatinosa, have
extensive projections to the brain. In primates, the majority
project through the spinothalamic tract, while some appear to
project through the dorsolateral and dorsal column systems. Although the deeper laminae (6 to 10) have not been examined as
extensively as lamina 5, there is evidence that they also contribute to the pattern of afferent pain signals (16).

The mechanism of the inhibition produced by the large fibres
and the facilitation produced by the small fibres is unknown,
but Hillman and Wall (23) suggest that it may be due to pre- and
post-synaptic effects produced by the small cells of laminae 2
and 3. A similar effect has been observed by Mendell and Wall
(38). They found that a single electrical pulse delivered to
small fibres produces a burst of nerve impulses followed by repetitive discharges in spinal cord cells. Successive pulses, if
delivered at sufficiently high frequency, produce a "wind-up"
effect--a burst followed by a discharge of increasing duration
after each stimulation. In contrast, successive pulses delivered
to large fibres produce a burst of impulses followed by a "turn-
off" or period of silence after each pulse. These opposing
effects of facilitation and inhibition after small and large
fibre stimulation are believed (60) to be mediated by the substantia gelatinosa, and provide the physiological basis of the
gate-control theory.

The Gate-Control Concept

The conceptual model that underlies the gate-control theory of
pain is based on the following propositions:
1. The transmission of nerve impulses from afferent fibres to
spinal cord transmission (T) cells is modulated by a spinal gating
(SG) mechanism in the dorsal horns.

2. The spinal gating mechanism is influenced by the relative
amount of activity in large-diameter (L) and small-diameter (S)
fibres: activity in large fibres tends to inhibit transmission

(close the gate) while small-fibre activity tends to facilitate transmission (open the gate).

3. The spinal gating mechanism is influenced by nerve impulses that descend from the brain.

4. A specialized system of large-diameter, rapidly conducting fibres (the Central Control Trigger) activates selective cognitive processes that then influence, by way of descending fibres, the modulating properties of the spinal gating mechanism.

5. When the output of the spinal cord transmission (T) cells exceeds a critical level, it activates the Action System--those neural areas that underlie the complex, sequential patterns of behaviour and experience characteristic of pain.

The small (A-delta and C) fibres, in this conceptual framework, play a highly specialized and important role in pain processes. They activate the T-cells directly and contribute to their output. The activity of high-threshold small fibres, during intense stimulation, may be especially important in raising the T-cell output above the critical level necessary for pain. But the small fibres are believed (37) to do much more than this. They facilitate transmission ("open the gate") and thereby provide the basis for summation, prolonged activity, and spread of pain to other body areas. This facilitatory influence provides the small fibres with greater power than any envisaged in the concept of "pain fibres". Yet at the same time the small-fibre impulses are susceptible to modulation by activities in the whole nervous system. This multi-faceted role of the small fibres is consistent with the psychological, clinical, and physiological evidence.

The substantia gelatinosa (laminae 2 and 3) appears to be the most likely site of the spinal gating mechanism (37,60). It receives axon terminals from many of the large- and small-diameter fibres and the dendrites of cells in deeper laminae project into it. The substantia gelatinosa, moreover, forms a functional unit that extends the length of the spinal cord on each side. Furthermore, its rostral extension is continuous with the substantia gelatinosa of the trigeminal system. Its cells connect with one another by short fibres, and influence each other at distant sites on the same side by means of Lissauer's tract and on the opposite side by means of commissural fibres that cross the cord (58). The substantia gelatinosa, then, consists of a highly specialized, closed system of cells throughout the length of the spinal cord on both sides; it receives afferent input from large and small fibres, and is able to influence the activity of cells that project to the brain.

We have already noted that cognitive or "higher central nervous system processes" exert a powerful influence on pain processes. It is also firmly established that stimulation of several different brain regions activates descending efferent fibres

which can influence afferent conduction at the earliest synaptic
levels of the somesthetic system. Thus it is possible for brain
activities subserving attention, emotion and memories of prior
experience to exert control over the sensory input. This control
of spinal cord transmission by the brain may be exerted through
several systems.

Reticular projections. The brainstem reticular formation, particularly the midbrain reticular areas (see 16), exert a powerful
inhibitory control over information projected by the spinal
transmission cells. The inhibition of activity in lamina 5 cells
by descending fibres from the brain is at least partly due to
reticulo-spinal influences on the dorsal horn gating system.
This descending inhibitory projection is itself controlled by
multiple influences. Somatic projections comprise the largest
input to the midbrain reticular formation. There are also projections from the visual and auditory systems (47). In this way,
somatic inputs from all parts of the body, as well as visual and
auditory inputs, are able to exert a modulating influence on
transmission through the dorsal horns.

Cortical projections. Fibres from the whole cortex, particularly
the frontal cortex, project to the reticular formation. Cognitive processes such as past experience and attention, which are
subserved at least in part by cortical neural activity, are
therefore able to influence spinal activities by way of the
reticulo-spinal projection system. Cognitive processes can also
influence spinal gating mechanisms by means of pyramidal (or
cortico-spinal) fibres, which are known to project to the dorsal
horns as well as to other spinal areas. These are large, fast-
conducting fibres so that cognitive processes can rapidly and
directly modulate neural transmission in the dorsal horns.

Concept of a central control trigger. It is apparent that the
influence of cognitive "central control" processes on spinal
transmission are mediated, in part at least, through the gate-
control system. While some central activities, such as anxiety
or excitement, may open or close the gate for all inputs from
any part of the body, others obviously involve selective, localized gate activity. Melzack and Wall (37) have therefore proposed that there exists in the nervous system a mechanism, which
they have called the central control trigger, that activates the
particular, selective brain processes. These brain activities,
they suggest, do not give rise to sensory experience, but instead
act, by way of central-control efferent fibres, on the gate-
control system. Part, at least, of their functions, then, could
be to activate selective brain processes such as memories of
prior experience and pre-set response strategies that influence
information which is still arriving over slowly conducting fibres
or is being transmitted up more slowly conducting pathways.
These functions will be discussed in more detail in the next
section.

THE DIMENSIONS OF PAIN EXPERIENCE

The problem of pain, since the beginning of this century, has been dominated by the concept that pain is purely a sensory experience. Yet pain also has a distinctly unpleasant, affective quality. It becomes overwhelming, demands immediate attention, and disrupts ongoing behaviour and thought. It motivates or drives the organism into activity aimed at stopping the pain as quickly as possible. To consider only the sensory features of pain, and ignore its motivational-affective properties, is to look at only part of the problem. Even the concept of pain as a perception, with full recognition of past experience, attention, and other cognitive influences, still neglects the crucial motivational dimension.

The motivational-affective dimension of pain is brought clearly into focus by clinical studies on frontal lobotomy, congenital insensitivity to pain, and pain asymbolia. Patients who have undergone a frontal lobotomy (which severs the connections between the prefrontal lobes and the thalamus) rarely complain about severe clinical pain or ask for medication (20). Typically, these patients report after the operation that they still have pain but it does not bother them. When they are questioned more closely, they frequently say that they still have the "little" pain, but the "big" pain, the suffering, the anguish are

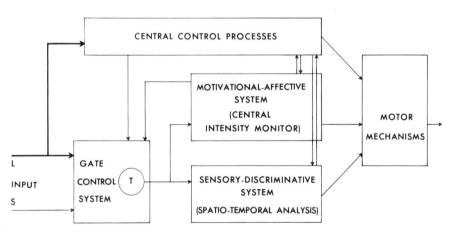

FIG. 1. Conceptual model of the sensory, motivational and central control determinants of pain. The output of the T (transmission) cells of the gate control system projects to the sensory-discriminative system and the motivational-affective system. The central control trigger is represented by a line running from the large fibre system to central control processes; these, in turn, project back to the gate control system, and to the sensory-discriminative and motivational-affective systems. All three systems interact with one another, and project to the motor system.

gone. It is certain that the sensory component of pain is still present because these patients may complain vociferously about pin prick and mild burn. The predominant effect of lobotomy, in relation to pain, appears to be on the motivational-affective dimension. The aversive quality of the pain and the drive to seek pain relief both appear to be diminished.

People who are congenitally insensitive to pain also are able to feel pricking, warmth, cold, and pressure. They give accurate reports of increasing intensity of stimulation, but the input, even at intense, noxious levels, seems never to well up into frank pain. The evidence (56) suggests that it is not the sensory properties of the input but rather the motivational-affective properties that are absent. Similarly, patients exhibiting "pain asymbolia" (48) after lesions of portions of the parietal lobe or the frontal cortex are able to appreciate the spatial and temporal properties of noxious stimuli but fail to withdraw or complain about them.

These considerations suggest that there are three major psychological dimensions of pain: sensory-discriminative, motivational-affective, and cognitive-evaluative. Melzack and Casey (32) have proposed that they are subserved by physiologically specialized systems in the brain (Fig. 1).

Physiological Mechanisms

The Sensory-Discriminative Dimension

Physiological and behavioural studies suggest that several rapidly conducting systems--the neospinothalamic tract, the spinocervical tract and possibly the postsynaptic elements in the dorsal column system contribute to the sensory-discriminative dimension of pain. Neurons in the ventrobasal thalamus, which receive a large portion of their afferent input from these systems, show discrete somatotopic organization. Studies in human patients and in animals (see 61) have shown that surgical section of the dorsal columns, long presumed to subserve virtually all of the discriminative capacity of the skin sensory system, produces little or no loss in fine tactile discrimination and localization. Furthermore, Semmes and Mishkin (50) found marked deficits in tactile discriminations that are attributable to injury of the cortical projection of the neospinothalamic system. These data, taken together, suggest that the rapidly conducting projection systems have the capacity to process information about the spatial, temporal, and magnitude properties of the input. It is possible, of course, that information from these rapidly conducting systems may reach reticular and limbic structures via several indirect routes.

The Motivational-Affective Dimension

There is convincing evidence (32) that the brainstem reticular formation and the limbic system, which receive projections from the spinoreticular and paleo-spinothalamic components of the anterolateral somatosensory pathway, play a particularly important role in the motivational-affective dimension of pain. These medially coursing fibres, which comprise a "paramedial ascending system" (32), tend to be short and connect diffusely with one another during their ascent from the spinal cord to the brain. They are not organized to carry discrete spatial and temporal information. Their target cells in the brain usually have wide receptive fields, sometimes covering half or more of the body surface. In addition to the convergence of somatosensory fibres, inputs from other sensory systems, such as vision and audition, also arrive at many of these cells.

Reticular formation. It is now well established that the reticular formation is involved in aversive drive and similar pain-related behaviour. Stimulation of nucleus gigantocellularis in the medulla (10) and the central grey and adjacent areas in the midbrain (14) produces strong aversive drive and behaviour typical of responses to naturally occurring painful stimuli. In contrast, lesions of the central grey or spinothalamic tract produce marked decreases in responsiveness to noxious stimuli (36). Similarly, at the thalamic level, "fear-like" responses associated with escape behaviour have been elicited by stimulation in the medial and adjacent intralaminar nuclei of the thalamus (46). In the human, lesions in the medial thalamus (parafascicular and centromedian complex) and intralaminar nuclei have provided relief from intractable pain (63).

Although these reticular areas are clearly involved in pain, they may also play a role in other somatosensory processes. Casey (10) found that sixteen out of twenty cells in nucleus gigantocellularis responded to tapping or moderate pressure on the skin. The response pattern of the cells, moreover, was a function of the intensity of stimulation; the cells responded with a more intense and prolonged discharge to stimuli (pinch, pin prick) that elicited withdrawal of the tested limb. Similarly, Becker et al. (5) found that many cells in the midbrain central grey and tegmentum responded to electrical stimulation of large, low-threshold fibres. An increase in the stimulus level in order to fire the small, high-threshold fibres produced distinctively patterned responses showing high discharge rates, prolonged afterdischarges for several seconds, and the "wind-up" effect (increasing neural response to repeated intense stimuli).

Limbic system. The reciprocal interconnections between the reticular formation and the limbic system is of particular importance in pain processes (32). The midbrain central grey, which is traditionally part of the reticular formation, is also a major gateway to the limbic system. It is part of the "limbic midbrain area" (39) that projects to the medial thalamus and hypothalamus which in turn project to limbic forebrain structures. Many of these areas also interact with portions of the frontal cortex that are sometimes functionally designated as part of the limbic system.

It is now firmly established (see 32) that the limbic system
plays an important role in pain processes. Electrical stimulation of the hippocampus, amygdala, or other limbic structures may
evoke escape or other attempts to stop stimulation (15). After
ablation of the amygdala and overlying cortex, cats show marked
changes in affective behaviour, including decreased responsiveness to noxious stimuli (49). Surgical section of the cingulum
bundle, which connects the frontal cortex to the hippocampus,
also produces a loss of "negative affect" associated with intractable pain in human subjects (17). This evidence indicates that
limbic structures, although they play a role in many other functions, provide a neural basis for the aversive drive and affect
that comprise the motivational dimension of pain.

These data show clearly that the neural areas comprising the
paramedial, reticular, and limbic systems are involved in the
motivational and affective features of pain. The manner in which
these areas are brought into play will be discussed shortly.

The Cognitive-Evaluative Dimension

We have already noted that cognitive activities such as cultural values, anxiety, attention and suggestion all have a profound
effect on pain experience. These activities, which are subserved
in part at least by cortical processes, may affect the sensory-
discriminative dimension or the motivational-affective dimension.
Thus, excitement in games or war appears to block both of these
dimensions of pain, while suggestion and placebos may modulate
the motivational-affective dimension and leave the sensory-
discriminative dimension relatively undisturbed.

Cognitive functions, then, are able to act selectively on sensory processing or motivational mechanisms. In addition, there
is evidence that the sensory input is localized, identified in
terms of its physical properties, evaluated in terms of past
experience, and modified before it activates the discriminative
or motivational systems. Men wounded in battle may feel little
or no pain from the wound but may complain bitterly about an in-
ept vein puncture (6). Dogs that repeatedly receive food immediately after the skin is shocked, burned, or cut soon respond to
these stimuli as signals for food and salivate, without showing
any signs of pain, yet howl as normal dogs would when the stimuli
are applied to other sites on the body (42).

The neural system that performs these complex functions of
identification, evaluation, and selective input modulation must
conduct rapidly to the cortex so that somatosensory information
has the opportunity to undergo further analysis, interact with
other sensory inputs, and activate memory stores and pre-set
response strategies. It must then be able to act selectively on
the sensory and motivational systems in order to influence their
response to the information being transmitted over more slowly
conducting pathways. Melzack and Wall (37) have proposed that
the dorsal-column and dorsolateral projection pathways act as the

"feed-forward" limb of this loop. The dorsal column pathway, in particular, has grown apace with the cerebral cortex (7), carries precise information about the nature and location of the stimulus, adapts quickly to give precedence to phasic stimulus changes rather than prolonged tonic activity, and conducts rapidly to the cortex so that its impulses may begin activation of central control processes.

Influences that descend from the cortex are known to act, via pyramidal and other central-control fibres, on portions of the sensory-discriminative system such as the ventrobasal thalamus (51). Moreover, the powerful descending inhibitory influences exerted on dorsal-horn cells in the spinal cord (23) can modulate the input before it is transmitted to the discriminative and motivational systems (Fig. 1). These rapidly conducting ascending and descending systems can thus account for the fact that psychological processes play a powerful role in determining the quality and intensity of pain.

The frontal cortex may play a particularly significant role in mediating between cognitive activities and the motivational-affective features of pain. It receives information via intracortical fibre systems from virtually all sensory and association-al cortical areas and projects strongly to reticular and limbic structures. The effects of lobotomy, which are characterized by lowered affect and decreased drive for narcotics and other methods of pain relief, could be due to disruption of the regulating effects of central control processes on activity in the reticular and limbic systems.

The Conceptual Model

The physiological and behavioural evidence described above led Melzack and Casey (32) to extend the Gate Control Theory to include the motivational dimension of pain (Fig. 1). They proposed that:

1. The sensory-discriminative dimension of pain is influenced primarily by the rapidly conducting spinal systems.

2. The powerful motivational drive and unpleasant affect characteristic of pain are subserved by activities in reticular and limbic structures which are influenced primarily by the slowly conducting spinal systems.

3. Neocortical or higher central nervous system processes, such as evaluation of the input in terms of past experience, exert control over activity in both the discriminative and motivational systems.

It is assumed that these three categories of activity interact with one another to provide <u>perceptual information</u> regarding the location, magnitude, and spatiotemporal properties of the noxious stimulus, <u>motivational tendency</u> toward escape or attack, and <u>cognitive information</u> based on analysis of multi-modal information, past experience, and probability of outcome of different response strategies. All three forms of activity could then influence motor mechanisms responsible for the complex pattern of overt responses that characterize pain.

A crucial question still remains. The somatic input has access to reticular and limbic areas involved in both approach and avoidance, and stimulation of some areas can produce either kind of response. On what basis, then, are aversive rather than approach mechanisms triggered by the input?

Melzack and Casey propose that portions of the reticular and limbic systems function as a <u>central intensity monitor</u>: that their activities are determined, in part at least, by the intensity of the T-cell output (the total number of active fibres and their rate of firing) after it has undergone modulation by the gate-control system in the dorsal horns. The cells in the midbrain reticular formation are capable of summation of input from spatially separate body sites; furthermore, the post-stimulus discharge activity of some of these cells lasts for many seconds, so that their activity may provide a measure of the intensity of the total T-cell output over relatively long periods of time. Essentially, both kinds of summation transform discrete spatial and temporal information into intensity information. Melzack and Casey propose that the output of these cells, up to a critical intensity level, activates those brain areas subserving positive affect and approach tendency. Beyond that level, the output activates areas underlying negative affect and aversive drive. They suggest, therefore, that the drive mechanisms associated with pain are activated when the somatosensory input into the motivational-affective system exceeds the critical level. This notion fits well with observations (21) that animals seek low-intensity electrical stimulation of some limbic system structures, but avoid or actively try to stop high-intensity stimulation of the same areas. Signals from these limbic structures to motor mechanisms, together with the information derived from sensory and cognitive processes, could selectively activate neural networks that subserve adaptive response patterns.

The complex sequences of behaviour that characterize pain are determined by sensory, motivational, and cognitive processes that act on motor mechanisms. By "motor mechanisms" (Fig. 1), Melzack and Casey mean all of the brain areas that contribute to overt behavioural response patterns. These areas extend throughout the whole of the central nervous system, and their organisation must be at least as complex as that of the input systems we have primarily dealt with so far.

CHRONIC AND ACUTE PAIN

The time-course of pain is profoundly important in determining its psychological effects on an organism. Acute pain, which is usually associated with a well-defined cause (such as a burned finger or a ruptured appendix), normally has a characteristic time-course and vanishes after healing has occurred. The pain usually has a rapid onset--the phasic component--and then a subsequent tonic component that persists for variable periods of time. Chronic pain states--such as low back pain, the neuralgias, or phantom limb pain--may begin as acute pain and pass through both the phasic and tonic phases. The tonic pain, however, may persist long after the injury has healed. It is then labelled as "chronic pain" and appears to involve neural mechanisms that are far more complex than those of acute pain. The pain not only persists but may spread to adjacent or more distant body areas. It is resistant to surgical control and its prolonged time-course is characteristically associated with high levels of anxiety and depression.

We will first deal with the neural mechanisms of acute pain and then briefly examine some of the properties of chronic pain.

Acute Pain

We noted above that acute pain is characterized by phasic and tonic components. This simple statement belies the enormous complexity of the neural mechanisms that underlie the two components and their interactions in even relatively "simple" behaviour patterns.

Dennis and Melzack (16) recently reviewed the properties of the spinal cord pain-signalling pathways and speculated on some of their possible functions. One set of pathways—the dorsal-column post-synaptic (DCPS) system, the spino-cervical tract (SCT), and the neospinothalamic tract (nSTT)--are all rapidly conducting and seem to be particularly well suited to convey phasic information. The value of rapidly conducting, direct pain-signalling systems is obvious: unless an organism reacts quickly, a stimulus which only threatens tissue damage may become overtly damaging. But why three rapidly conducting systems?

The Rapidly Conducting Systems

Injurious stimulation may occur under many circumstances. An animal may be attacked by another when it is awake or asleep. If asleep, the attack could occur during any of the various stages of sleep. If awake, the attack could come while it is food-gathering, drinking, nest-building, exploring a novel or familiar environment, grooming, copulating, and so forth. Similarly, objects which are sharp or at an extreme temperature may be accidentally encountered during any of the organism's waking behaviour patterns. The key to minimizing the damage done by these stimuli is for the animal to perform appropriate motor responses which, in a purely mechanical sense, may need to be different depending on what the animal is doing at the time. It is conceivable, then, that the fast nociceptive pathways represent different sensory channels which are individually inhibited or facilitated depending on the ongoing behaviour or behavioural state of the

animal. The same noxious stimulus, occurring during different
behaviour patterns, might evoke impulses in different pathways.
Depending on the pathway(s) by which it arrives, the nociceptive
message may be treated differently by the information-processing
and response selection mechanisms of the brain. Thus, a nociceptive message ascending in one pathway may trigger different
responses than the same message ascending in another pathway.

An important factor which may contribute to this process is
the brain's need to obtain light tactile or proprioceptive information from these multi-modal systems. None of the three systems
is purely nociceptive. Each has a complement of cells responsive
only to light tactile stimuli, and, perhaps more importantly, each
has a significant population of multi-modal cells--units that
respond both to light tactile and nociceptive stimuli. There is
some evidence that there are qualitative differences in the types
of innocuous information carried by the systems (9). Perhaps
during a particular behaviour pattern, the brain selects one type
of information from a system and filters out the other types such
as nociceptive inputs. Thus, when a system is functioning in a
proprioceptive capacity, or monitoring light tactile stimuli, it
cannot simultaneously act as a nociceptive system for that part
of the body. However, the enormous biological importance of
nociception makes it essential that this modality be operative in
some form at all times. Therefore, one of the other systems must
provide the necessary pain-signalling function for the duration
of the behaviour. When the ongoing behaviour or behavioural state
changes, the brain selects other classes of tactile information,
perhaps from other systems. When this occurs, a new pattern of
differential inhibition and facilitation is imposed on the systems, such that the previously suppressed nociceptive capacity of
one system may now be facilitated. In this way, the brain can
always extract necessary tactile information from peripheral systems, and still maintain vigilance regarding sudden injury or
threat of injury. The possibility that the DCPS, SCT and nSTT
systems can be independently switched between nociceptive and
light tactile modalities is consistent with this kind of model.
Moreover, there is evidence for behaviour-dependent inhibition of
transmission through the medial lemniscus (see 16).

There is an alternative model of the functions of the 3 lateral
projection systems. The components of the lateral group could be
viewed as behaviour-dependent "amplifiers" of nociceptive messages. One pathway (e.g., the nSTT) may be used as the primary
rapid pain-signalling system, while the nociceptive impulses
carried in the other systems are used to amplify or modulate the
primary message in much the same manner as innocuous stimuli have
been proposed to do (32,37). The difference is that under this
formulation, nociceptive information in one pathway is used to
modulate nociceptive information in another pathway. This modulation could be either inhibitory or excitatory. The ongoing
behaviour pattern or behavioural state might determine whether
these supplementary pathways are open or closed, and thus indirectly affect the primary nociceptive message. However, the form

of the reaction to noxious stimuli is determined primarily by the
responses triggered by the primary pain-signalling system, and by
the complex response selection mechanisms of the brain.

A factor which may be of critical importance in determining
how the lateral pain projection pathways are used is whether the
animal has already sustained some serious injury. Tactile stimuli which would be innocuous to normal tissue might be painfully
damaging if applied to an existing wound. Escape mechanisms must
therefore be activated in response to such stimuli. However, it
may also be advantageous for the animal to tend the wound
(cleaning, covering, and so forth). Such activities would also
produce light tactile stimuli. Thus, the same stimulus (for
example, licking) would have very different effects depending on
whether it is self-induced or coming from another animal. How
does the nervous system tell the difference? While it is possible that such decisions are made by the brain, it may also be
that the nervous system actually "anticipates" such situations at
the spinal cord level. Thus, in a wounded, <u>resting</u> animal, a
"licking" message is, from the outset, channeled into systems
which rapidly trigger escape reactions. However, in a wounded,
<u>grooming</u> animal, the message may take an alternative route which
does not provoke escape reactions as readily.

There are, of course, other possible roles for the fast, direct,
multimodal systems, and there are other explanations for the
presence of several such systems. The above speculations, however, suggest new behavioural experiments and re-evaluations of
present physiological data.

The Slower Projection Systems

The slowly conducting systems of the spinal cord--the spinoreticular tract (SRT) and the paleospinothalamic tract (pSTT) in
particular--are unlikely to signal the need for immediate action.
Instead, it is more likely that they play a role in chronic,
deeply unpleasant and diffuse pain, as well as contributing to
the longer lasting motivational-affective dimension of pain.
While the dorsal cord pathways and nSTT appear eminently suited
for rapid transmission of <u>phasic</u> information, such as the threat
or onset of injury, or sudden changes in a damaged area, the
other ventral pathways seem best adapted to carrying <u>tonic</u> information on the state of the organism. Thus, an important, although perhaps not exclusive, role for these ventral systems may
be to signal the actual presence of peripheral damage, and to continue to send that message as long as the wound is susceptible to
re-injury. In this way, the slow nociceptive pathways may in part
determine the level of arousal or the general behavioural state
necessary to prevent further damage, and to foster rest, protec-
tion, and care of the damaged areas, thereby promoting healing
and recuperative processes.

Activity in the SRT and pSTT may also affect the switching
mechanisms which operate on the fast systems. Perhaps they "set
the bias" on the DCPS, SCT, and nSTT systems, influencing them

more toward the selection of nociceptive information from a
damaged area. As healing proceeds, activity in the medial systems decreases and the normal balance between light tactile and
nociceptive inputs in the lateral projection systems is restored.

An experimental approach for determining the type of mechanism
which may be involved in these interactions is suggested by the
effects of morphine, which appears to act at various sites in the
central nervous system, including the dorsal part of the spinal
grey matter (27,28). Morphine generally diminishes tonic postsurgical pain, but has less effect on the pain produced by sudden
movements or removal of stitches. In contrast, nitrous oxide at
analgesic dosages seems to diminish both the phasic and the tonic
pain. Thus, the major ascending systems may be subserved or controlled by different neurochemical mechanisms which are selectively affected by different pharmacological agents.

Chronic Pain

So far in this section we have dealt with tonic pain--that is,
pain that persists for the duration of injury until healing has
occurred. However, some kinds of clinical pain, such as post-
herpetic neuralgias, may occur long after healing has been completed. Livingston (24) and Melzack (30) have suggested that prolonged intense pain or even low-level abnormal inputs may produce
reverberatory or other self-sustaining neural activity that sub-
serves memory-like processes related to pain.

This speculation is crucially important because a memory-like
mechanism may account for pain in the absence of a detectable
lesion or any other peripheral input that can account for the
pain. A patient in whom a memory-like mechanism such as this is
active may be diagnosed as a malingerer or a conversion hysteric
when, in fact, a central neural mechanism, such as self-sustaining
neural activity, may be the major underlying cause of the pain.

The concept of a memory-like mechanism in pain is supported by
convincing experimental evidence obtained in both man and animals.
After teeth on both sides of the mouth were drilled and filled
without local anaesthetic, pin-pricks of the nasal mucosa, as long
as seventy days later, produced pain in the treated teeth on the
stimulated side. The effect was permanently abolished on one
side by a single novocaine block of the trigeminal nerve, but
persisted in the opposite, non-blocked side (45). These referred
pains necessitate the assumption of a long-term central neural
change. The data suggest that the treatment of the teeth evoked
inputs that produced changes in firing patterns in the central
nervous system. These changes, once initiated, were somehow capable of summating the continuous, low-level input from the treated
teeth with inputs from more distant sources. The single block of
a peripheral nerve, which could not have affected the teeth, permitted resumption of normal neural activity and the end of pain.
That the input as such, rather than conscious awareness, was essential in initiating the abnormal central activity is evident in

the observation that a subject who had four teeth extracted under nitrous oxide anaesthesia felt pain referred to the jaw when the nasal mucosa was pricked thirty-three days after treatment.

Similar observations were made by Cohen (13) who studied patients that had anginal-effort syndrome, with pain referred only to the left side. He injected a small amount of hypertonic saline under the skin of the right side of the back which gave rise to a diffuse, deep-seated pain that soon disappeared. Two hours later, long after the pain had passed, exertion and anginal pain again caused its appearance.

Comparable conclusions can be drawn from experiments with animal subjects. Injection of turpentine under the skin of a cat's paw produces a temporary inflammation and a tendency to flex the paw. After the inflammatory process has healed completely and the animal walks normally, an abnormal flexion-extension pattern is seen in the limbs when the animal is decerebrated (19). Similarly, postural asymmetries produced by cerebellar lesions persist after transection of the spinal cord only if they are maintained for at least forty-five minutes before the cord section (11). Impulses descending from the cerebellum for 45 minutes or longer thus appear to bring about a permanent change in spinal neuron networks.

The neural mechanisms that subserve long-term memory of any sensory experience are not understood. Indeed, the neural basis of memory remains as one of the key problems of psychology. Even studies (33,55) in which activity is recorded directly from neural structures for prolonged periods of time--as long as several hours--after a brief sensory input fail to reveal the basis of the memory trace. At best, it is only possible to speculate about reverberatory neuron loops (24) or a simpler two-neuron circuit (2) capable of producing rhythmic, sustained activity for long periods of time. These kinds of circuits could underlie prolonged, yet reversible changes in the spinal cord or brain. They could play a role, as we shall see in the next section, in prolonged pathological pain which is permanently relieved by either blocking or intensifying the sensory input.

HYPERSTIMULATION ANALGESIA

It is an assumption that memory-like circuits play a role in pain. However, it is a fact that chronic pain can be controlled by relatively brief decreases or increases of the sensory input. This clinical fact can be explained in terms of a disruption of memory-like mechanisms.

It is well known that short-acting, local anesthetic blocks of trigger points often produce prolonged, sometimes permanent relief of some forms of myofascial or visceral pain (24,59). Astonishingly, brief, intense stimulation of trigger points by dry needling (59), intense cold (59), or injection of normal saline (54) often produces prolonged relief of some forms of myofascial or visceral pain. This type of pain relief, which may be generally labelled as <u>hyperstimulation analgesia</u> (30), is one of the oldest methods used for the control of pain. It is sometimes known as "counter-irritation", and includes such methods of folk-medicine as application of mustard plasters, ice packs, hot cups, or blistering agents to parts of the body. Some of these methods are still frequently used although there has not been (until recently) any theoretical or physiological explanation for their effectiveness. Suggestion and distraction of attention are the usual mechanisms invoked, but neither seems capable of explaining the power of the methods or the long duration of the relief they may afford.

This interest in folk-medicine gained enormous impetus in recent years by the re-discovery of the ancient Chinese practice of acupuncture--inserting needles into specific body sites and twirling them manually. More recently, the Chinese have prac- ticed electro-acupuncture, in which electrical pulses are passed through the needles. We now know that the original claims that acupuncture can always produce surgical analgesia (or anesthesia) have not been borne out by later investigation. However, acupunc- ture stimulation has recently been shown in several well-control- led clinical, and experimental investigations (12) to provide substantial relief of pain. This is not surprising because it is now evident that there is nothing mysterious or magical about acupuncture; it is a form of <u>hyperstimulation analgesia</u> compara- ble to cupping or blistering the skin.

Transcutaneous electrical nerve stimulation has recently been found to provide a powerful technique for the control of pain. When it is administered the same way as acupuncture--for brief periods of time at moderate-to-high stimulation intensities (just below painful levels), it frequently produces pain relief that outlasts the 20-minute period of stimulation by several hours, occasionally for days or weeks (31). Daily stimulation carried out at home by the patient sometimes provides gradually increasing relief over periods of weeks or months.

A recent study (18) compared the relative effectiveness of transcutaneous stimulation and acupuncture on low back pain. The results showed that both forms of stimulation at the same points produce substantial decreases in pain intensity but neither pro- cedure is statistically more effective than the other. Most pa- tients were relieved of pain for several hours, and some for one or more days. Statistical analysis also failed to reveal any differences in the duration of pain relief between the two pro- cedures.

Another recent study (35) examined the correlation between trigger points and acupuncture points for pain. The results of the analysis showed that every trigger point reported in the Western medical literature has a corresponding acupuncture point. Furthermore, there is a close correspondence —— 71%——between the pain syndromes associated with the two kinds of points. This close correlation suggests that trigger points and acupuncture points for pain, though discovered independently and labelled

differently, represent the same phenomenon and can be explained
in terms of the same underlying neural mechanisms.

Physiological Basis of Hyperstimulation Analgesia

There are three major properties of hyperstimulation analgesia:
(1) a moderate-to-intense sensory input is applied to the body to
alleviate pain, (2) the sensory input is sometimes applied to a
site distant from the site of pain, and (3) the sensory input,
which is usually of brief duration (ranging from a few seconds to
20 or 30 minutes) may relieve chronic pain for days, weeks, sometimes permanently.

The relief of pain by brief, intense stimulation of distant
trigger points (or acupuncture points) can be explained in terms
of the gate control theory. The most plausible explanation (30)
seems to be that the brainstem areas which are known to exert a
powerful inhibitory control over transmission in the pain signalling system may be involved. These areas, which may be considered to be a "central biasing mechanism" (30), receive inputs
from widespread parts of the body and, in turn, project to widespread parts of the spinal cord and brain (Fig. 2). The stimulation of particular nerves or tissues by transcutaneous electrical stimulation or any other form of stimulation that activates
small fibers could bring about an increased input to the central
biasing mechanism, which would close the gates to inputs from
selected body areas. The cells of the midbrain reticular formation are known to have large receptive fields, and the electrical
stimulation of points within the reticular formation can produce
analgesia in discrete areas of the body (3). It is possible,
then, that particular body areas may project especially strongly
to some reticular areas, and these, in turn, could "close the
gate" to inputs from particular parts of the body.

There has been recent support for this hypothesis. Direct
electrical stimulation of the brainstem areas which produce behavioural analgesia inhibits the transmission of nerve impulses in
dorsal horn cells that have been implicated in gate-control mechanisms (41). Bilateral lesions of the dorsolateral spinal cord
abolish these inhibitory effects and also abolish or reduce the
analgesia produced by brainstem stimulation and morphine (4).
Furthermore, the analgesia-producing brainstem areas are known to
be highly sensitive to morphine, and the effect of stimulation is
partially reduced by administration of naloxone, an opiate antagonist (1). The demonstration that naloxone also reduces the
analgesic effects of transcutaneous electrical stimulation (52)
and acupuncture (29) is consistent with the hypothesis that intense stimulation activates a neural feedback loop through the
brainstem analgesia-producing areas. The analgesia-producing
areas have also been found to contain endogenous morphine-like
compounds (endorphins) and electro-acupuncture reportedly produces an increase in endorphins in cerebrospinal fluid in patients
treated for chronic pain (53).

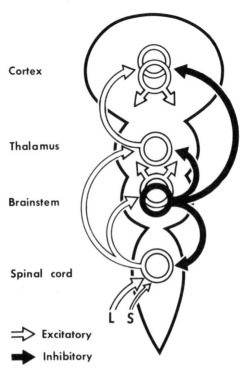

FIG. 2. Schematic diagram of the central biasing mechanism. Large and small fibres from a limb activate a neuron pool in the spinal cord, which excites neuron pools at successively higher levels. The central biasing mechanism, represented by the inhibitory projection system that originates in the brainstem reticular formation, modulates activity at all levels. When sensory fibres are destroyed after amputation or peripheral nerve lesion, the inhibitory influence decreases. This results in sustained activity at all levels that can be triggered repeatedly by the remaining fibers. L, large fibres; S, small fibres.

The prolonged relief of pain after only brief stimulation requires the additional postulation of prolonged, reverberatory activity in neural circuits which may underlie "memories" of earlier injury (24). These reverberatory circuits may be facilitated by low-level inputs, such as those from the pathological structures or processes that subserve trigger points or acupuncture points, and is disrupted for long periods of time(perhaps) permanently) by a massive input produced by electrical or other intense stimulation. Furthermore, when pain is blocked, even briefly, the patient tends to become physically active and carry out normal motor activities such as walking and working. The normal, patterned proprioceptive inputs that result from these activities may prevent the resumption of the abnormal reverberatory neural activity that underlies prolonged pain.

INTERACTING DETERMINANTS OF PAIN

The complexity of the interacting sensory and psychological factors in pain and its management is highlighted by studies of chronic phantom body pain in paraplegics with total spinal cord lesions. Melzack and Loeser (34) recently reviewed cases of patients who had sustained total spinal cord sections at thoracic or lumbar levels, yet continued to suffer severe pain in the abdomen, groin or legs. The completeness of the lesion was verified visually during surgical removal of injured tissue or as a result of segmental cordectomy (the removal of an entire section of the spinal cord) to prevent nerve impulses produced by injured tissues from reaching the brain. Nevertheless, pain returned immediately or as long as 11 years later. The pain was usually felt in definite parts of the body phantom and was often described as burning, crushing or cramping. The sympathetic ganglia— the only other possible route for nerve impulses from the legs — were also blocked in several patients without effect on the pain. Since there is no known anatomical substrate for sensory input from the lower abdomen or legs entering the spinal cord above mid-thoracic levels, it is evident that peripheral input from levels below the total transection is not the cause of pain in these patients. Although many of the patients were severely depressed by their physical status as paraplegics, there was no evidence that the pain was caused by depression or neurosis. On the basis of the clinical data, Melzack and Loeser proposed that the loss of input to central structures after deafferentation may play an important role in producing pain.

The effects of deafferentation on the activity of central neurons have been investigated in several contexts. Loeser and Ward (25) showed that cutting several dorsal roots in the cat produces abnormal bursts of firing in dorsal horn cells that persist for as long as 180 days after the root section. Furthermore, single shock pulses to adjacent intact roots produce prolonged firing that persists for hundreds of milliseconds. These abnormal patterns are commonly seen after deafferentation. Non-noxious input has the ability to trigger the high-frequency burst firing patterns. It is of particular interest that this abnormal activity has been recorded from lamina 5 cells, which are known to be involved in sensory transmission processes related to pain. Similar abnormal activity in trigeminal cells in the cat is also seen after extraction of all the teeth on one side (8).

The abnormal firing patterns observed in the deafferented spinal cord in cats have also been observed in man (26). In one case, just prior to cordectomy, the deafferented cord was examined physiologically with microelectrodes. The cells showed abnormal bursting activity which resembled that seen after chronic deafferentation in the cat spinal cord.

These observations led Melzack and Loeser to suggest a concept (Fig. 3) of pain to explain the clinical data. They proposed that neuron pools at many levels of the spinal cord and brain can act as pattern generating mechanisms. These neuron pools are assumed

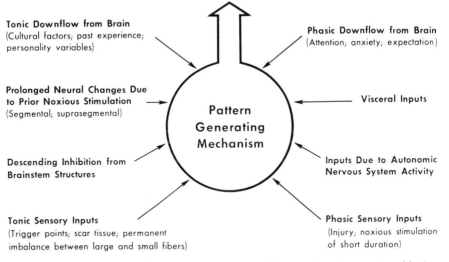

FIG. 3. Concept of a pattern generating mechanism controlled by multiple inputs.

to comprise the dorsal horns (i.e., the entire gate system) in the spinal cord and the homologous interacting systems associated with the cranial nerves. They proposed that other nuclei along the course of the major somatosensory projection systems can act as pattern generating mechanisms. These cells are normally under sensory and downstream control. When deafferentation occurs, however, the cells fire spontaneously in abnormal bursts for prolonged periods of time. They proposed that the pattern generating mechanisms, in paraplegics, must lie above the level of spinal transection or cordectomy. Furthermore, those regions responsible for pattern generation are assumed to project to the regions of the brain involved in precise localization of sensory inputs— that is, those neural areas that subserve the body schema—as well as to the areas that subserve pain experience.

The concept suggests that the prolonged bursting activity generated by the deafferented neuron pools can be modulated by somatic, visceral and autonomic inputs as well as by inputs from neural mechanisms that underlie personality and emotional variables. Brain stem inhibitory areas are also assumed to modulate activity in the neuron pools. The loss of segmental input would lead to a decreased input to brain stem mechanisms that normally exert an inhibitory downstream influence on sensory transmission. The loss of descending inhibition would make it easier for non-noxious inputs to trigger the abnormal bursting patterns. Furthermore, the neural substrates of memories of prior pains, at spinal and supraspinal levels, may become active and also trigger abnormal firing patterns. The release from inhibition, moreover, in addition to

the sensory deafferentation, would allow unchecked abnormal bursting activity so that the pain would persist for indefinitely long periods of time. The diminished inhibition would also allow recruitment of additional neurons into the abnormally firing pools and, thereby, underlie the intensification and spread of pain.

The phantom pain itself, however, may inhibit other types of pain. Thus, paraplegics with pain generally have a higher pain threshold than those without pain (22). In these cases, the increased output of the pattern generating mechanisms could increase the descending inhibition and shut the gates to input from peripheral nociceptors above the cord section.

Thus Melzack and Loeser conceive of the phantom body pain reported by paraplegics to be based upon the abnormal activity of neuron pools that lie rostral to the cord transection. This abnormal activity can be gated by visceral and somatic inputs from areas below and above the level of the section as well as by neural activities that descend from the brain. All of these contributions modulate activity in the deafferented pools, but no one of them appears to be the major cause of the phantom pain.

Implications of the Concept of a Central Pattern Generating Mechanism

The concept of a central pattern generating mechanism underscores central factors in pain and places peripheral contributions where they should be —at the periphery. There is no denying the role of neuromas, nerve injury, herniated intervertebral discs and so forth as major contributions to pain or as initiators of abnormal central processes. But once the abnormal central pattern generating processes are underway, the peripheral contributions may assume less importance. They are, to be sure, avenues for modulating the activities in the pattern generating mechanisms, but their removal may not stop pain once it is established. The proof of this statement lies in the countless patients who continue to suffer severe phantom limb, neuralgic, and back pain after removal of neuromas, nerves, and protruding discs, after extensive rhizotomies and multiple cordotomies, and even after total spinal cord transection.

Once the pattern generating mechanisms become capable of producing patterns for pain, any input may act as a trigger. Thus, the emphasis for therapy lies in the modulation by inputs that affect the pattern generating mechanisms. Decreasing the input by anesthetic blocks or increasing it by electrical stimulation may be efficacious. Psychotherapeutic methods or drugs such as mood elevators and antidepressants may also be helpful. Aims and goals in life that make life worth living in spite of the pain may diminish both anxiety and pain.

The concept of central pattern generating mechanisms provides an explanation for those pain states which are characterized by degeneration of sensory nerve fibers, dorsal root pathology, or spinal injury. Many of the neuralgias occur after partial nerve injury, and causalgia occurs more frequently after partial than

after total peripheral nerve lesions (57). Even phantom limb pain is associated with partial nerve damage since a portion of the fibres in a nerve bundle degenerates after total section, while the remainder regenerates into the stump tissue (57). Partial deafferentation, therefore, may alter the activity of cells in the spinal cord and brain. Moreover, the diminished input to areas that comprise the "central biasing mechanism" that inhibits inputs at all levels would further release cells in pattern generating areas (such as the dorsal horns, thalamus, sensory cortex) from sensory and central control. Thus, the "free wheeling" cells could be triggered by the remaining neurons into producing abnormal, prolonged bursting activity that could evoke pain. Gentle sensory input from distant areas, sympathetic activity, and psychoneural activities could all trigger or augment abnormal activity. Intense somatic stimulation or temporary anesthetic blocks at trigger points or appropriate nerves could disrupt the abnormal patterns. The prolonged relief produced by such therapy could be due to the time required to recruit sufficient numbers of active cells to exceed the critical level for pain. The normal motor activity of the person when pain-free would tend to maintain normal patterning and to occlude or inhibit the abnormal bursting activity that produces pain.

The concept of pattern generating mechanisms which are triggered and modulated by multiple inputs has important therapeutic implications. Therapy at present is often predicated on a one cause—one effect relationship. In contrast, Fig. 3 indicates multiple interactions that determine the nature of the pattern which is generated. Attempts can therefore be made to change the pattern by simultaneous use of several procedures. Thus, it is plausible to provide patients with an antidepressant drug, electrical stimulation at trigger points and anesthetic blocks all at the same time. Therapeutic procedures in combination are sometimes more effective than the mere additive effects of each presented by itself (60). This kind of approach is reasonable in terms of pattern generating mechanisms as the cause of chronic pain.

REFERENCES

1. Akil, H., Mayer, D.J., and Liebeskind, J.C. (1976): Science, 191:961-962.
2. Anderson, P. and Eccles, J.C. (1962): Nature, 196:645-647.
3. Balagura, S. and Ralph, T. (1973): Brain Res., 60:369-379.
4. Basbaum, A.I., Marley, N.E.J., O'Keefe, J., and Clanton, C.H. (1977): Pain, 3:43-56.
5. Becker, D.P., Gluck, H., Nulsen, F.E., and Jane, J.A. (1969): J. Neurosurg., 30:1-13.
6. Beecher, H.K. (1959): Measurement of Subjective Responses. Oxford Univ. Press, New York.
7. Bishop, G.H. (1959): J. Nerv. Ment. Dis., 128:89-114.
8. Black, R.G. (1970): In: Pain and Suffering, edited by B.L. Crue. Thomas, Springfield.

9. Brown, A.G. (1973): In: Somatosensory System, Handbook of Sensory Physiology, edited by A. Iggo. Springer, Berlin.
10. Casey, K.L. (1971): Science, 173:77-79.
11. Chamberlain, T.J., Halick, P., and Gerard, R.W. (1963): J. Neurophysiol., 26:662-676.
12. Chapman, C.R., Chen, A.C., and Bonica, J.J. (1977): Pain, 3:213-228.
13. Cohen, H. (1944): Trans. Med. Soc. London, 64:65-74.
14. Delgado, J.M.R. (1955): J. Neurophysiol., 18:261-275.
15. Delgado, J.M.R., Rosvold, H.E., and Looney, E. (1956): J. comp. physiol. Psychol., 49:373-380.
16. Dennis, S.G. and Melzack, R. (1977): Pain, 4:97-132.
17. Foltz, E.L. and White, L.E. (1962): J. Neurosurg., 19: 89-100.
18. Fox, E.J. and Melzack, R. (1976): Pain, 2:141-148.
19. Frankstein, S.A. (1947): Science, 106:242-244.
20. Freeman, W. and Watts, J.W. (1948): Ann. Internal. Med. 28: 747-754.
21. Grastyan, E., Czopf, J., Angyan, L., and Szabo, I. (1965): Acta Physiol. Acad. Sci. Hung., 26:9-46.
22. Hazouri, L.A. and Mueller, A.D. (1950): Arch. Neurol. Psychiat., 64:607-613.
23. Hillman, P. and Wall, P.D. (1969): Exper. Brain Res., 9: 284-306.
24. Livingston, W.K. (1943): Pain Mechanisms. MacMillan, New York.
25. Loeser, J.D. and Ward, A.A. (1967): Arch. Neurol. (Chic.), 17:629-636.
26. Loeser, J.D., Ward, A.A., and White, L.E. (1968): J. Neurosurg., 29:48-50.
27. Mayer, D.J. and Hayes, R. (1975): Science, 188:941-943.
28. Mayer, D.J. and Liebeskind, J.C. (1974): Brain Res., 68: 73-93.
29. Mayer, D.J., Price, D.D., Barber, J. and Rafii, A. (1976): In: Advances in Pain Research and Therapy, Vol. 1, edited by J.J. Bonica and D. Albe-Fessard. Raven Press, New York.
30. Melzack, R. (1973): The Puzzle of Pain. Basic/Harper Torchbooks, New York.
31. Melzack, R. (1975): Pain, 1:357-373.
32. Melzack, R. and Casey, K.L. (1968): In: The Skin Senses, edited by D. Kenshalo. Thomas, Springfield.
33. Melzack, R., Konrad, K., and Dubrovsky, B. (1969): Exp. Neurol., 25:416-428.
34. Melzack, R. and Loeser, J.D. (1978): Pain 4:195-210.
35. Melzack, R., Stillwell, D.M., and Fox, E.J. (1977): Pain, 3:3-23.
36. Melzack, R., Stotler, W.A. and Livingston, W.K. (1958): J. Neurophysiol., 21:353-367.
37. Melzack, R. and Wall, P.D. (1965): Science, 150:971-979.
38. Mendell, L.M. and Wall, P.D. (1965): Nature, 206:97-99.
39. Nauta, W.J.H. (1958): Brain, 81:319-340.
40. Noordenbos, W. (1959): Pain, Elsevier Press, Amsterdam.

41. Oliveras, J.L., Besson, J.M., Guilbaud, G., and Liebeskind, J.C. (1974): <u>Exp. Brain Res.</u>, 20:32-44.
42. Pavlov, I.P. (1928): <u>Lectures on Conditioned Reflexes</u>. International Publishers, New York.
43. Perl, E.R. (1971): <u>J. psychiat. Res.</u>, 8:273-287.
44. Pomeranz,B., Wall, P.D., and Weber, W.V. (1968): <u>J. Physiol. (Lond.)</u>, 199:511-532.
45. Reynolds, O.E. and Hutchins, H.C. (1948): <u>Amer. J. Physiol.</u>, 152:658-662.
46. Roberts, W.W. (1962): <u>J. comp. physiol. Psychol.</u>, 55: 191-197.
47. Rossi, G.F. and Zanchetti, A. (1957): <u>Arch. ital. Biol.</u>, 199-435.
48. Rubins, J.L. and Friedman, E.D. (1948): <u>Arch. Neurol. Psychiat.</u>, 60:554-573.
49. Schreiner, L. and Kling, A. (1953): <u>J. Neurophysiol.</u>, 16: 643-659.
50. Semmes, J. and Mishkin, M. (1965): <u>J. Neurophysiol.</u>, 28: 473-486
51. Shimazu, H., Yanagisawa, N., and Garoutte, B. (1965): <u>Jap. J. Physiol.</u>, 15:101-115.
52. Sjolund, B. and Eriksson, M. (1976): <u>Lancet</u>, 2:1085.
53. Sjolund, B., Terenius, L., and Eriksson, M. (1977): <u>Acta Physiol. scand.</u>, 100:382-384.
54. Sola, A.E. and Williams, R.L. (1956): <u>Neurology</u>, 6:91-95.
55. Spencer, W.A. and April, R.S. (1970): In: <u>Short-term Changes in Neural Activity and Behaviour</u>, edited by G. Horn and R.A. Hinde. Cambridge Univ. Press, Cambridge.
56. Sternbach, R.A. (1963): <u>Psychol. Bull.</u>, 60:252-264.
57. Sunderland, S. (1968): <u>Nerves and Nerve Injuries</u>. Livingstone, Edinburgh.
58. Szentogathai, J. (1964): <u>J. comp. Neurol.</u>, 122:219-239.
59. Travell, J. and Rinzler, S.H. (1952): <u>Postgrad. Med.</u>, 11: 425-434.
60. Wall, P.D. (1964): <u>Progr. Brain Res.</u>, 12:92-115.
61. Wall, P.D. (1970): <u>Brain</u>, 93:505-524.
62. Wall, P.D. (1976): In: <u>Advances in Pain Research and Therapy</u>, Vol. 1, edited by J.J. Bonica and D. Albe-Fessard. Raven Press, New York.
63. White, J.C. and Sweet, W.H. (1969): <u>Pain and the Neuro-surgeon</u>. Thomas, Springfield.

The Psychology of Pain, edited by R. A. Sternbach.
Raven Press, New York © 1978.

Neural and Neurochemical Mechanisms of Pain Inhibition

J. Timothy Cannon, John C. Liebeskind, and Hanan Frenk*

*Department of Pyschology, University of California, Los Angeles, Los Angeles,
California 90024; and *Department of Psychology, Tel Aviv University,
Ramat Aviv, Israel*

INTRODUCTION

Responsiveness to painful stimulation is notoriously variable,
much to the frustration and dismay of all workers in this field.
This variability can probably be attributed to the complex and·
little understood interactions which occur among sensory inputs
and between such inputs and on-going emotional and cognitive
processes. In the past few years, considerable information has
been gathered suggesting the existence of powerful, endogenous
pain-inhibitory mechanisms in the brain and spinal cord. It may
be that fluctuations in the activity of these systems account for
some of the variability in pain perception, and very recent
studies are providing the first clues that this is so. In this
brief chapter we will broadly review the relevant literature,
focusing on the major observations and conceptual issues within
it. For more detailed treatment of one or another of these
points, the reader may refer to other recent review articles in
this area (36,42,77,89,91,101,142,150,165).

STIMULATION-PRODUCED ANALGESIA: BEHAVIORAL OBSERVATIONS

The first solid experimental evidence that the central nervous
system possesses a pain-suppressive capacity derived from
behavioral studies employing electrical stimulation of discrete
brain regions. The early report by Reynolds (125) that such
stimulation applied to the midbrain periaqueductal gray matter
(PAG) rendered rats sufficiently analgesic to permit abdominal
surgery without drugs is difficult to improve upon as a dramatic
demonstration of the analgesic potency of central stimulation.
Subsequent studies have shown that brief trains of PAG stimulation in rats can induce a degree of analgesia in quantitative
pain tests comparable to that requiring up to 50 mg/kg of morphine, without producing the muscular rigidity associated with

such high doses of that drug (99). Stimulation-produced analgesia (SPA) from the PAG has been reported capable of totally
blocking behavioral responses, including even spinally or tri-
geminally mediated withdrawal reflexes, to extremely intense
pinch (99,125), tissue damaging heat (99,103,146), electrical
tooth pulp stimulation (114), and the application of algesic
chemicals to subcutaneous (105) and visceral (49) tissues. SPA
has now also been reported in cats (105,112), monkeys (53,133),
and most significantly in man (1,23,59,69,127,128). In pain
patients, acute experimental pain may be reduced as well as
various chronic pain syndromes (69,127,128; c.f., however 59).

Typically, SPA can be measured after only a few seconds of
central stimulation (e.g., 103). Its post-stimulation duration,
however, may be of the order of minutes or even hours (e.g., 99,
103). Long-duration analgesic effects have been especially
evident in pain patients, where several minutes of stimulation
can provide clinical pain relief for up to a day (128). In man,
it has been reported that clinical pain is more readily blocked
by brain stimulation and blocked for a longer time than are
responses to experimentally applied noxious stimuli (69).
Whether this difference reflects simple quantitative or more
complex qualitative differences between acute and chronic pain
is not known but would be an important question to address in
future research as better animal models of chronic pain states
become available.

Despite its impressive potency, evidence from several sources
clearly indicates that SPA is not the result of more general
disruptive influences caused by the electrical stimulation.
Perhaps the clearest demonstration of this fact is the observation that in many rats (11,99,103) and sometimes in the cat (112)
the analgesic effect is restricted to one body region while
noxious stimulation delivered elsewhere evokes normal defensive
and escape responses. SPA has been measured during the course
of normal eating and locomotion (103,130,146) in laboratory
animals; and in pain patients, as in primates (53), analgesia
has been reported to occur in the absence of undesirable side
effects. At many stimulation sites other behaviors can be
evoked, but in general it has been observed that none of these
are uniformly associated with the analgesic effect. For example,
self-stimulation has often been reported at the same brain loci
and stimulation parameters as SPA in the rat; yet other self-
stimulation sites do not consistently yield SPA and many non-
rewarding, in fact, some aversive sites do (99,103,156). Even
when self-stimulation and SPA are seen together, these phenomena
can be dissociated pharmacologically (2,92,170). Therapeutic
central stimulation in man has not been reported to induce pleasure or other psychological effects. Perceptual deficits in
other sense modalities, although not often assiduously investigated, have generally not been seen to accompany SPA (103,105,
115).

RELATION OF SPA TO OPIATE ANALGESIA: HISTORICAL OVERVIEW

Perhaps the most significant theme to have emerged from the SPA literature is that, to a remarkable degree, SPA seems to share with opiate analgesia both common sites and mechanisms of action (90,103). Dramatically rapid progress has been made in the past few years in our understanding of SPA and opiate mechanisms in large part because advances in each line of research have importantly contributed to advances in the other.

Lim and his colleagues (93) were among the first to establish with certainty that opiate compounds, in contrast to the salicylates, exert their analgesic action via the central nervous system. At about that time and subsequently, others showed that injections of even minute quantities of opiates into or near the periaqueductal gray matter or more rostral or caudal periventricular structures induced a strong general analgesic effect (64, 155). It was also found that similarly small amounts of an opiate antagonist drug delivered to these regions blocked the analgesic action of systemically administered morphine (154).

Since then, a number of studies have mapped the brain for effective analgesic sites with focal electrical stimulation and with opiate microinjections. This work has recently been reviewed (101,165) and need, therefore, be summarized here only briefly. To be noted is the fact that a great deal of overlap exists between effective loci mapped by these two methods. Sites throughout the PAG support SPA (11,99,126), although morphine analgesia is best seen from injections in the ventrocaudal portion of this structure (75,138,167). The diencephalic periventricular gray, the pretectal nucleus, and at least certain hypothalamic areas have also consistently yielded SPA (11,99,126, 130), and many of the same sites provide opiate analgesia as well (74,119). Medial periventricular thalamic structures are the targets of choice among neurosurgeons (69,128) since PAG stimulation in some patients has been reported to induce unpleasant sensations (127). The nucleus raphe magnus (NRM) of the medulla yields excellent SPA in the rat and cat (111,113,114,124). This structure, like the dorsal raphe nucleus in ventrocaudal PAG, is rich in serotonin-containing cell bodies. Morphine microinjections in this region have been less clearly successful, although slightly more lateral sites are reported to be particularly sensitive (147). In sum, medial portions of the brain stem extending from the rostral medulla to the diencephalon contain SPA and opiate analgesia sites. The degree of overlap, while impressive, is not perfect (169). Much has yet to be learned about the full extent of this anatomical system and the functional interconnections among its parts.

Another theme of particular importance which was recognized early in the emerging SPA and opiate literature (103) is that although the medial brain stem appears to serve as the initiating or original site of analgesic action, the spinal cord and trigeminal nucleus are the ultimate loci of this pain inhibition. Thus, the anti-nociceptive effect underlying the SPA and opiate analgesia is seen to an important extent at least as a descending or centrifugal one. This theme had its origins in several early studies of opiate action. Irwin et al. (72) reported that spinal transection reduced the analgesic effectiveness of morphine. They noted as well that certain spinal nociceptive reflexes were enhanced after transection and attributed this finding to the presence of a tonically active, descending path with control over pain reflexes. More recently, Satoh and Takagi (135) found that high spinal transection also blocked the suppressive effect of morphine on pain-evoked potentials in the cord. Such findings, coupled with the observation that PAG stimulation inhibited the spinally mediated tail-flick response, a reflex known to be resistant to all but opiate drugs (56), led Mayer et al. (103) to suggest that SPA and opiate analgesia share a common substrate in the medial brain stem and in descending pathways from the brain stem to the spinal cord. It was proposed (103) that this substrate represents a natural or endogenous pain suppressive system which is activated by electrical stimulation and by opiate drugs and which, by energizing descending controls, blocks transmission of pain information through spinal cord neurons participating in the projection of pain messages to the brain. Since that time, an outpouring of new and extremely exciting information has occurred which serves to confirm and enrich this concept. Some of the most salient of these findings will be reviewed in the remaining portions of this chapter.

SELECTIVITY OF THE ENDOGENOUS ANALGESIA SYSTEM

Behavioral studies have been successful to varying degree in showing that SPA, like opiate analgesia, can exert a selectively anti-nociceptive effect. In a particularly powerful demonstration, Oliveras et al. (115) showed that SPA in the cat blocked the jaw-opening reflex to noxious tooth pulp stimulation without affecting a similar response evoked by innocuous tooth tap. It has also been reported (103) that SPA may be accompanied by hyper-responsiveness to light touch, just as another study has shown that responsiveness to tactile stimuli is augmented following opiate administration (29). Electrophysiological investigations have been more telling in this regard. PAG and NRM electrical stimulation and morphine administered systemically or into the PAG have all been shown to cause powerful and, in many instances, preferential inhibition on those particular dorsal horn interneurons involved in pain mechanisms (18,19,43,78,85, 112). Similar findings have been made at the level of the trigeminal nucleus (133,137). In one early study examining the effects of PAG stimulation on dorsal horn cells in the cat (112), it was found that central stimulation reduced the responsiveness of only 5 of 30 neurons responding maximally to innocuous peripheral stimuli (lamina 4-type cells) but reduced the responsiveness of 93 of 102 neurons responding differentially to noxious stimuli (lamina 5-type cells), often blocking completely the vigorous discharge of such cells to tissue damaging mechanical or thermal stimuli. Still more importantly, PAG stimulation was observed to block the response to noxious but not innocuous stimuli in 9 of 17 lamina 5-type cells. Many of these cells are known to project to the brain (8,153). In the monkey, NRM stimulation has been seen to exert this kind of descending inhibitory control on interneurons antidromically identified as projecting in the spinothalamic tract (15,160).

Unfortunately, electrophysiological studies of the sort described above have uniformly been conducted in anesthetized animals. Although the brain stem sites at the origin of this descending inhibition have in some animals been previously confirmed to elicit behaviorally measured analgesia, in other animals behaviorally ineffective sites nonetheless later proved capable of inhibiting spinal cord interneurons under conditions of anesthesia (112). It will be important in future work to confirm the neurophysiological effects in awake animals with concurrent analgesia testing in order to assess the degree to which the behavioral phenomenon of SPA can be understood in terms of dorsal horn inhibition.

In other studies (108,111), single or multiple unit recording was used to investigate the effects of SPA and morphine on responses in different brain areas evoked by noxious and non-noxious stimuli. Both unanesthetized and lightly anesthetized preparations were employed. Again, these analgesic manipulations were shown to exert good specificity in blocking preferentially the nociceptively evoked cellular activity. Whether this inhibition occurred locally in the brain or was merely a reflection of inhibition occurring at lower (presumably spinal) levels is not known.

INVOLVEMENT OF SEROTONIN

Drugs affecting serotonin, as well as drugs affecting norepinephrine and dopamine, have been shown to alter SPA much as they alter opiate analgesia (2,4,35,123,134). The special significance of the fact that analgesia can be altered by drugs which influence synaptic transmission in the central nervous system, and the fact that this can be accomplished at doses which do not change baseline pain sensitivity, was recognized by Mayer et al. (103) who suggested that the dependence of analgesic mechanisms on the integrity of a neurotransmitter implied that analgesia was an active process exciting pathways in which such transmitters are released. Particular interest has focused on serotonin since the cell bodies of the dorsal raphe nucleus and the NRM are serotonin-containing and these nuclei appear to be integral parts of the endogenous analgesia system. An extensive review of this topic has recently appeared (106). Drugs which interfere with serotonin's action have been found to reduce the potency of SPA and morphine analgesia (2,4,148,162) as well as to block the efficacy of such analgesic procedures in inhibiting spinal cord nociceptive interneurons (57). Destruction of NRM, whether accomplished electrolytically (124,163) or by administration of a serotonin neurotoxin (158), has been shown to reduce or abolish morphine analgesia. In an important and related series of studies it has been shown that selective lesions of the spinal cord dorsolateral funiculus abolish the analgesic effect of PAG stimulation in the rat (14). They similarly block the inhibitory effect of NRM stimulation on spinal cord interneurons in the cat and monkey (43,160). Even more dramatically, these same lesions block the analgesic effects of morphine, whether administered locally into the PAG (109) or even systemically in doses up to moderate levels (14,62). Dorsolateral funiculus lesions are known to interrupt the serotonin-containing fibers descending to the cord from the NRM. In fact, recent autoradiographic data show that fibers from NRM terminate especially in those regions of the dorsal horn (marginal zone, substantia gelatinosa, lamina 5) where pain modulation is thought to occur (13). Analogous projections have also been found to the trigeminal nucleus caudalis (13). These particular findings, taken together with those described in the preceding section, illustrate the importance of descending or centrifugal pathways underlying the analgesic effect of medial brain stem stimulation and opiate administration and illustrate as well the close parallels between the two forms of analgesia with regard to both site and mechanism of action. Since, as will be recalled, opiate microinjections into NRM are apparently not successful in causing analgesia (147), yet this nucleus and its fiber pathway are important for opiate analgesia and PAG SPA, it may well be that NRM serves as a relay between more rostral analgesia-initiating brain stem centers and the final sites of inhibitory action in the trigeminal nucleus and spinal cord. The finding that the PAG sends projections to the NRM (132) supports this view.

That serotonin plays an important but surely not unique role in these anti-nociceptive systems is illustrated by the following experiments: Stimulation in or near the dorsal raphe nucleus and stimulation at sites more distant from these cells can both inhibit spinal cord interneurons (57) and cause analgesia (4). Administration of anti-serotonergic drugs, however, blocks the inhibitory effects provoked by raphe stimulation without blocking the inhibitory effects derived from stimulation elsewhere (4,57). Clearly, non-serotonergic pathways exist for mediating SPA.

OPIATE AND NON-OPIATE MECHANISMS

Considerable import has been ascribed to the observation that naloxone, a specific opiate antagonist drug, can at least partially block SPA in the rat (5,6). This finding greatly reinforced the view expressed earlier by Mayer et al. (103) that SPA and opiate analgesia share an underlying mechanism of action, a common neurochemistry, and lent credence to their contention that the common substrate activated by SPA and opiate drugs was a normal or endogenous pain-inhibitory system. This finding apparently also served to stimulate other workers (c.f., 80) in their search for an endogenous morphine-like substance in the brain (see below). More recently it has been shown that naloxone can also powerfully interfere with SPA from NRM stimulation in the cat (113,114) and completely block the pain-attenuating effect of medial diencephalic stimulation in chronic pain patients (1,69,128). In other important and conceptually related experiments (98,100), it has been reported that SPA in the rat manifests tolerance and cross-tolerance with morphine. Similar observations have again been made in man (69).

On the other hand, Akil et al. (5,6) found that naloxone only partially blocks SPA in the rat, and some investigators have failed to demonstrate an SPA-suppressive effect of this drug (110,118,168). Similarly, tolerance to SPA and cross-tolerance between SPA and morphine are also seen to be incomplete (98). Such findings suggest that non-opiate mechanisms of analgesia also exist in the brain. Several additional studies support this idea: Naloxone has been reported to block the analgesic effect of acupuncture in man without affecting hypnotic analgesia (12,102; c.f., also 51). Moreover, subjecting rats to certain highly stressful procedures induces analgesia in standard pain tests which according to some authors is (3,22,33), and to others is not (61) antagonized by naloxone. In one study, although complete spinal transection blocked stress-induced analgesia, dorsolateral funiculus lesions did not (62). Again, it seems evident that multiple descending analgesia systems exist, some possessing an opiate and/or serotonergic link, and some not. Certainly much work remains to be done to sort out the apparently separate anatomy, physiology, and neurochemistry underlying these different analgesia systems.

OPIATE RECEPTORS AND ENDOGENOUS OPIOID PEPTIDES

Among the most dramatic events in the recent history of neuroscience research has been the discovery of stereospecific opiate binding sites in the central nervous system (117,143,149) and the subsequent discovery and chemical identification of endogenous peptides which appear to be the natural ligands of these opiate receptors (37,58,70,71,117,141,151,152). Obviously, these findings have had enormous impact on the development of thinking and research in relation to mechanisms of pain modulation. The first of the endogenous opioids found in the brain and sequenced by Hughes and Kosterlitz and their colleagues (70,71) were the pentapeptides, methionine- and leucine-enkephalin, which differed from each other only in the presence of methionine or leucine in the fifth amino acid position. More recently, other larger peptides have been found in the brain and pituitary with similar opiate action (37,58,152). The generic term "endorphins" was coined by E.J. Simon (c.f., 50) to encompass all such endogenous morphine-like peptides. Shortly after the original sequencing of the enkephalins it was noted that the structure of methionine-enkephalin occupied positions 61 to 65 within a 91-amino acid pituitary prohormone, β-lipotropin (80), discovered some years earlier by Li et al. (88). It has now been shown that the entire fragment 61 to 91 of β-lipotropin is itself a potent opiate receptor agonist (24,25). This peptide has been labeled "C-fragment" or "β-endorphin". According to some workers (c.f., 50), β-lipotropin may be enzymatically cleaved in the pituitary or brain to form β-endorphin and, in turn, methionine-enkephalin. On the other hand, it has recently been shown (34,131,159) that the quantity and distribution of these endorphins in the brain is unaffected by hypophysectomy, suggesting that the pituitary and brain are separate compartments with respect to these substances. Also, no prohormone or other precursor has yet been disclosed for leucine-enkephalin; so the possibility remains that β-endorphin and the enkephalins, all of which have been found to exist intra-neuronally in the brain with separate but partially overlapping distributions (7, 20,40,66), are synthesized de novo and do not result from cleavage of larger peptide chains.

That these discoveries bear importantly on the findings and concepts discussed in earlier portions of this chapter is assured by the following observations:

1. Opiate binding sites and endorphin-containing cell bodies and/or terminals have been found to be distributed in the brain in close proximity to each other and to medial brain stem sites known to support SPA and opiate analgesia following microinjections (7,10,20,40,66,140). For example, the PAG contains opiate binding sites (10,82), enkephalin cell bodies and terminals (40, 66), and β-endorphin terminals (7,20). The NRM, on the other hand, appears to be very low in opiate binding sites (9), no doubt explaining the previously noted failure of opiate microinjections here to elicit analgesia; yet this structure is rich in enkephalin-containing cell bodies and, paradoxically, in enkephalin terminals as well (66).

2. β-endorphin and the enkephalins have been shown to induce analgesia following intraventricular injection (16,21,27,54,104, 157) or administration directly into the PAG (31,46,76,96,136). Some authors, however, have failed to find analgesia with enkephalin (21,76,87). Although a definitive explanation is lacking, it seems likely that these negative results are attributable to the fact that the enkephalins (unlike β-endorphin) are rapidly destroyed enzymatically in the brain, and that to be effective they must be administered with sufficient accuracy, in sufficient quantity, and within a sufficiently compressed time period to permit the requisite degree of mass action on appropriate receptor sites.

3. Akil et al. (7) reported that in pilot work continuous electrical stimulation at SPA sites in the PAG of rats altered the amount of enkephalin-like material which could be detected

in this region of the brain. Either an increase or decrease in such material was produced depending upon the duration of prior stimulation. These investigators also found increases in enkephalin-like material in the cerebrospinal fluid (CSF) of chronic pain patients after the delivery of analgesic central stimulation (7).

4. Several groups have reported that baseline CSF endorphin levels are lower than normal in chronic pain patients (7,139, 145,151). These levels may be increased, however, by trans-cutaneous electrical stimulation at acupuncture points (145). Notably, this restoration did not occur in those patients successfully treated for pain localized above the lumbar dermatomes. Since CSF was withdrawn from a lumbar puncture, these findings were taken to indicate that changes in endorphin levels are not a general response to percutaneous stimulation, but rather an effect specifically associated with the region of the nervous system in which analgesia is produced.

5. In man, naloxone has been shown to diminish the analgesic effect of transcutaneous electrical stimulation (32) as well as the analgesic effect of acupuncture (102,144). Electrophysio-logical and behavioral data derived from animal models of these analgesic procedures have been consistent with the human findings. For example, Woolf et al. (161) found that electroanal-gesia was almost completely reversed by naloxone in both intact and spinal rats. Pomeranz et al. (121) showed that naloxone antagonized the suppressive effect of electroacupuncture on nociceptively activated spinal cord neurons in the cat. Electroacupuncture analgesia in mice was similarly blocked by this drug (122). Furthermore, Pomeranz (120) has reported preliminary findings that a selectively bred line of mice showing low sensitivity to morphine in vivo and low opiate receptor binding activity in vitro exhibit little to no analgesia from electroacupuncture. Finally, the fact that electroacupuncture analgesia in mice could be abolished by hypophysectomy led Pomeranz et al. (121) to suggest that pituitary endorphins may also play a role in this form of analgesia.

6. A final note of particular interest is the recent report by Dehen et al. (39). These investigators found in a human subject congenitally insensitive to pain that naloxone restored pain sensitivity, as measured by the flexion reflex threshold, to approximately normal levels.

ACTIVATION OF THE MEDIAL BRAIN STEM ANALGESIA SYSTEM

Although it was suggested some time ago by Mayer et al. (103) that SPA and opiate drugs cause analgesia by activating the medial brain stem, since then relatively little direct evidence has become available concerning this point. First to be noted is that analgesia has been reported in rats following chemical stimulation of the PAG by local application of glutamate (G. Urca, manuscript in preparation) or tetanus toxin (81), but not when

this structure is blocked by locally administered dibucaine
(166). Several recent electrophysiological investigations provide additional support for this view (111,156,157). In the
first of these (111), it was shown that analgesia from PAG
stimulation and from systemic morphine administration was accompanied by significantly augmented spontaneous multiple unit
activity (MUA) in the dorsal raphe nucleus, and especially in
the nucleus raphe magnus, of awake, chronically prepared rats.
Subsequently, it was found (157) that MUA in the dorsal raphe
region of the PAG in similarly prepared rats was again powerfully increased not only by systemic injections of morphine, but
also by analgesic doses of morphine and methionine-enkephalin
injected into the lateral ventricle. Notably, rats not showing
enkephalin analgesia also failed to demonstrate the multiple
unit effect. In several animals, MUA increases were not seen in
simultaneous recordings from another brain region, indicating
that this effect is, to some degree at least, area-specific.
MUA increases were at least partly reversed by naloxone in all
animals.

In a recently completed study, Urca (156) has pursued this
line of research in greater detail, examining morphine's effect
on MUA recorded from a variety of brain stem sites established
as supporting SPA, self-stimulation, or neither behavior. Virtually all SPA sites manifested the MUA increase to systemically
administered morphine, considerably fewer sites did which supported self-stimulation but not SPA, and fewer still of the sites
supporting neither behavior showed this effect. A statistically
significant correlation was seen between the latencies to onset
of morphine analgesia and to onset of MUA increases. Tolerance
developed both to the behavioral and electrophysiological effects
of morphine with repeated administration of this drug. Throughout these studies, then, an excellent relationship is found
between the occurrence of analgesia and the activation of PAG
MUA.

By contrast, other investigators using single neuron recording
methods and systemic or iontophoretic injections of opiates have
generally reported inhibition of spontaneous firing rates (45,
48,60,63). The reason for this display is not clear. It may be
that single and multiple unit recording techniques exert different biases in the cell types (e.g., small versus large) from
which they preferentially record. It is also true that the
single unit studies have generally been performed in anesthetized
or decerebrate preparations, whereas the multiple unit studies
were all conducted in awake, intact animals. Importantly, Urca
(156) has now shown that whereas increased MUA following morphine
is found uniformly in PAG of the awake rat, decreased MUA is
routinely observed in this same brain region when recordings are
made under urethane anesthesia. More evidence will be required
to resolve this question, especially microelectrode data in
awake, chronically prepared animals. Until such evidence is
forthcoming, it cannot be determined what is the immediate effect

of opiate drugs on cells involved in the mediation of pain inhibition. Nonetheless, whether opiates directly excite such neurons or, by inhibiting them, release others farther along in the
modulation path from tonic inhibition, it seems abundantly clear
from the preponderance of evidence reviewed in this chapter that
an essential excitation occurs somewhere in the descending path
which permits pain modulation to be conveyed from the brain stem
to the cord.

CONCLUDING REMARKS

The findings summarized in this review clearly and consistently support the conclusion that portions of the medial brain stem
mediate SPA and opiate analgesia by actively imposing an ultimate
inhibitory effect on neurons early in the ascending pain path.
Many of us have, explicitly or otherwise, assumed this substrate
to possess a normal pain-inhibitory function, a view made more
compelling by the discovery of endogenous opioid peptides in all
the places in the central nervous system where from other lines
of evidence they might have been expected to occur. Yet reason
and historical perspective suggest caution. Much of the evidence
reviewed above suffers from insufficient opportunity to be
extended and confirmed. Simple ideas can appear simplistic in
the light of new information. Already it has been seen that
multiple paths of modulation exist, some apparently opiate-
related, others not. Similarly, the causal link between analgesia and dorsal horn inhibition has yet to be established, and
a great deal of circuitry and synaptic neurochemistry in the
modulation paths has yet to be worked out.

At least three other major issues have arisen which require
comment:

1. The first bears upon the question of whether the medial
brain stem system mediating SPA and opiate analgesia actually
serves to inhibit pain under biologically meaningful conditions.
Evidence has already been reviewed at least suggesting that
endorphin levels are low in chronic pain patients, high in those
congenitally insensitive to pain, and brought towards normal in
the former by analgesic central, cutaneous, and acupunctural
stimulation. Do we then have an endogenous analgesia system
which is somehow dulled or depleted by persistent pain? Evidence
has also been mentioned briefly that some severe stresses can
induce analgesia which according to certain authors at least is
reversed by naloxone. Do endogenous systems exist to block pain
during dire emergencies when unmodulated pain perception might
prove maladaptive by distracting the organism from finding or
executing coping strategies or, under more severe circumstances,
by causing shock?

Is the putative pain-inhibitory system tonically active? The
obvious approach to addressing this question has been to study
the effect of naloxone on normal pain responsiveness. Jacob et
al. (73) originally showed that naloxone increased pain respon-

siveness of rodents in the hot plate test. Since then, some studies have (26,44,79) and others have not (41,52,55) made similar observations in rodents and in man using a variety of pain assessment methods. Other findings suggest, however, that inter- and intra-individual variations in naloxone sensitivity occur which may at least partly account for the disparity among these naloxone studies. For example, it has recently been shown (44) that naloxone increases pain in rats to a greater or lesser degree as a function of a daily rhythm, suggesting that endorphin release co-varies diurnally with sensitivity to this drug. In another report (30), a direct relationship was suggested between normal variations in anti-nociception and brain endorphin activity. Thus, pain sensitivity (tail-flick latency) in normal rats predicted the degree to which binding of labeled enkephalin later occurred; that is, the brains of animals who were more sensitive to pain exhibited higher binding of labeled enkephalin, presumably indicating lower occupation of their receptor sites by an endogenous ligand. It has similarly been reported (26) that naloxone increased pain perception and somatosensory evoked potentials recorded from the scalp in human subjects below the mean on pain sensitivity, but reduced these behavioral and electrophysiological responses in other subjects with higher than average sensitivity to pain. Once again, these results were taken to indicate that individual differences in pain sensitivity may reflect differences in the endogenous opiate system. Finally, it has recently been shown (86) that naloxone can increase the perception of pain in placebo-responsive human subjects without affecting those unresponsive to placebo (c.f., however 107). It seems evident from these reports that endorphin-related differences do occur within and between normal individuals which can importantly influence the outcome of studies in this area and badly confuse the interpretation of their findings if not adequately controlled.

What other circumstances or stimuli have access to the supposed endogenous analgesia substrate? It has been reported that the duration of "animal hypnosis" which provides analgesia in the rabbit is curtailed by naloxone administration (28). On the other hand, analgesia accompanying vaginal cervix probing in rats is not affected by this drug (38). Are there other situations which actually block this system and hence exacerbate pain? Is analgesia the only or even the most important function of this system, or might more subtle modulations than pain control be the system's usual role? The questions raised in this section are but a few of the important ones in this area awaiting definitive answers. Until such are forthcoming, the nature and even the existence of a normal pain-inhibitory system in the brain must remain hypothetical.

2. Although great emphasis has been placed in preceding sections of this chapter on descending control mechanisms of brain stem origin, in fact excellent evidence exists that opiate drugs and endorphins can also exert a direct anti-nociceptive influence

in the spinal cord. First to be noted in this regard is that opiate binding sites (9,83) and endorphins (66) are found in great density in those regions of the dorsal horn where pain modulation is thought to occur. Second, it has been known for some time that spinal reflexes can still be attenuated by morphine after spinal transection, although sensitivity to the drug is reduced in this preparation (72). Nociceptive responding in dorsal horn interneurons is readily blocked by opiates in the spinal cat (19,78,84,85). Finally, very recent evidence shows that small quantities of opiates delivered into the subarachnoid space over the lumbar cord produce analgesia in rats, and similar injections of naloxone antagonize analgesia from systemically administered morphine (164). It appears that opiate receptors in the spinal cord as well as those in the brain stem are both necessary and sufficient to mediate the analgesic action of opiate drugs injected systemically. Yaksh and Rudy (165) provide a provocative discussion of the implications of these findings in their recent and extensive review of opiate mechanisms.

3. Finally, it is known that opiate binding sites (9,10,65, 82) and endorphins (7,20,66) are located in brain areas apparently unrelated to pain inhibition. It is generally assumed that such sites must be involved in mediating other well known opiate effects such as respiratory, pupillary, and thermoregulatory changes, euphoria and dysphoria, and perhaps the motor and pathological electrographic signs of opiate abstinence. Some data are available to suggest this is so. For example, cortical EEG recordings from awake rats reveal that a distinctive pattern of seizures is obtained following enkephalin injections into the lateral ventricle (157). It has more recently been shown that such seizures result from doses of methionine- or leucine-enkephalin well below those required to produce analgesia from the ventricle, as well as from morphine injected in a similar fashion but at doses greatly exceeding the analgesic dose (47). Such seizures are blocked by prior administration of naloxone, suggesting their mediation by opiate binding sites (47). The location of these sites and their anatomical dissociation from others mediating analgesia is suggested by the demonstration that enkephalin injected into dorsomedial thalamus can yield seizures without analgesia, whereas similar injections into the periaqueductal gray matter can provide analgesia without seizures (46). It has further been suggested (46) that the analgesic and epileptic effects of the enkephalins are not only mediated by opiate binding sites in different brain areas but by sites which differ from each other in their pharmacological properties. This suggestion is in accord with a growing body of evidence pointing to the existence of pharmacologically different opiate receptor types (94,97).

One might wonder what normal function is served by an endogenous opioid system which can elicit seizures under pathological circumstances. Several lines of evidence suggest an attractive hypothesis: Belluzzi and Stein (17) first reported that rats self-administer the enkephalins into the lateral ventricle at doses just below those which Frenk et al. (47) found produced seizures. They further reported that naloxone could block electrical self-stimulation from the PAG, and concluded that enkephalin might serve normally as a drive-reduction reward transmitter or endogenous euphorigen (17). Rogers et al. (129; c.f., also 67,68,95) found that naloxone blocks food and water consumption in deprived rats, a finding taken to indicate that normal rewards may be at least partly mediated by endorphins, just as brain-stimulation reward appears to be.

The relation of such findings to the subject of this review is at least two-fold: On the one hand, it is evident that endorphins cannot be assigned a role exclusively in anti-nociception. On the other hand, it seems likely, if subsequent research confirms the euphorigenic properties of endogenous opioids, that close ties will be found between the substrates of analgesia and reward since mechanisms serving pain inhibition and pleasure must surely interact. The development of new pharmacological and biochemical tools will be enormously helpful in resolving the problems introduced by the presence of qualitatively different opiate binding sites in the brain. The imagination and special talents of behavioral scientists, however, will clearly be required to dissect out and re-integrate the functional characteristics of these no doubt complex and subtly active systems.

REFERENCES

1. Adams, J.E. (1976): Pain, 2:161-166.
2. Akil, H., and Liebeskind, J.C. (1975): Brain Res., 94:279-296.
3. Akil, H., Madden, J., Patrick, R.L., and Barchas, J.D. (1976): In: Opiates and Endogenous Opioid Peptides, edited by H.W. Kosterlitz, pp. 63-70. Elsevier, Amsterdam.
4. Akil, H., and Mayer, D.J. (1972): Brain Res., 44:692-697.
5. Akil, H., Mayer, D.J., and Liebeskind, J.C. (1972): C. R. Acad. Sci. (Paris), 274:3603-3605.
6. Akil, H., Mayer, D.J., and Liebeskind, J.C. (1976): Science, 191:961-962.
7. Akil, H., Watson, S.J., Berger, P.A., and Barchas, J.D. (1978): In: The Endorphins, edited by E. Costa, and M. Trabucchi, pp. 125-140. Raven Press, New York.
8. Albe-Fessard, D., Levante, A., and Lamour, Y. (1974): Brain Res., 65:503-509.
9. Atweh, S.F., and Kuhar, M.J. (1977): Brain Res., 124:53-67.
10. Atweh, S.F., and Kuhar, M.J. (1977): Brain Res., 129:1-12.
11. Balagura, S., and Ralph, T. (1973): Brain Res., 60:369-379.
12. Barber, J., and Mayer, D. (1978): Pain, 4:41-48.
13. Basbaum, A.I., Clanton, C.H., and Fields, H.L. (1978): J. Comp. Neurol., 178:209-224.

14. Basbaum, A.I., Marley, N., O'Keefe, J., and Clanton, C.H. (1977): Pain, 3:43-56.
15. Beall, J.E., Martin, R.F., Applebaum, A.E., and Willis, W.D. (1976): Brain Res., 114:328-333.
16. Belluzzi, J.D., Grant, N., Garsky, V., Sarantakis, D., Wise, C.D., and Stein, L. (1976): Nature (London), 260:625-626.
17. Belluzzi, J.D., and Stein, L. (1977): Nature (London), 266:556-558.
18. Bennett, G.J., and Mayer, D.J. (1976): Proc. Soc. Neurosci., 2:928.
19. Besson, J.M., Wyon-Maillard, M.C., Benoist, J.M., Conseiller, C., and Hamann, K.F. (1973): J. Pharmacol. Exp. Ther., 187:239-245.
20. Bloom, F.E., Rossier, J., Battenberg, E.L.F., Bayon, A., French, E., Henriksen, S.J., Siggins, G.R., Segal, D., Browne, R., Ling, N., and Guillemin, R. (1978): In: The Endorphins, edited by E. Costa, and M. Trabucchi, pp. 89-109. Raven Press, New York.
21. Bloom, F., Segal, D., Ling, N., and Guillemin, R. (1976): Science, 194:630-632.
22. Bodnar, R.J., Kelly, D.D., Spiaggia, A., and Glusman, M. (1977): Fed. Proc., 36:3.
23. Boethius, J., Lindblom, U., Meyerson, B.A., and Widén, L. (1976): In: Sensory Functions of the Skin in Primates, edited by Y. Zotterman, pp. 531-548. Pergamon Press, Oxford.
24. Bradbury, A.F., Smyth. D.G., Snell, C.R., Birdsall, N.J.M., and Hulme, E.C. (1976): Nature (London), 260:793-795.
25. Bradbury, A.F., Smyth, D.G., Snell, C.R., Deakin, J.I.W., and Wendlandt, S. (1977): Biochem. Biophys. Res. Commun., 74:748-752.
26. Buchsbaum, M.E., Davis, G.C., and Bunney, W.E. (1977): Nature (London), 270:620-622.
27. Büscher, H.H., Hill, R.C., Römer, D., Cardinaux, F., Closse, A., Hauser, D., and Pless, J. (1976): Nature (London), 261:423-425.
28. Carli, G., Farabollini, G., and Fontani, G. (1978): Pain Abst., 1:000-000.
29. Carrol, M.N., Jr., and Lim, R.K.S. (1960): Arch. Int. Pharmacodyn., 125:383-403.
30. Chance, W.T., White, A.C., Krynock, G.M., and Rosecrans, J.A. (1978): Brain Res., 141:371-374.
31. Chang, J.K., Fong, B.T.W., Pert, A., and Pert, C.B. (1976): Life Sci., 18:1473-1482.
32. Chapman, C.R., and Benedetti, C. (1977): Life Sci., 21:1645-1648.
33. Chesher, G.B., and Chan, B. (1977): Life Sci., 21:1569-1574.
34. Cheung, A.L., and Goldstein, A. (1976): Life Sci., 19:1005-1007.
35. Cicero, T.J., Meyer, E.R., and Smithloff, B.R. (1974): J. Pharmacol. exp. Ther., 189:72-82.

36. Costa, E., and Trabucchi, M., editors (1978): The Endorphins. Raven Press, New York.
37. Cox, B.M., Goldstein, A., and Li, C.H. (1976): Proc. Natl. Acad. Sci. (U.S.A.), 73:1821-1823.
38. Crowley, W.R., Rodriguez-Sierra, F.J., and Komisaruk, B.R. (1977): Psychopharmacology (Berlin), 54:223-225.
39. Dehen, J., Willer, J.C., Boureau, F., and Cambier, J. (1977): Lancet, 2:293-294.
40. Elde, R., Hökfelt, T., Johansson, O., and Terenius, L. (1976): Neuroscience, 1:349-351.
41. El-Sobky, A., Dostrovsky, J.O., and Wall, P.D. (1976): Nature (London), 263:783-784.
42. Fields, H.L., and Basbaum, A.I. (1978): Ann. Rev. Physiol., 40:217-248.
43. Fields, H.L., Basbaum, A.I., Clanton, C.H., and Anderson, S.D. (1977): Brain Res., 126:441-453.
44. Frederickson, R.C.A., Burgis, D., and Edwards, J.D. (1977): Science, 198:756-759.
45. Frederickson, R.C.A., and Norris, F.H. (1976): Science, 194:440-442.
46. Frenk, H., McCarty, B.C., and Liebeskind, J.C. (1978): Science, 200:335-337.
47. Frenk, H., Urca, G., and Liebeskind, J.C. (1978): Brain Res., 150:000-000.
48. Gent, J.P., and Wolstencroft, J.H. (1976): In: Opiates and Endogenous Opioid Peptides, edited by H.W. Kosterlitz, pp. 217-224. Elsevier, Amsterdam.
49. Giesler, G.J., Jr., and Liebeskind, J.C. (1976): Pain, 2:43-48.
50. Goldstein, A. (1976): Science, 193:1081-1086.
51. Goldstein, A., and Hilgard, E.R. (1975): Proc. Natl. Acad. Sci. (U.S.A.), 72:2041-2043.
52. Goldstein, A., Pryor, G.T., Otis, L., and Larsen, F. (1976): Life Sci., 18:599-604.
53. Goodman, S.J., and Holcombe, V. (1976): In: Advances in Pain Research and Therapy, Vol. 1, edited by J.J. Bonica, and D. Albe-Fessard, pp. 495-502. Raven Press, New York.
54. Graf, L., Szekely, J.I., Ronai, A.Z., Dunai-Kovacs, Z., and Bajusz, S. (1976): Nature (London), 263:240-242.
55. Grevert, P., and Goldstein, A. (1978): Science, 199:1093-1095.
56. Grumbach, L. (1966): In: Pain, edited by R.S. Knighton, and P.R. Dumke, pp. 163-182. Little, Brown and Co., Boston, Mass.
57. Guilbaud, G., Besson, J.M., Oliveras, J.L., and Liebeskind, J.C. (1973): Brain Res., 61:417-422.
58. Guillemin, R., Ling, N., Burgus, R. (1976): C. R. Acad. Sci. (D) (Paris), 282:783-785.
59. Gybels, J., and Cosyns, P. (1978): In: Sensory Functions of the Skin in Primates, edited by Y. Zotterman, pp. 521-530. Pergamon Press, Oxford.

60. Haigler, H.J. (1976): Life Sci., 19:841-858.
61. Hayes, R.L., Bennet, G.J., Pauline, N.G., and Mayer, D.J. (1978): Brain Res., (in press).
62. Hayes, R.L., Price, D.D., Bennet, G.J., Wilcox, G.L., and Mayer, D.J. (1978): Brain Res., (in press).
63. Henry, J.L. (1976): In: Advances in Pain Research and Therapy, Vol. 1, edited by J.J. Bonica, and D. Albe-Fessard, pp. 615-620. Raven Press, New York.
64. Herz, A., Albus, K., Metys, J., Schubert, P., and Teschemacher, H. (1970): Neuropharmacology, 9:539-551.
65. Hiller, J., Pearson, J., and Simon, E.J. (1973): Res. Commun. Chem. Pathol. Pharmacol., 6:1052-1062.
66. Hökfelt, T., Ljungdahl, A., Terenius, L., Elde, R., and Nilson, G. (1977): Proc. Natl. Acad. Sci. (U.S.A.), 74:3081-3085.
67. Holtzman, S.G. (1974): J. Pharmacol. Exp. Ther., 189:51-60.
68. Holtzman, S.G. (1975): Life Sci., 16:1465-1470.
69. Hosobuchi, Y., Adams, J.E., Linchitz, R. (1977): Science, 197:183-185.
70. Hughes, J. (1975): Brain Res., 88:295-308.
71. Hughes, J., Smith, T.W., Kosterlitz, H.W., Fothergill, L.A., Morgan, B.A., and Morris, H.R. (1975): Nature (London), 258:577-579.
72. Irwin, S., Houde, R.W., Bennett, D.R., Hendershot, L.C., and Seevers, M.H. (1951): J. Pharmacol. Exp. Ther., 101:132-143.
73. Jacob, J.J., Tremblay, E.C., and Colombel, M. (1974): Psychopharmacologia (Berlin), 37:217-223.
74. Jacquet, Y.F., and Lajtha, A. (1973): Science, 182:490-492.
75. Jacquet, Y.F., and Lajtha, A. (1976): Brain Res., 103:501-513.
76. Jacquet, Y.F., and Marks, N. (1976): Science, 194:630-632.
77. Kerr, F.W.L., and Wilson, P.R. (1978): Ann. Rev. Neurosci., 1:83-102.
78. Kitahata, L.M., Kosaka, Y., Taub, A., Bonikos, K., and Hoffert, M. (1974): Anesthesiology, 41:39-48.
79. Kokka, N., and Fairhurst, A.S. (1977): Life Sci., 21:975-980.
80. Kosterlitz, H.W., and Hughes, J. (1978): In: The Endorphins, edited by E. Costa, and M. Trabucchi, pp. 31-44. Raven Press, New York.
81. Kryzhanovsky, G.N. (1978): Pain Abst, 1:000-000.
82. Kuhar, M.S., Pert, C.B., and Snyder, S.H. (1973): Nature (London), 245:447-450.
83. LaMotte, C., Pert, C.B., and Snyder, S.H. (1976): Brain Res., 112:407-412.
84. LeBars, D., Menétrey, D., and Besson, J.M. (1976): Brain Res., 113:293-310.
85. LeBars, D., Menétrey, D., Conseiller, C., and Besson, J.M. (1975): Brain Res., 98:261-277.
86. Levine, J.C., Gordon, N.C., and Fields, H.L. (1978): Pain Abst., 1:000-000.

87. Leybin, L., Pinsky, C., LaBella, F.S., Havlicek, V., and
    Rezek, M. (1976): Nature (London), 264:458-459.
88. Li, C.H., Barnafi, L., Chrétian, M., and Chung, D. (1965):
    Nature (London), 208:1093-1094.
89. Liebeskind, J.C., Giesler, G.J., Jr., and Urca, G. (1976):
    In: Sensory Functions of the Skin in Primates, edited by
    Y. Zotterman, pp. 561-573. Pergamon Press, New York.
90. Liebeskind, J.C., Mayer, D.J., and Akil, H. (1974): In:
    Advances in Neurology, Volume 4: Pain, edited by J.J.
    Bonica, pp. 261-268. Raven Press, New York.
91. Liebeskind, J.C., and Paul, L.A. (1977): Ann. Rev. Psychol.,
    28:41-60.
92. Liebman, J.M., and Butcher, L.L. (1973): Naunyn-
    Schmiedeberg's Arch. Pharmacol., 277:305-318.
93. Lim, R.K.S., Guzman, F., Rodgers, D.W., Goto, K., Braun, C.,
    Dickerson, G.D., and Engle, R.J. (1964): Archs. Int.
    Pharmacodyn., 152:25-58.
94. Lord, J.A.H., Waterfield, A.A., Hughes, J., and Kosterlitz,
    H.W. (1977): Nature (London), 267:495-499.
95. Maickel, R.P., Braude, M.C., and Zabik, J.E. (1977):
    Neuropharmacology, 16:863-866.
96. Malick, J.B., and Goldstein, J.M. (1977): Life Sci., 20:
    827-832.
97. Martin, W.R., Eades, C.G., Thompson, J.A., Huppler, R.E.,
    and Gilbert, P.E. (1976): J. Pharmacol. Exp. Ther., 197:
    517-532.
98. Mayer, D.J., and Hayes, R. (1975): Science, 188:941-943.
99. Mayer, D.J., and Liebeskind, J.C. (1974): Brain Res., 68:
    73-93.
100. Mayer, D.J., and Murphin, R. (1976): Fed. Proc., 35:385.
101. Mayer, D.J., and Price, D.D. (1976): Pain, 2:379-404.
102. Mayer, D.J., Price, D.D., Rafii, A., and Barber, J. (1976):
     In: Advances in Pain Research and Therapy, Vol. 1, edited
     by J.J. Bonica, and D. Albe-Fessard, pp. 751-754. Raven
     Press, New York.
103. Mayer, D.J., Wolfle, T.L., Akil, H., Carder, B., and
     Liebeskind, J.C. (1971): Science, 174:1351-1354.
104. Meglio, M., Hosobuchi, Y., Loh, H.H., Adams, J.E., and Li,
     C.H. (1977): Proc. Natl. Acad. Sci. (U.S.A.), 74:774-776.
105. Melzack, R., and Melinkoff, D.F. (1974): Exp. Neurol., 43:
     369-374.
106. Messing, R.B., and Lytle, L.D. (1978): Pain, 4:1-21.
107. Mihic, D., and Binkert, E. (1978): Pain Abst., 1:000-000.
108. Morrow, T.J., and Casey, K.L. (1976): In: Advances in Pain
     Research and Therapy, Vol. 1, edited by J.J. Bonica, and
     D. Albe-Fessard, pp. 503-510. Raven Press, New York.
109. Murfin, R., Bennett, G.J., and Mayer, D.J. (1976): Neurosci.
     Abst., 2:946.
110. Oleson, T.D., and Liebeskind, J.C. (1976): In: Advances
     in Pain Research and Therapy, Vol. 1, edited by J.J.
     Bonica, and D. Albe-Fessard, pp. 487-494. Raven Press,
     New York.

111. Oleson, T.D., Twombly, D.A., and Liebeskind, J.C. (1978): Pain, 4:211-230.
112. Oliveras, J.L., Besson, J.M., Guilbaud, G., and Liebeskind, J.C. (1974): Brain Res., 20:32-44.
113. Oliveras, J.L., Hosobuchi, Y., Redjemi, F., Guilbaud, G., and Besson, J.M. (1977): Brain Res., 120:221-229.
114. Oliveras, J.L., Redjemi, F., Guilbaud, G., and Besson, J.M. (1975): Pain, 1:139-145.
115. Oliveras, J.L., Woda, A., Guilbaud, G., and Besson, J.M. (1974): Brain Res., 72:328-331.
116. Pasternak, G.W., Goodman, R., and Snyder, S.H. (1975): Life Sci., 16:1765-1769.
117. Pert, C.B., and Snyder, S.H. (1973): Science, 179:1011-1014.
118. Pert, A., and Walter, M. (1976): Life Sci., 19:1023-1032.
119. Pert, A., and Yaksh, T. (1974): Brain Res., 80:135-140.
120. Pomeranz, B. (1978): In: The Endorphins, edited by E. Costa, and M. Trabucchi, pp. 351-360. Raven Press, New York.
121. Pomeranz, B., Cheng, R., and Law, P. (1977): Exp. Neurol., 54:172-178.
122. Pomeranz, B., and Chiu, D. (1976): Life Sci., 19:1757-1762.
123. Price, M.T.C., and Fibiger, H.C. (1975): Brain Res., 99:189-193.
124. Proudfit, H.K., and Anderson, E.G. (1975): Brain Res., 98:612-619.
125. Reynolds, D.V. (1969): Science, 164:444-445.
126. Rhodes, D.L., and Liebeskind, J.C. (1978): Brain Res., 143:521-532.
127. Richardson, D.E., and Akil, H. (1977): J. Neurosurg., 47:178-183.
128. Richardson, D.E., and Akil, H. (1977): J. Neurosurg., 47:184-189.
129. Rogers, G.H., Frenk, H., Taylor, A.N., and Liebeskind, J.C. (1978): Proc. West. Pharmacol. Soc., 21:000-000.
130. Rose, M. (1974): J. Comp. Physiol. Psychol., 87:607-617.
131. Rossier, J., French, E.D., Rivier, C., Ling, N., Guillemin, R., and Bloom, F.E. (1977): Nature (London), 270:618-620.
132. Ruda, M. (1975): Autoradiographic Study of the Efferent Projections of the Midbrain Central Gray of the Cat. Ph.D. Dissertation, University of Pennsylvania.
133. Ruda, M., Hayes, R.L., Dubner, R., and Price, D.D. (1976): Neurosci. Abst., 2:952.
134. Saarnivaara, L. (1969): Ann. Med. exp. Fenn., 47:113-123.
135. Satoh, M., and Takagi, H. (1971): Europ. J. Pharmacol., 14:60-65.
136. Segal, D.S., Browne, R.G., Bloom, F., Ling, N., and Guillemin, R. (1977): Science, 198:411-414.
137. Sessle, B.J., Dubner, R., Greenwood, L.F., and Lucier, G.E. (1975): Canad. J. Physiol. Pharmacol., 54:66-69.
138. Sharpe, L.G., Garnett, J.E., and Cicero, T.J. (1974): Behav. Biol., 11:303-314.

139. Sicuteri, F., Anselmi, B., Curradi, C., Michelacci, S.,
     and Sassi, A. (1978): In: The Endorphins, edited by
     E. Costa, and M. Trabucchi, pp. 363-366. Raven Press,
     New York.
140. Simantov, R., Kuhar, M.J., Uhl, G.R., and Snyder, S.H.
     (1977): Proc. Natl. Acad. Sci. (U.S.A.), 74:2167-2171.
141. Simantov, R., and Snyder, S.H. (1976): Life Sci., 18:
     781-787.
142. Simon, E.J., and Hiller, J.M. (1978): Ann. Rev. Pharmacol.
     and Toxicol., 18:371-394.
143. Simon, E.J., Hiller, J.M., and Edelman, I. (1973): Proc.
     Natl. Acad. Sci. (U.S.A.), 70:1947-1949.
144. Sjölund, B., and Eriksson, M. (1976): Lancet, 2:1085.
145. Sjölund, B., Terenius, L., Eriksson, M. (1977): Acta
     Physiol. Scand., 100:382-384.
146. Soper, W.Y. (1976): J. comp. physiol. Psychol., 90:91-101.
147. Takagi, H., Satoh, M., Akaike, A., Shibata, T., and
     Kuraishi, Y. (1977): Europ. J. Pharmacol., 45:91-93.
148. Tenen, S.S. (1968): Psychopharmacologia (Berlin), 12:278-
     285.
149. Terenius, L. (1972): Acta Pharmacol., 31, Suppl. I:50.
150. Terenius, L. (1978): Ann. Rev. Pharmacol. and Toxicol.,
     18:189-204.
151. Terenius, L., and Wahlström, A. (1975): Life Sci., 16:
     1759-1764.
152. Teschemacher, H., Opheim, K.E., Cox, B.M., and Goldstein,
     A. (1975): Life Sci., 16:1771-1776.
153. Trevino, D.L., Coulter, J.D., and Willis, W.D. (1973):
     J. Neurophysiol., 36:750-761.
154. Tsou, K. (1963): Acta physiol. Sin., 26:332-337.
155. Tsou, K., and Jang, C.S. (1964): Sci. Sinica, 13:1099-1109.
156. Urca, G. (1978): Electrophysiological Correlates of Opiate
     Action in the Central Nervous System of the Rat. Ph.D.
     Dissertation, University of California, Los Angeles.
157. Urca, G., Frenk, H., Liebeskind, J.C., and Taylor, A.N.
     (1977): Science, 197:83-86.
158. Vogt, M. (1974): J. Physiol. (London), 236:483-498.
159. Wesche, D., Höllt, V., and Herz, A. (1977): Naunyn-
     Schmiedeberg's Arch. Pharmacol., 301:79-82.
160. Willis, W.D., Haber, L.H., and Martin, R.F. (1977): J.
     Neurophysiol., 40:968-981.
161. Woolf, C.J., Barrett, G.D., Mitchell, D., and Myers, R.A.
     (1977): Europ. J. Pharmacol., 45:311-314.
162. Yaksh, T.L., DuChateau, J.C., and Rudy, T.A. (1976): Brain
     Res., 104:367-372.
163. Yaksh, T.L., Plant, R., and Rudy, T.A. (1976): Europ. J.
     Pharmacol., 41:399-408.
164. Yaksh, T.L., and Rudy, T.A. (1977): J. Pharmacol. Exp.
     Ther., 202:411-428.
165. Yaksh, T.L., and Rudy, T.A. (1978): Pain, 4:299-359.

166. Yaksh, T.L., Rudy, T.A., and Yeung, J.C. (1975): Neurosci. Abst., 1:283.
167. Yaksh, T.L., Yeung, J.C., and Rudy, T.A. (1976): Brain Res., 114:83-103.
168. Yaksh, T.L., Yeung, J.C., and Rudy, T.A. (1976): Life Sci., 18:1193-1198.
169. Yeung, J.C., Yaksh, T.L., and Rudy, T.A. (1977): Pain, 4:23-40.
170. Yunger, L.M., Harvey, J.A., and Lorens, S.A. (1973): Physiol. Behav., 10:909-913.

The Psychology of Pain, edited by R. A. Sternbach.
Raven Press, New York © 1978.

Learning Processes in Pain

Wilbert E. Fordyce

*Department of Rehabilitation Medicine, University Hospital, University of Washington,
Seattle, Washington 98195*

INTRODUCTION

The purpose of this chapter is to present a behavioral analysis of chronic pain and to describe methods of evaluating and managing chronic pain problems derived from the behavioral perspective.

A behavioral approach has two essential conceptual features. One is that behavior (i.e., "behavior" is defined here as the observable, measurable, overt actions of the organism) has significance in its own right. Behavior is not to be understood solely as an automatic extension or overt expression of some underlying causative factor within the organism. Stated another way, behavior does not have a simple 1:1 linkage to alleged or inferred internal events. Behavior is subject to influence by a variety of factors, a major one of which is learning/conditioning effects. It follows that when one is concerned about behavior or actions of, for example, pain patients, an understanding of what is going on requires considering the spectrum of factors which influence that behavior.[1]

The second conceptual underpinning to a behavioral approach is the emphasis on operationalizing measurement and observations. The phenomena of interest is behavior. To assess behavior, and changes in it, it

---

[1] For those less familiar with behavioral perspectives, it is pertinent to note that the behavioral model presented here does not seek to deny existence of mental events "within the black box", nor even to avoid concern with them. The point is that one need not resort to considering those mental events in order to study, understand, or modify behavior. The reverse, however, is not considered here to be true; namely, that one cannot study, understand, or modify behavior by focusing on mental events.

is essential to develop methods for measurement of
behavior. Moreover, in an intervention program
designed to change behavior, the criterion of change
or success/failure is to be found in the measurement
of changes in behavior; i.e., in what the person does.
    It is necessary also for the purposes of this
chapter to consider some of the differences between
acute and chronic illness. These differences assume
paramount importance in dealing with pain.
    Acute illness ("acute here is a time related
statement referring simply to recent onset) presents
a different set of circumstances from chronic illness
(illness which has persisted consistently for extended
periods; e.g., 4-6 months or more). A brief
examination of some of these will aid in clarifying
the relevance of a behavioral approach to chronic
pain.
    When, for whatever reason, an illness and the
associated symptom complex persist for long intervals,
there is inherently present an increased opportunity
for learning/conditioning effects to exert influence.
Some parts of the set of symptoms associated with the
illness are behavior. In the case of pain, for
example, such actions as grimacing, moaning, verbal-
izing the experience of somatic distress, limping,
asking to be helped with or relieved of a pain-
aggravating task, are all forms of behavior. Those
behaviors are subject to influence by learning/
conditioning effects, just as is true for other kinds
of behavior. The originating "cause" for these
symptom behaviors to begin to occur is not important
to the point. What is important is that the symptoms
persist across time and that they occur in a set of
circumstances conducive to learning/conditioning. The
fact of chronicity of illness provides two of the
three essentials for conditioning; namely, that
symptom behaviors occur and that they continue to
occur for a few weeks, months, or years. The third
essential of conditioning, circumstances conducive to
conditioning, may or may not exist in the context of a
given person's chronic illness. It is enough for now
to note that if those circumstances do exist, they
will have opportunity to exert influence.
    A second distinction between acute and chronic
illness should also be noted. When an illness is
short lived, there is little need for the patient, or
those around him/her, to make major or lasting
changes in their behavioral repertories. A fractured
ankle, for example, requires for a few days or weeks
crutch ambulation or use of a walking cast, but it
does not require that the person make major and
enduring changes in the type of work or play engaged

in or in the major methods for mobility. Moreover, vocational, avocational, and social behaviors are still at hand and can be readily resumed. In acute illness, the reduction of illness behavior (i.e., symptoms and their associated "causes") leads virtually automatically to a return to well behaviors.

The situation in chronic illness is often quite different. The fact of chronicity means that both the patient and those around him/her will have had to establish and persist in the exercise of many illness related behaviors. If, for example, instead of a relatively simple ankle fracture, the injury had been a severe shattering of the ankle and foot requiring multiple surgeries and many months of relative immobilization, the patient will have had to develop various illness-related behaviors (e.g., wheelchair mobility, methods for occupying one's time when unable to go to work or to move about). Family members will have had to shift their repertoires, as well, to accomodate the demands of the illness and the changes in social, avocational, and household maintenance activities produced by the injury. Concomitantly, both patient and family members will have, to some extent, not been engaging in or practicing many of the things they did before but which are no longer accessible because of the injury. The longer the duration of the injury, the greater the amount of disuse of elements of pre-onset repertoires and the greater the rehearsal of and reinforcement of illness-related repertoires. When healing has occurred and the disability has run its course, the process of shifting back to a resumption of the well behavior repertoire can be and often is a formidable task. When illness has persisted for several years, the pre-onset repertoire will have become quite remote. In such a situation, reduction of symptoms or illness behavior by no means leads automatically to replacement by effective well behavior. It follows that effective treatment of chronic illness, including chronic pain, must address both the task of reducing illness behavior and that of increasing or reestablishing effective well behavior.

Definitions of Pain

Much confusion has arisen from the tendency of many to try to encompass many divergent and only loosely related phenomena under one term: pain. We shall not attempt here to carry out a full review of the problem of definition. Liebeskind (10) states the problem well. He says, in part, "Pain means many different things; and the variables which correlate with, inhibit or enhance one kind of pain, and the neural mechanisms which underlie it, may not be associated with or influence other kinds. Thus one must distinguish between the normal perception of noxious stimuli and pain of pathological origin, and between acute pathological pain and chronic, intractable pain conditions . . . While it is often useful to distinguish between various aspects of pain experience (e.g., 'sensory-discriminative' versus 'motivational-affective' components) other dichotomus terms used in an attempt to specify the origin of pain ('physiological' versus 'psychological', 'organic' versus 'functional') connote a Cartesian dualism and should have been discarded long ago."

Pain as a clinical entity has typically been viewed from a bio-medical or Medical/Disease Model perspective. The assumption has been made that the observable indicators of the problem (i.e., signs or symptoms) are but an extension or reflection of underlying causative factors: in the case of pain, a nociceptive stimulus impinging on some free nerve ending or other pain receptor. This view of pain has all too often been accepted as a statement of facts. The model has considerable descriptive and predictive power in relation to acute or recent onset illness but the mere existence of many persisting pain problems when treatment was based on assumptions of the Disease Model perspective, is itself an indicator of limitation of the model. In addition, however, treatment of chronic pain problems derived from markedly different conceptual bases, and which has enjoyed considerable success with patients previously treatment failures by traditionally derived methods, lends further evidence to the limitations of reliance solely on a Disease Model perspective Roberts (17) Swanson et al (21) Sternbach (20) Fordyce (3) Fordyce et al (4) and to the credibility of alternatives.

Loeser (11) has organized an approach to the definitional problem which appears to handle well the diverse phenomena with which one is confronted in clinical pain, acute and chronic. There is as a starting basis, as shown in Figure 1, nociception, defined as, "potentially tissue-damaging thermal or mechanical energy impinging upon specialized nerve endings of A delta and C fibers." Next, there is pain. Pain is defined as "perceived nociceptive input to the nervous system." In this schema, the term "pain" is reserved for a sensory experience. That sensory experience is defined tautologically in that the "experience" must be perceived in order for it to be said to have occurred. But it is not necessary

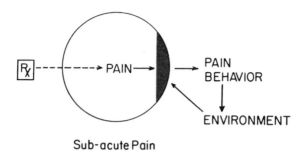

Sub-acute Pain

FIG. 1. The dimensions of chronic pain. This figure, the conceptualization which underlies it, and the definitions of terms
were developed by and are used with permission of John D. Loeser,
M.D., Associate Professor, Neurological Surgery, University of
Washington School of Medicine, Seattle. (The terms are defined
in the text.)

that there be nociceptive input in order for "pain",
as defined, to occur, for it is entirely conceivable
an organism may perceive an experience ordinarily
associated with nociceptive stimuli in the absence
of such stimuli. Similarly, the presence of a
nociceptive stimulus does not insure there will be an
experience of "pain", as defined. Neurological
defect, analgesia, and other factors make it
possible for the stimulus to occur without the
response. Thus, the association between nociception
and pain, while close, is not 1:1.
    The next level is "suffering", defined as,
"negative affective response generated in higher
nervous centers by pain and other situations; loss of
loved objects, stress, anxiety, etc." This suffering
component corresponds to what Merskey (14) was
referring to in his definition of pain: ". . . an
unpleasant experience which we primarily associate
with tissue damage or describe in terms of tissue
damage or both." Loeser's (11) term directs our
attention to the involvement of higher nervous
centers including the cortex. The fact of higher
nervous center influence has many important
implications, not the least of which is that cross
currents within that system make it possible for a
diversity of factors, simultaneously or consecutively,
to influence the suffering experience. Nociception,
and from it, pain, as defined, is not necessary to
induce suffering. Thus, the linkage between
nociception and suffering is even less compelling than
between nociception and "pain."
    In the clinical setting, an addition to Merskey's
(14) definition is appropriate. To restate the

amended definition, "Pain[2] is an unpleasant experience which we primarily associate with tissue
damage or describe in terms of tissue damage or both,
and the presence of which is signaled by some form of
visible or audible behavior." That is, in the
context of clinical pain, suffering becomes an issue
because it leads to pain behavior, defined by
Loeser (11) as, "All forms of behavior generated by
the individual commonly understood to reflect the
presence of nociception, including speech, facial
expression, posture, seeking health care attention,
taking medications, refusing to work." If there were
no pain behavior, there would be no pain problem.

Lazarus (8) has stated, "Of course, nearly everyone, apart from ESP enthusiasts, will agree that the
only way we can know anything about another person is
through his or her behavior (verbal and non-verbal
responses). . ." In regard to clinical pain, the
essence of the problem is that there is pain behavior.
It is through the person's pain behavior that we
come to know about and perhaps eventually to understand that person's pain problem, or even that she/he
has one. It is the pain behavior we observe, whether
it be such autonomically mediated responses as
changes in heart rate or palmar sweating; verbal
descriptions of a suffering experience; or striated
musculature movements such as a limp, reaching for
medications, rubbing a sore shoulder, reclining in a
time and place where ordinarily one might expect the
person to be engaging in some other activity. Thus,
we have come full cycle and are back to the starting
point of this chapter; namely that behavior, in this
case, pain behavior, has significance in its own
right and is not to be understood solely as an
automatic extension or overt expression of some
underlying causative factor within the organism.

Behavioral Analysis of Pain

In the special case of chronic clinical pain, we
have a situation in which the problem is identified
from and manifested by pain behaviors. Moreover,
those pain behaviors will have been occurring for
extended intervals. It becomes a matter of
paramount importance to the understanding of the
chronic clinical pain problem to consider the array

---

[2]The intent here is not to depart from the Loeser
scheme but to relate it to the more common parlance of
the clinical setting by using "pain" for the moment as
a generic term.

of factors which may be exerting influence on the
occurrence of those pain behaviors.

B.F. Skinner (19) many years ago drew the
distinction between two classes of organism actions
or behaviors: respondents and operants. For the
purposes of this paper, the distinction can be
summarized briefly. Respondents are organism actions
which occur in response to antecedent, stimuli
("antecedent stimulus" here refers to an event
preceding in time occurrence of the respondent. The
"stimulus" might be within or without the organism).
If there is an adequate antecedent stimulus, in an
intact organism, the response occurs and without an
adequate stimulus, it does not. Respondents can be
said to be controlled by antecedent stimuli; i.e.,
are reflexive in nature. Respondents typically
involve glandular or smooth muscular actions; i.e.,
autonomically mediated actions.

Operants are actions of the organism which
typically involve striated or voluntary musculature.
Operants are given that term because they are overt
or visible/audible and thereby have an effect on or
operate on the environment. Operants are capable of
being elicited by antecedent stimuli. Operants,
however, have an additional and critically important
characteristic: sensitivity to the influence of
consequences. An operant which occurs and is
followed in systematic fashion by a reinforcing
consequence, is thereby influenced in the direction
of becoming more likely to occur again. Repeated
contingent reinforcement of an operant can result in
that operant coming under essential control of the
reinforcing consequence. The organism, upon
anticipating occurrence of the consequence, likely
will emit the operant. Conversely, withdrawal or
termination of previously established contingent
reinforcement pattern leads to reduction and ultimate
disappearance of the operant. An operant may also
be reduced or eliminated by effective contingent
reinforcement of a behavior incompatible with it,
i.e., conditioning a substitute behavior.

The validity of the observation that operants are
subject to influence by contingent reinforcement has
been verified by literally millions of observations.
(Ferster and Skinner (2)).

Studies subsequent to Skinner's formulations have
led to at least one modification of the original
formulation. Work on autonomic conditioning in the
past 15-20 years indicates that autonomically
mediated responses or organisms, human and other, are
also sensitive to the conditioning effects of
contingent reinforcement. Many "respondents" have

now been shown to function as "operants" in the sense that they can be conditioned.

The importance of the consideration of respondents and operants is that pain behaviors are operants. The visible/audible communications to the environment by a pain patient are operants which are sensitive to the influence of contingent environmental reinforcement. When considering chronic clinical pain, the question arises of whether the pain behaviors observed or reported are automatic extensions or reflections of an antecedent nociceptive stimulus or occur, altogether or in part, because of contingent environmental reinforcement. Experience with behavioral methods for evaluating and treating selected chronic pain problems Fordyce et al (4), Roberts (17) Sternbach (20) Swanson et al (21) supports the thesis that pain behaviors may come under control of and be influenced by environmental contingencies. Treatment based on modification of the relationships between pain and well behaviors, on the one hand, and environmental contingencies, on the other, is capable of leading to marked improvement in the pain problem, and, in some instances, total resolution.

One implication of a behavioral perspective on chronic pain is that evaluation must attend to what the person does, actions or behavior, and not be guided principally by what the patient says he/she is experiencing "inside". This point is so basic it is easy to overlook. Pain behaviors are not necessarily intimately--or, as is sometimes the case-- even loosely linked to alleged, inferred, or patient-reported events or experiences invisible to the observer but said to exist within the organism. It follows that pain problems cannot be understood without studying what the person does.

When, for example, a person, while exercising reports he/she cannot continue because of pain, the statement "I cannot continue because I hurt" is behavior. Stopping the exercise to do something else (e.g., sit quietly) is also behavior. The reported experience is implied by the communication, ". . . I cannot continue <u>because I hurt</u>. . ." is not behavior. The <u>essence</u> of the person's problem is that he/she cannot continue. That is what needs to be changed. The effectiveness of treatment is to be found in whether or not that behavior does change; i.e., the person's activity level expands. One treatment strategy to bring about the change is to do something designed to eliminate or reduce the reported inner experience of "pain". That choice should be followed if one is confident the pain behaviors ("I cannot continue. . .") are controlled by some underlying or within-the-organism event or experience.[3] But there is an alternative. If the pain behaviors have come under control of such other factors as environmental contingencies, treatment may proceed by whatever means seem helpful in changing those behaviors; i.e., helping the person to do more exercises and to expand activity. The essence of the problem has become the pain behaviors. Whichever alternative is followed, the criterion for progress is a change in activity or behavior. Both the nature of the problem (diagnosis or evaluation) and the criterion of improvement (assessing effects of treatment) inevitably must consider what the person actually does.

In problems of chronic pain there are at least two sets of factors which may play major roles. One is where the pain behaviors continue to be influenced substantially by or are under control of some under-lying nociceptive stimulus. That may be said to be a problem of respondent pain as the pain behaviors are essentially controlled by antecedant stimuli and occur in response to them. The second is where the pain behaviors, having persisted for many weeks and months in an environment providing suitable contingent reinforcement, have been conditioned to respond in anticipation of that reinforcement. In that case, the pain behaviors are functioning as operants. The problem may be said to be one of operant pain. Those alternatives are not mutually exclusive. Clinical experience indicates that some mixture of the two is common. A given patient's pain behaviors occur in part in response to residuals of the originating "cause" of the pain problem, or the effects of surgi-cal efforts to treat it, and in part because of influence of environmental contingencies those behaviors meet.

The evolution or development of a problem of operant pain relates mainly to the interaction be-tween the patient's pain behaviors and events in his/her environment. Therefore, operant pain is not particularly related to a given body site or body system involvement. Operant pain may evolve from problems of low back pain, leg pain, chest pain, or whatever.

---

[3]That choice represents viewing the pain problem in medical/disease or biomedical model terms.

Evolution of Operant Pain

Pain problems initially are virtually all respondent in character. A nociceptive stimulus leads to pain and thence on to suffering, which in turn elicits pain behaviors. If early evaluation and treatment are effective, the problem is resolved and there is no chronicity. If, however, that is not the case, and the problem persists, there is always the risk that contingent environmental reinforcement will influence. If the chronic pain problem, and the person who has it, exists in an environment which indeed delivers effective pain contingent reinforcement, a problem of operant pain, may evolve.

It is beyond the scope of this paper to deal in detail with either the technology of operant conditioning or the myriad ways in which that conditioning may occur to bring a pain problem under operant control. There appear to be three major ways in which that may occur. They will be described briefly.

Direct Reinforcement of Pain Behavior

Some reinforcing, environmentally situated, events may be pain contingent. The reinforcing events do not occur unless preceded by pain behaviors. Two examples illustrate. Pain medications are often prescribed on a take-only-as needed or prn basis. There must be an indication from the patient by some form of pain behavior that medication is needed. When that happens, the medication is provided. If it does not happen, no medication is provided. The medication is pain contingent.

For some people, pain medications are not reinforcers or positive consequences. Some people find sedating effects aversive. They tend to under-utilize prescribed medications. They are recalcitrant with respect to compliance with a medication regimen. For those people, pain contingent medications are not likely to lead to conditioning the pain behaviors to occur in anticipation of additional medications. Other people, however, find the chemotherapeutic effects of pain medications very reinforcing. They feel better when sedated or analgesic. For them, medications are positive consequences or effective reinforcers. Placing that kind of person on a long-enduring prn regimen risks promoting conditioning effects, both in the sense of physiological addiction and in the sense that the pain behaviors necessary and sufficient to lead to delivery of medications may come to occur in anticipation of medications long after the original nociceptive stimulus has resolved. The problem has become one of operant pain. In similar fashion, the attention of significant and influential people around the patient may tend to become pain contingent. At the least, that attention may increase in intensity and promptness in response to patient pain behaviors. Physicians, spouses, and others may let that potentially influential attention serve as a pain behavior contingent consequence. Direct reinforcement of pain behavior may be paraphrased as, "Good things happen when I hurt that otherwise would not".

Indirect Reinforcement of Pain Behavior

Indirect reinforcement of pain behavior may occur when pain behavior leads to effective avoidance of some aversive or unpleasant consequence. When the person engages in pain behavior, she/he is thereby able to avoid or reduce aversive consequences which likely would have to be met were there no pain behavior. To paraphrase briefly, "when I (hurt), bad things don't happen which otherwise would". A person who spends the day reclining because of back pain, thereby eases the pain which would be experienced were she/he up doing things. In addition, however, spending the day on the couch may also effectively avoid some other aversive events, such as an unpleasant job, a threatening social encounter, an aversive set of chores or responsibilities.

The arrangement just described illustrates avoidance learning. One learns to engage in a behavior which effectively avoids or minimized an aversive consequence. Avoidance learning has long been recognized as highly persistent. Once established, little additional reinforcement is required to maintain it. The phenomenon corresponds approximately to the long-used term, secondary gain.

Examples of indirect reinforcement are commonplace. A construction worker with limited education and vocational options may sustain a back sprain. When put on bed rest or "light duty status", he thereby eases pain but also avoids the arduous job which advancing age has made more and more aversive. His pain behavior of hurting and requiring bed rest may become highly aversive if there is not replacement income in the form of compensation funding. But if there is that income, the aversiveness cost of being on light duty may be diminished. The result may be a persistence of pain long after the originating sprain had resolved. Another example in a different context concerns the elderly housewife who has had a minor stroke or some cortical deficit from arteriosclerosis. She may find it increasingly difficult to perform recent memory tasks. Participating in a bridge club may become aversive for that reason. Some pain episode or illness event then occurs, for which she stays home. Staying home not only may ease pain in a direct sense but also in an indirect sense of helping to avoid the aversive consequences of revealing memory deficits to old friends and being unable to play her cherished bridge game with anything near her previous effectiveness.

Punishment of Activity or Well Behavior

Occasionally militantly supportive family members will admonish a pain patient against undertaking physically demanding activity. They wish to protect the person from aggravating the pain problem. But they may do so long after healing has occurred. If the patient ventures into activity, she/he may receive a form of punishment from people close to them. It seems unlikely this source of maintenance of pain behavior plays a major role but it does seem to be a factor in some chronic pain problems.

The Concept of Psychogenic Pain

Traditionally, the alternative to a "physical finding" or "organic" or, in the terms of this paper, "respondent" explanation to a pain problem has been that there is a discrepancy between physical findings and amount of pain behavior observed. That is but another way of stating a disease model perspective has failed to account for the pain behaviors. In that use of the term, traditionally, efforts may then be made to account for the pain behaviors in other ways. That use of the term raises few problems so long as it is understood to be based on an observed or inferred discrepancy and not on some specific characteristic of the patient. The second use of "psychogenic" is to imply the person who displays a discrepancy between physical findings and pain behaviors therefore has some emotional, motivational, or personality disturbance problem. The person may receive some such label as "hypochrondriac", "conversion hysteric", "malingerer,", etc.

The second use of the term raises problems which must be considered briefly. The alternative to "respondent" pain is not "psychogenic" in the sense of some personality aberration. Many chronic pain patients having much operant pain indeed have personality or motivational problems, but not all do, nor is it inevitably necessary to postulate that they do in order to understand the nature of the pain problem.

The essence of the point is that traditional psychiatric evaluation and treatment is not the sole alternative and often is irrelevant when dealing with pain behaviors in the relative absence of currently active and sufficient nociceptive stimuli. A detailed analysis of the interaction between pain behaviors and environmental contingencies may lead to identification of an emotional or personality problem but may, instead, lead to other environmental factors which play key roles. One cannot therefore simply dismiss what here has been termed "operant pain" as a psychological problem which somehow then belongs in some other domain.

Depression and Pain

A number of authors such as Merskey and Spear (15) have noted the frequent association of pain and depression in patients. Depressed patients frequently complain of pain problems and most chronic pain patients are depressed. It is often difficult to distinguish which is the major problem: pain or depression. Depression is often mis-labelled as pain by the patient, family, and health care professionals.

The functionally impaired pain patient is often saddened by his/her plight and is therefore depressed. In that instance the depression is a product of the pain problem. In addition, prior associations between pain and depression may have become conditioned such that cues or stimuli for one produce the other as well resulting in a labelling problem. Depression and other members of the response class of distress may elicit pain behaviors. Insofar as the patient may be perceiving a depression problem as "pain", it is a problem of labelling, or mis-labelling. The essence of the point is that "suffering", as defined by Loeser (11), leads to behaviors. Those behaviors are often recognized as "pain behaviors" but they may occur for a variety of reasons, one of which is depression, or some other form of emotional distress.

Seen behaviorally, depression is often considered as a deprivation of reinforcers Lewinsohn (9) or as a state of learned helplessness Seligman (18). In either case, we have a person whose behavioral output or repertoire is excessively restricted from productive activity. In either case, any program having the effect of re-establishing activity and providing for re-engagement in those activities which

lead to effective reinforcement from the natural
environment, is helpful. In many instances, therefore, in the context of chronic pain, whether the
problem is accurately or inaccurately labelled as a
problem of operant pain or depression, as the case
may be, an important part of treatment is the
restoration of activity level and a re-engagement in
reinforcing activities. Treatment might then be said
to aim at reducing pain or distress behaviors and at
helping to replace them with effective well behaviors.
We may also, therefore, now consider depression-
related distress behaviors as having highly similiar
implications for treatment as operant pain behaviors.

Implications for Evaluation and Management of Chronic Clinical Pain

Before proceeding, one more thread must be added
to the tapestry, albeit briefly. In recent years a
series of studies and theoretical papers has emerged
which have had enormous impact on and importance for
clinical pain. These papers may be clustered under
the term of stimulus produced analgesia (SPA) or
endogenous mechanisms of pain inhibition. An
excellent review of this work is found in Liebeskind
(10). The subject will also be dealt with elsewhere
in this volume, hence the brevity of the comments
here, which do not reflect by their brevity, the
significance of this work.

No review of the evolution of our understanding of
pain could suffice without mention of the Gate
Control Theory of Pain first advanced by Melzack and
Wall (13). Their work was a landmark in synthesizing
what was then known about the subject and a beginning
at clarifying the function of endogenous, descending
pain suppression mechanisms within the organism. A
parallel root began with Reynolds (16), who found
that stimulation of small areas of the central gray
produced behavioral analgesia. Then, in more recent
work, Hughes, et al. (7) have by their work unleashed
a host of experiments by showing that there is within
the central nervous system the capability of generating biochemical analgesia.

Little is yet known about the time course of
these phenomena; i.e., the duration of SPA and of the
capacity of the organism to produce SPA effects
across extended time intervals. It is therefore
difficult to assess the role of SPA in chronic pain.
The implications of SPA for acute pain seem profound.
The implications for chronic pain are yet to be
articulated. For the purposes of this chapter, we
shall be content with observing that one logical

explanation for the persistence of pain behaviors is
an organism deficiency for one reason or another in
the ability to generate and/or maintain SPA. It may
also be the case that one remedy for an SPA deficiency is activation. That is, in the clinical
setting, the relatively immobilized and inactive
patient may, be increasing activity level, increase
SPA.

The foregoing analysis of chronic clinical pain
can now be summarized into the options shown in
Table 1.

TABLE 1. Factors Influencing Pain Behavior

SOURCE	EXPLANATION
A. Nociception	A problem of malignant (as dis-tinguished from benign) pain. The pathogenic factor continues to be active. It is a problem of res-pondent pain. There are two sub-alternatives: - the nociceptive stimulus is so strong it over-rides SPA -there is a deficiency in SPA capability
B. Mis-labelled Suffering	Suffering induced by emotional/ situational factors (e.g., depression, anxiety) is mis-labelled by the patient or others as 'pain'. Pain behaviors or suffering-like behaviors are emitted but are mistakenly attrib-uted to nociception.
C. Contingent Reinforcement	Pain behaviors are emitted and have come largely or partially under control of contingent reinforcement. It is a problem of operant pain. Principle sub-types are: -direct or pain contingent reinforcement. -indirect reinforcement (avoid-ance learning) in which pain behaviors lead to "time out" from other aversive consequences. -activity or well behaviors are punished.

Generalization or Maintenance of Performance

Treatment of chronic pain is not effective if the changes brought about do not persist into other times and other environments. This is a problem of generalization. The objective is to optimize the extent to which the increases in activity level expand in scope and persist across time and into a variety of settings. The problem of generalization is a central one in chronic illness, including chronic pain. The guiding principle is that behaviors (now the concern is with activity and well behaviors) will occur and will persist only insofar as they meet supportive reinforcement.

There are three general strategies for promoting generalization. One is to help the patient to develop self control techniques. These techniques have the basic effect of teaching the patient how to avoid or abort situations or emotional states which inhibit the desired activities or well behaviors and to direct her/his behavior toward effective incentives. No attempt will be made here to describe the variety of techniques by which those objectives are pursued. One major source for more detail is Meichenbaum (12).

A second strategy to promote generalization is to work with the natural environment of the patient to maximize the ability of that environment to reinforce effectively the desired behaviors and to avoid effective reinforcement of pain behaviors. That objective is pursued mainly by working with the immediate family, as noted above.

The third strategy for optimizing generalization and maintenance of performance is to seek to engage the patient in post-treatment activities which elicit naturally occurring reinforcement from which performance may be sustained. One essential dimension of treatment then becomes that of assisting the patient to become involved in, as may be indicated, vocational and avocational pursuits. These are selected with patient and family. They are designed to maintain the activity gains of treatment or, in other terms, to reinforce the well behavior alternatives to the pain behaviors reduced by treatment.

It is beyond the scope and mission of this chapter to attempt to set forth detailed methods for pursuing these objectives. But the importance of the generalization issue can hardly be over-stated. Generalization should be an integral part of treatment planning. During the evaluation phase, attention should be directed to the question of what post treatment activities are anticipated. Treatment should then be designed specifically to prepare for those activities and to ready the family unit to support and facilitate participation in them.

A particularly lucid discussion of the concept of generalization can be found in Baer & Wolf (1). More detailed consideration of tactical approaches to the generalization problem can be found in Fordyce (3).

Treatment Methods

The rationale for treating chronic pain via behavioral methods is based on several assumptions. First, the pain behaviors may now be occurring for reasons partially or totally unrelated to nociceptive stimuli arising from a site of body damage, irrespective of what may have initiated those pain behaviors at time of onset. Secondly, evaluation through behavioral analysis must indicate systematic relationship between pain behaviors and contingent reinforcement. Thirdly, what the patient needs (i.e., the objectives of treatment) are to increase activity level (or, decrease functional impairment); to diminish such pain behaviors as seeking treatment, taking analgesics or other pain-related medications, behaving in ways causing others to take protective actions which inhibit activity; and to resume activity patterns characterizing adequate performance prior to onset of the pain problem. One of the most powerful ways to help a person change behavior is through contingent reinforcement, the technology for which is known as operant conditioning.

One additional premise underlies a behavioral approach which was stated previously. Conceptually, the desired alternative to pain behaviors is activity or well behaviors. But the reduction or elimination or one does not automatically lead to an increase of the other. It follows that treatment of chronic pain must aim at two general targets; the reduction or elimination of pain behavior and the restoration or establishment of effective well behaviors.

Reduced to bare essentials, the conditions necessary and usually sufficient to help a person bring about significant and lasting behavior change are that: (a) the changes to be brought about can and must be specified in terms of what behaviors are to be increased and what are to be decreased; (b) increases in a behavior occur when that behavior is systematically, contingently, and promptly followed by effective positive reinforcement; (c) decreases or elimination of a behavior occurs when the positive reinforcers previously sustaining that behavior are

now withdrawn or no longer occur contingent upon
occurrence of the behavior or where behaviors
incompatible with the behavior to be reduced are
contingently reinforced to the point where they
effectively replace the unwanted behaviors; and
(d) behavior changes brought about by modifying
reinforcing contingencies will persist only to the
extent that either the special reinforcing arrange-
ments set up to bring about change are continued or
the environment of the person provides naturally
occurring sustaining reinforcement for the new
behavior patterns and not the old.

Proceeding with behaviorally based treatment
assumes full discussion and informed consent prior to
beginning. There are ethical and legal reasons for
that and no process or pragmatic reasons for not
having a full discussion of all aspects of the
process at the outset.

Evaluation and Selection of Patients

Patient selection is preceded by a thorough
medical evaluation, though in chronic pain evaluation
from a biomedical perspective alone has usually been
found wanting. Behavioral analysis of chronic pain
typically consists of interviews with patient and
spouse; an MMPI, and a sample (e.g., two weeks) of
diaries recorded by patients to show when they are
sitting, standing/walking, or reclining; medications
taken; and hourly ratings of subjective pain. Those
data are used to assess, to paraphrase, "what good
things happen when pain behaviors occur", ie., are
pain contingent; and "what bad things don't happen
when pain behaviors occur;" i.e., what aversive
events are avoided pain contingently. If those data
indicate a probable problem of operant pain,
additional assessment is needed to judge the
likelihood that change can be effected and to
identify treatment objectives; i.e., the behaviors to
be increased and decreased by treatment.[4]

TREATMENT

Objectives of Treatment

Objectives of treatment in behavioral terms,
while varying from patient to patient according to

---

[4]Detailed methods for evaluating and selecting patients, using a behavior approach, have been set forth
in Fordyce (3) pp. 103-146.

immediate circumstances, usually are encompassed in the following:

1. increase in activity level, both generally and in regard to specific exercise or activity constraints; i.e., reduction in functional impairment;
2. reduction of pain behaviors evocative of protective actions by others;
3. reduction in pain-related medication consumption;
4. restoration or establishment of effective well behaviors, including remediation of social skill and interpersonal problems previously limiting the ability to be effectively well;
5. modification of the reinforcing contingencies to pain and well behavior extant in the patient's immediate milieu.
6. reduction in health care utilization related to the pain problem, including particularly the continued fruitless pursuit of additional diagnostic and treatment procedures;

There is no mention of the reduction of pain, only of pain behaviors, for conceptual reasons. A given patient may at the outset of treatment be able to do only x amount and require y amount of medications to accomplish that. At the end of the treatment, he/she may be able to do much more than was possible before and may be consuming zero medication. It is moot as to whether there has been a corresponding reduction in "pain," as defined by Loeser (11).

A brief description of behaviorally-based treatment methods and strategies will be presented, organized in the sequence of objectives listed.

Reduction in pain behaviors and increases in activity level

Exercise lies at the core of treatment. Exercise programs are individualized according to the particulars of each patient. Basically, the procedure is first to establish tolerance for each prescribed exercise by direct observations. There is then a shift from exercising until pain, weakness or fatigue encourage one to stop (exercising to tolerance) wherein rest is pain contingent, to a quota system in which rest becomes work contingent. Initial quotas are well within the patient's demonstrated current capabilities but are raised systematically on a pre-set basis; e.g., one additional repetition per

session until a pre-determined ceiling is reached.
Concomitantly, those around the patient (e.g.,
nurses, physical therapists, physicians) adopt an
interactional style in which pain behaviors receive
minimal social attention while activity, exercise or
attempts at well behavior, are responded to with
appropriate social reinforcement. The combination
of shifting social reinforcement from pain behavior
and inactivity to exercise and expanding activity
and of systematically working to replace immobilization and constrained motion with vigorous and
expanding motion aims at replacing pain behavior
with well behavior.

Medication reduction

Patients toxic and addicted cannot be evaluated
adequately until that problem is cleared. An
accelerated version of the pain cocktail regimen now
to be described is used to cope with that problem.
(Halpern, L. (5)).

Two methods have been used. In both cases, there
is first a period of direct observation (pain patients
with significant medication abuse or addiction should
be treated on an inpatient basis) during which
current medication consumption and needs are identified precisely by giving the patient free access to
pain related medication; i.e., a medication baseline
is obtained. One method is then to take the medications the patient uses and incorporate them into a
single mix, eliminating redundancies and potentiating
mixes. This mix, known as the pain cocktail,
consists of the patient's active ingredients plus a
color and taste masking vehicle (e.g., cherry syrup).
This mix is delivered at fixed time intervals
(i.e. is time contingent) approximating those time
frequencies the patient has displayed during
observation. Twenty four hours totals of each
ingredient start at the same level observed during
baselines. Active ingredients are reduced
systematically, typically at a rate close to 10%
per week or 10 days, while exercise and activity level
is expanding. Usually zero levels can be achieved in
appropriately selected patients.

The second method follows the same time and time
contingent patterns but substitutes equivalent amounts
of slow acting Methadone for all narcotics and
equivalent amounts of phenobarbital for all
barbiturates. Tranquillizers are simply eliminated
at the outset.

In either method, an anti-depressant (e.g. Sinequan) is often added to the mix either as a remedy for depression or to help with sleep disturbance.

The regimen is explained fully to patient and spouse at the outset, except for the precise schedule of decreases in active ingredients.

Remediating or establishing effective well behavior

This is the most difficult part of the process and the mission most likely to fail. Most chronic pain patients have significant problems or gaps in their ability to be effectively well. That is so for two reasons. One is that these problems made it more likely a problem of operant pain would evolve once a pain episode began because the pain behaviors had the additional effect of providing a haven from the aversive consequences they met when they were involved fully in work and social responsibilities. The second is that the long intervals between onset and effective treatment, through sheer disuse likely produces deficiencies in a person's ability to cope effectively with the responsibilities of daily living.

It is not appropriate that this chapter attempt to catalog either the problems encountered or the treatments applied. It should suffice simply to note that evaluation of chronic pain patients must examine the issue of problems or gaps in well be-havior repertoires and of identification of post-treatment activities the patient can be expected to be involved in. In light of that evaluation, treatment must do what it can to take effective action to remediate, as needed. Clinical experience indicates that pain treatment programs which do not come to grips with this issue tend to produce many short term successes and long term failures of treatment.

Modification of social contingencies to pain and well behavior

Significant family members (usually working with the spouse alone is sufficient) are trained in how to identify pain and well behaviors, to become aware of their own responses to these, and, as needed, to acquire and practice more effective alternatives.

Reduction in pain-related health care utilization

Effective treatment is the remedy to this problem.

CONCLUSION

The major points of this chapter can be reduced to four.

The first point is that acute and chronic illness, including pain, present very different phenomena and problems. Concepts and methods appropriate to one may not be effective with the other. In fact, treatment methods for one may make the other worse.

The second point is that chronic pain cannot be understood without consideration and analysis of the pain behaviors manifested by the person and of the array of factors which may influence those behaviors.

The third point is that treatment of chronic pain by behavioral methods deals with specific target behaviors (e.g., exercise, pain behaviors, post-treatment activity plans) and environmental contingencies which may influence them.

Finally, in chronic illness and chronic pain, the reduction of symptoms does not inevitably lead to an ascension of health and well behaviors. For adequate treatment, one must aim at both the reduction of symptoms and the enhancement of effective alternative well behaviors.

REFERENCES

1. Baer, D. and Wolf, M., The Entry Into Natural Communities of Reinforcement, Symposium presented at American Psychological Association, National Convention, Washington D.C., September, 1967.

2. Ferster, C.B., and Skinner, B.F., Schedules of Reinforcement, New York: Appleton-Century-Crofts, 1957.

3. Fordyce, W.E., Behavioral Methods in Chronic Pain and Illness. St. Louis: C.V. Mosby Company, February, 1976, 236 pages.

4. Fordyce, W.E., Fowler, R., and Lehmann, J.R., DeLateur, B.J., Sand, P.L., and Trieschmann, R.: Operant Conditioning in the Treatment of Chronic Clinical Pain, Arch. Phys. Med. 54:9:399-408 Sept.) 1973.

5. Halpern, L., Analgesic Drugs in the Management of Pain, Arch. Surg. 112: 861-9, 1977.

6. Hughes, J. "Isolation of an Endogenous Compound from the Brain with Pharmacological Properties Similar to Morphine" Brain Research, 88:295-308, 1975.

7. Hughes, J., Smith, T.W., Kosterlitz, H.W., Fothergill, L.A., Morgan, B.A., Morris, H.R., "Identification of two related pentapeptides from the brain with potent opiate against activity" Nature 258:577-79, 1975).

8. Lazarus, Arnold A.: "Has Behavior Therapy Out-lived its Usefullness?", American Psychologist, Vol 32, No. 7, July, 1977, p. 553.

9. Lewinsohn, P., Biglan, A., and Zeiss, A., Behavioral Treatment of Depression, in Davidson, P.O., (ed) The Behavioral Management of Anxiety, Depression, and Pain, Brunner/Mazel, NYC, 1976, pp. 91-146.

10. Liebeskind, J., Paul, L., Psychological and Mechanisms of Pain. Annual Review of Psychology Vol. 28, 1977: pp. 41-60.

11. Loeser, J. D., Personal Communication, University of Washington Department Neurol. Surg., Seattle, WA 1978.

12. Meichenbaum, D., Cognitive Behavior Modification Plenum Press, N.Y., 1977, 293 pages.

13. Melzack, R. and Wall, P., Pain Mechanisms: A New Theory, Science 150:971-79, 1965.

14. Merskey, H., in Weisenberg, M. (ed.), 1975 Pain: Clinical and Experimental Perspectives, St. Louis: Mosby, p. 6.

15. Merskey, H. and Spear, F.G., Pain: Psychological and Psychiatric Aspects, Baltimore, 1967, The Williams & Wilkens Co.

16. Reynolds, D.B., "Surgery in the Rat During Electrical Analgesia Induced by Focal Brain Stimulation", Science, 164:444-45, 1969.

17. Roberts, Allen, Behavioral Treatment in Pain in Ferguson, J.M., and Taylor, C.B., (ed.) Advances in Behavior. New York Spectrum, in press, 1978.

18.   Seligman, M.E.P. Helplessness: On depression,
      development, and death. San Francisco: W.H.
      Freeman, 1975.

19.   Skinner, B.F., "Science and Human Behavior"
      New York, 1953, the McMillan Co.

20.   Sternbach, R.A., Pain Patients: Traits and
      Treatment, Academic Press, New York, 1974.

21.   Swanson, D., Swenson, W., Maruta, T., and
      McPhee, M.: Program for managing Chronic Pain.
      I Program description and characteristics of
      patients. Mayo Clinic. Proc. 51: 401-411, 1976.

The Psychology of Pain, edited by R. A. Sternbach.
Raven Press, New York © 1978.

Social Modeling Influences on Pain

Kenneth D. Craig

*Department of Psychology, University of British Columbia,
Vancouver, B.C., Canada, V6T 1W5*

Witnessing the distress of another person in pain tends to
be a compelling experience that potentially has dramatic
effects on the observer's behaviour. Ongoing activity almost
invariably will be interrupted when others suffer unexpected
injuries or complain of pain. A variety of immediate reactions
may be provoked, ranging from fear of similar threat to
oneself, and efforts at self-protection, to empathic distress
and caretaking designed to relieve the other's distress or to
encourage recovery. Displays of pain and suffering and other
person's reactions provide powerful examples of interpersonal
behavior with the immediate and long term effects on the
observer potentially of considerable importance.

The command that expressions of pain have over the
observer's attentional behaviour is well-illustrated in popular
experience. Some people actively seek out opportunities to
view or hear real or dramatically portrayed incidents of injury
and suffering. The purposeful development of scenarios
portraying physical assault and injury in the visual arts and
communications industries capitalizes, for commercial reasons,
on the capacity of these events to attract our attention.
Interest in sporting events where participants are at risk of
personal injury can be characterized for some spectators as
the result of a fascination with injury or death. While many
people dislike viewing violence-produced pain, others derive
satisfaction from watching it, and most people feel compelled
to attend to it, at least initially.

More formal evidence of the compelling qualities of viewing
others in pain and distress is available from research
laboratories. The pattern of physiological arousal identified
with strong emotional reactions (18,85) and with attention to
the external environment (40,79) is provoked by real or filmed
presentations of victims who are, or have been, subjected to
pain and injury. In fact, the attention demanding qualities of
physically harmful events is so considerable that observers
have described their reaction as one of morbid fascination
(47). Of course, there are substantial individual differences
in observers' emotional reactions to another persons' suffering
and anguish, which range from sadistic pleasure to sorrow and

horror (18,40). Even though many people purposefully avoid attending to evidence of the distress of others, those who divert attention still display strong emotional arousal (84). The strength of the act of avoidance itself frequently signifies how powerful the response to another's distress can be.

Not only the immediate effects of observing another in pain can be dramatic and substantial but the experience may have durable consequences. This chapter reviews available evidence of the longterm impact of opportunities to witness response patterns of others to noxious stimulation. The emphasis is on isolating the influence of exposure to models from the complex amalgam of factors that must be included in a comprehensive formulation of pain. Initially, the immediate effects of viewing others in distress on verbal and nonverbal observable behavior, cognitive processes and emotional experiences are examined from the perspective of the general literature on observational learning processes. Accounts of persisting effects of modeling influences that were available in the clinical and research literatures are described subsequently. These include well-documented and presumptive evidence that suggests modeling influences were at least partially responsible for cross-cultural differences in pain behavior and for individual differences among patients suffering from diverse complaints such as dental, abdominal, and phantom limb pain. Pain control strategies including modeling components provided more direct evidence of patient responsivity to social models. The modeling components of several conventional and innovative treatment programs, including hypnoanalgesia, acupuncture analgesia, and milieu therapy for burn patients, are described along with several modeling therapies purposefully developed to control pain behavior and behavior problems arising from pain-producing dental and medical care. The final section reviews experimental investigations of critical questions arising from clinical practice. Research evidence is examined considering issues such as the extent to which pain behavior is subject to the control of the social environment and whether modeling intervention strategies for pain affect sensory experiences as well as observable behavior.

OBSERVATIONAL LEARNING PROCESSES

Why are we so attracted to and curious about the painful experiences of other people? The most reasonable explanation would be that this information has considerable adaptive value for the observer. Detailed knowledge of dangerous circumstances, how pain is best expressed, whether the reaction is socially appropriate, and the circumstances associated with its prolongation or relief, may be very useful.

After a review of the relevant literature Bandura (9) concluded that observational learning was the principle mode of acquiring new patterns of behavior. The benefits of observing and understanding what happens to others experiencing injury or some painful condition are readily understood. Vicarious experience can substitute for direct experience without the observer suffering the intense or longterm distress of the direct experience. Indeed, knowing the circumstances associated with others' injuries and diseases allows avoidance not only of pain and injury but also of death. In some instances, however, matching the behavior of others may have maladaptive consequences for the individual. On occassion, modeling processes seem responsible for inappropriate pain complaints and other sick role behavior unrelated to verified organic pathology, or for avoidance of treatment that is in the best interests of the individual.

The following sections describe some of the behavioral, cognitive and affective consequences of opportunities to view the painful experiences of others.

Acquisition of Social Roles

Knowing how to communicate distress and pain may be crucial for the individual. When there is a risk that pain relief is not available without delay, either through self-limiting biological processes or self-administered treatment, the sufferer's success in soliciting help from others assumes considerable importance. Individuals who are competent in using health resources may protect themselves and avoid protracted or serious pathology.

A long developmental learning process seems to be involved. Attending to one's personal state of health, communicating important information within the constraints of social expectations, and complying with therapeutic regimens are all very complex tasks. Recent research on "illness behaviour", defined by Mechanic (90) as "the ways in which given symptoms may be differentially perceived, evaluated, and acted (or not acted) upon by different persons," helps in understanding the complex skills and decision-processes involved when people become ill. Of related interest are the phenomena of "abnormal illness behaviour," defined by Pilowsky (107) as persistent, maladaptive modes of perceiving, evaluating, and acting in relation to one's state of health, and described by him elsewhere in this volume.

The effects of pain on social performance and psychological well-being tend to be appreciated at a general level, but a great deal needs to be done in terms of recognizing the impact of different social, psychological and biological factors on individual variability. There is reason to believe that social competency prior to the onset of pain disorders

influences the severity of the response to the illness
(118,108). It seems unusual that the differences between
acute and chronic pain disorders have only been recognized
recently (21,118). Acute pains tend to be directly associated
with tissue damage resulting from disease or injury. They
usually provide warnings of destructive events and allow
preventive or remedial action. While acute pain can elicit a
dramatic reaction, it is subject to treatment, and is less
frequently destructive of social, familial and vocational
roles than chronic pain. On the other hand, chronic pain, as
Bonica (21) observed, has no biologic value, and imposes
severe ongoing stress on the patient and those who are
dependent on him or her. Reactive depression, withdrawal from
work and social activities, hypochondriasis, and inadequate,
dependent life styles often characterize chronic pain patients
(118,133), although Pilowsky and Spence (108) observed that
some patients do not adopt the role of an invalid or allow
intractable pain to disrupt every-day social commitments.
Patients of this type would appear to have personal and social
resources that prevent succumbing to invalid roles. The
origins of the individual differences in the pain patient's
ability to maintain healthy life styles and adaptive social
roles need to be further clarified.

The complex sequences of behaviour appropriate to either
the expression or suppression of pain and the impact of the
social environment are well illustrated by mutilative
religious rituals (96). High status may be earned by those
who subject themselves to self-injurious experiences without
expressions of suffering, or by displaying altered states of
consciousness or trance states during intense noxious
stimulation (14). Penitents, flagellators and others
participating in religious acts involving self-inflicted pain
require instruction if the roles are to be enacted properly.
The extent to which the individual matches societal standards
for these patterns of behavior would seem to be dependent in
part on observational learning.

Several unusual medical phenomena also illustrate how
deviant illness behavior can be modeled on legitimate
complaint patterns. The Couvade syndrome has as its major
feature a husband who complains of the symptoms from which
pregnant women commonly suffer (128). The behavioral pattern
can mimic the woman's symptoms during pregnancy or parturition
in varying degrees. The most dramatic examples are provided
by case reports describing fathers who complain of abdominal
pains and generally enact the role of a pregnant woman during
their wives' delivery of a child. In the Munchausen syndrome
the patient appears to purposefully feign severe illness of a
dramatic nature and may provide fictitious evidence of disease
by falsifying diagnostic information or evidence, or engaging
in self-mutilation. These patients usually have enough
medical information to convince health personnel of the

legitimacy of their complaints, at least initially, and not
infrequently receive surgery and are hospitalized for extended
periods of time (68). The extent to which this pattern of
behavior is purposefully simulated and is subject to voluntary
control is unknown. Confrontation of these patients with the
absence of organic pathology does not usually produce change.

These unusual syndromes and patient roles are dramatic in
appearance, but relatively infrequent. More common complaint
patterns may also be subject to modeling influences. Patients
may present to their physicians with particular complaint
patterns that represent the result of shaping and modeling
influences of others in the social environment, rather than
the exclusive report of somatic events. For example, Merskey
and Spear (101) observed that there appears to be a
substantial number of cases in which symptoms mimic
appendicitis, leading to apparently unneeded appendicectomies.

Once patterns of behavior appropriate to sickness and
health have been acquired, the social and environmental
constraints interact with biophysical factors to determine the
particular response patterns that are likely to appear.
People tend to be strikingly responsive to features of the
immediate social and physical environment when expressing pain
(17,53). Investigations of social modeling influences have
demonstrated considerable sensitivity to subtle nuances of the
immediate social context (35).

From the perspective of social learning theory, observing
the consequences of another person's actions may inhibit or
disinhibit well-established response patterns. In this
instance, the models signify whether particular patterns of
behavior are appropriate and likely to be reinforced, or are
socially unacceptable and likely to lead to punishment.
Consequently, the person in pain can be expected to behave in
either a stoical or histrionic manner if the observed
consequences for doing so represent incentives for the
observer. The operant approach to pain behaviour (53) has
documented how reinforcement contingencies such as sympathy,
medications, financial rewards and avoidance of
responsibilities can lead to and maintain pain disabilities.
Observation of these consequences for patterns of pain
behavior modeled by other persons would be expected to
influence whether the modeled pattern was matched.

Documentation of the effects of observing others suffering
punitive consequences for various patterns of pain behaviour
is not readily available. However, implicit social rules
specifying aversive consequences for failure to enact social
roles frequently seem to sanction stoical expressions in
response to noxious events. Soldiers and athletes would seem
to learn these rules from their compatriots. Descriptions of
Russian Cossack-soldiers, who purposefully subjected
themselves to wounds, and Roman legionnaires, who plunged
their arms into fire (20), illustrate the extreme of people

influenced to engage in self-mutilation without complaint
through exposure to others. Contemporary illustrations can be
found in self-injurious behavior which can be learned and
propagated in institutional settings. The disinhibitory
effects of viewing others who have engaged in suicide attempts
are well known in mental hospitals and prisons where one
dramatic suicidal effort greatly increases the probability of
attempts or gestures by other patients. Epidemics of
self-inflicted injuries ranging from slashing of wrists to
amputation of limbs have been described in general hospital
psychiatric wards, and involve not only patients but staff
members as well (116).

Private Behavior

It is generally understood that cognitive processes
critically determine the nature of the pain experience. The
individual in pain tends to interpret its source and personal
meaning in terms of the immediate environment, his or her past
history, and the future implications of an injury or disease
(17,96).

Information of critical interest to the person experiencing
or anticipating pain may be acquired through observational
learning. The experiences of others become particularly
important when the individual is in distress or at risk of
similar problems. Patients eagerly search to find out what is
the matter with them, or if the symptoms they experience
reflect a disease process, in terms understandable to them.
The course of the disease as it relates to organic damage,
subjective states, and behavioural deficits is critical.
Considerable effort may be devoted to discovering the
potential impact and risks of available treatments or
palliatives, no matter how conservative or radical. Existing
and potential consequences of the illness for personal, social
and vocational roles are important. Finally, patients want to
know how they can contribute to improving their own health.
Encouraging interaction among patients with identified
disorders through group therapy, self-help, and peer-support
groups can lead to beneficial information exchange (58).

Observational learning also influences the problem solving
strategies generated by observers regarding how they should
behave in similar circumstances (9,112) and is also a critical
determinant of perceived self-efficacy in coping with
stress-inducing situations (11). Chaves and Barber (29) have
shown that some subjects reported less pain as a consequence
of viewing experimenters modeling cognitive control strategies
while subjected to pain induced by a heavy weight applied to a
finger. Similarly, Neufeld and Davidson (103) demonstrated
that vicarious rehearsal produced by watching another person
experiencing noxious radiant heat without apparent distress
was as effective in reducing pain reactions as the cognitive

rehearsal of listening to the heat-induction procedure described in detail. Modeling strategies would seem to provide direct opportunities to influence cognitive coping strategies and judgmental processes.

While the origins of differences in pain behavior among cultural and ethnic groups are not well-understood, the consistencies within groups suggest that other members of the group model normative standards for both the degree to which suffering should be freely expressed or inhibited and the appropriate form for expressing complaints. Some crosscultural differences have been attributed to communalities in attitudinal patterns and cognitive styles. Sternbach and Tursky (119) concluded that attitudinal differences among subcultures in the United States accounted for major differences in psychophysical and psychophysiological reaction patterns to experimental pain. The culture-specific attitudes among groups of women were summarized as follows (126): Yankees had a phlegmatic, matter of fact, doctor-helping orientation, Jews were concerned about the implications of pain and distrusted palliatives, Italians readily expressed desires for pain relief, and Irish inhibited both expressions of suffering and their concern for the implications of pain.

Weisenberg et al. (131) reported socio-cultural differences in relative willingness to deny or to avoid dealing with pain. Dental patients in the United States with Puerto Rican backgrounds were reported to show strongest endorsement of cognitive denial and avoidance as strategies for coping with pain, whereas whites were least inclined to report these strategies and blacks were between these two groups. To account for the subculture differences, Weisenberg (130) has argued that pain may be a less well-defined experience than is commonly believed to be the case. The individual may have to turn towards his social environment for validation of his judgments. Through social comparisons the individual can decide what is appropriate behavior at a given time, and judge whether somatic events represent dysfunctions of organic processes.

Vicarious Emotional Processes

Observing the affective displays of others responding to painful stimulation also may provoke or reduce emotional arousal in the observer. As noted previously, studies of the patterns of physiological arousal provoked by witnessing others exposed to injury or pain typically suggest empathic emotional arousal (18,33). An early account of empathic communication of painful distress was provided by Breuer and Freud (24) in their 1895 monograph. They described a man's reaction to seeing his brother having a frozen (Ankylosed) hip joint broken open. At the instant the joint gave way with a crack, the watching brother reportedly felt a violent pain in his own hip joint, which persisted for nearly a year. Empathic emotional arousal may account, in part, for the stress experienced by hospital personnel in constant contact with patients suffering acute pain states.

It has been established that the emotional arousal instigated among observers when witnessing another persons' pain can be conditioned to initially neutral events (13,18,44,66). This evidence for vicarious classical conditioning suggests that the affective value of innocuous events may be changed by the emotional reactions of others to them. If another person reacts in a violently, distressed manner to events that would normally be judged to be neutral, the observing individual is likely to be apprehensive and wary. When the event has any risk of potential harm associated with it, the observer's vicarious emotional reaction is likely to be even more intense and persistent, despite efforts to reduce its severity (67). Children tend to share their parent's fears (12), and there is evidence indicating that the severity of children's affective reactions to pain are consistent with their parents (4,61). The child's reaction would seem to be governed more by the available information on the affective reaction of the parent than the actual nature of the noxious event (67,83).

The response to another person's injury or distress is not necessarily one of sympathetic distress. It appears to depend upon the degree of arousal and the affective state of the observer. Evidence to this effect has been observed in studies where observers were provided with an opportunity to engage in prosocial or antisocial behaviour towards an injured party. Krebs (78) demonstrated that those who were sympathetic to the suffering individual were inclined to help and intercede with the source of pain, whereas Baron (15) reported those who were initially angry with the suffering party appeared to be reinforced by their distress, and tended to intensify efforts to create harm. Extensive exposure to violence also appears to inure emotional responsibility to the plight of others (122).

Somewhat more speculative observations on the nature of vicarious emotional arousal to the pain of others derive from investigations of sadistic behavior (1,50). These studies suggest that the wounds and suffering of others may intensify sexual arousal in the observer. The exploitation of violence in the pornographic industry indicates that vicariously experiencing pain enhances sexual satisfaction. Case studies have suggested that sadistic tendencies have their origins in early experiences in which intense sexual arousal is associated with witnessing others who have been injured or are in pain (in reality or in fantasy). Later, sexual arousal induced through viewing erotic material or direct sexual stimulation is associated with fantasized or overt sadistic behavior thereby maintaining the association (1,50).

The extent to which an individual displays suffering while experiencing noxious stimulation can have an impact on the amount of emotional distress experienced by an observer to a similar painful event. Observing a dispassionate person exhibiting relatively good control over pain appears to have a calming effect on the observer. Under these circumstances, the autonomic response to noxious stimulation has been observed to be less intense (41,42). In part, this effect appears to be mediated by the model reducing the observer's anxiety about physical harm, but evidence also indicates that exposure to the model affects basic qualities of the sensory response to the noxious stimulation (42).

This analysis of observational learning processes represents only a brief introduction to a rapidly growing literature concerning many behavioral processes other than pain (9,10,89,112). A better understanding of social learning influences on pain processes and the individual's role as an active participant in determining the pain experience would be available if the life histories and current social environments of pain patients were explored using this perspective.

CLINICAL RESEARCH ANALYSES OF MODELING INFLUENCES

The social phenomena outlined to this point represent the expected consequences of exposure to others manifesting pain, as derived from studies of a wide range of social behaviour (9,10). Considerable evidence is available in the clinical and experimental research literature supporting the position that modeling processes are critical in the development of patterns of pain behaviour, the manner in which pain is experienced, and whether individuals display self-control, or uninhibited distress when in pain.

Three sources of evidence are reviewed. The first source involves studies of socialization processes in general. The following all appear subject to influence during the childhood years; one's interpretation of external and internal events as related to pain, the thoughts experienced when subjected to noxious events, the degree of emotional arousal that pain induces, the various cognitive strategies triggered by painful events, and willingness and skill in securing help from external resources. The second source derives from studies of a variety of techniques designed to produce pain tolerance which incorporate demonstrations by models manifesting minimal pain to noxious stimulation as one component of the intervention strategy. The third source comes from the development and purposeful application of therapies capitalizing upon modeling influences in the interests of patients.

Modeling of Pain During Socialization

The process whereby children acquire the attitudes, values, and behavioral skills needed to function as adults in society is to a considerable extent one of observational learning. Baron and Byrne's (16) recent social psychology text states, "It now appears that children can acquire everything from language to moral values, and from sexual identity to a knowledge of the social norms of their society through observational learning... (p. 315)." There is no reason to believe that the full range of pain and illness behavior is not also strongly affected by social modeling.

Injuries and sickness are inevitable for everyone, and during childhood, parents must help their children deal with them. The process of socialization necessarily involves teaching children how to avoid accidents and injury, how to discriminate signs of illness, the process of appropriately communicating states of health, and compliance with therapeutic regimens. The proper actions can lead to pain avoidance and relatively early relief, and most parents assume responsibility for instructing children in the appropriate skills.

Evidence of the impact of social models during the socialization of pain behavior comes from contrasts of a number of naturally occurring groups. Consistencies within groups, and differences between groups, indicate that parents and significant others serve as models and exert sanctions for what would be recognized as either adaptive cognitive, emotional or social coping strategies in response to actual or anticipated noxious stimulation, or for maladaptive behaviour inconsistent with organic pathology.

Crosscultural Differences

Several observations in the literature on crosscultural influences on pain emphasize the role of other members of the culture. Zborowski's (134) findings of changes in patterns of pain behaviour across generations as families move from one culture to another demonstrate aspects of an ongoing, observational learning process. Zborowski studied several groups of patients with common ethnic origins in a United States hospital. Successive generations beyond an initial immigrant family were found to increasingly resemble the host culture in their pain behavior. The description of the rationale for studying "Old Americans" suggests some of the pressures involved in assimilation: "The Old Americans were selected because...their behavior patterns are those of the social and cultural majority in this country. They seem to represent the cultural ideal that serves as an acculturation model for the descendants of immigrants who adopt the American way of life. As the preliminary interviews suggest, members of the medical and nursing professions tended to approve this kind of behavior and expected from their patients general conformity with such a model of behavior at home or in hospital (p. 6)."

Close identification with a cultural group was displayed in an investigation of reactions to instructions designed to provoke intergroup competitiveness among groups of women differing in religious affiliation (80). Jewish and Protestant groups did not differ on baseline measures of tolerance for pressure-induced pain. Information then was provided which implied that the religious group the subject identified with could not tolerate pain as well as members of the other religious group. This led to an increase in tolerance for the Jews, but not for the Protestants. In a followup study, in which religious affiliation was made even more salient, Protestants also significantly increased in pain tolerance when they were told that Christians tolerated less pain than Jews. Social comparisons in pain behavior clearly become important when group differences are made explicit and there is a risk that the group one identifies with compares unfavorably with others (25,80).

Evidence of consistent complaint and illness behavior patterns within subcultures, and differences between cultures, should be tempered by recognition of the considerable individual differences within any group, and the great overlap among groups. The consistent complaint patterns of subgroups within cultures provide additional evidence of socialization processes, including the impact of vicarious influences.

Patient Groups

A logical approach to isolating life history determinants of variability in pain reactions has involved the contrast between groups of patients who have objectively identified sets of symptoms and complaints and their appropriate control groups. Investigations using this strategy have suggested unique contributions from social modeling experiences.

Dental pain. The prevalence of dental fear strong enough to reduce the frequency of dental visits has been estimated at 5% to 6% in the general population and 16% among school-aged chilren (74). Fear of pain during treatment appears to represent the primary reason for avoiding dentists (110). Vicarious learning processes have been implicated by several investigations of fears of dental pain.

Shoben and Borland (115) attempted to identify the origins of individual differences in emotional response to dental procedures. A variety of hypotheses were evaluated, with data derived from structured interviews, comparing patients displaying strong, fearful behavior patterns toward dental treatment and patients who exhibited little or no objectively observable dental fear or distress. The hypotheses concerned

the effects of individual differences in pain tolerance, prior
traumatic experiences in dental and medical settings, parental
attitudes, family background, and personality factors.
Judges' ratings of the data led to the conclusion that dental
fear was related mainly to other family members' unfavorable
dental experiences and adverse attitudes. These appeared to
be more important determinants of anxiety over the prospect of
dental treatment, detrimental avoidance of dental care, and
poor cooperation during treatment than earlier personal
traumatic experiences, and individual differences in pain
tolerance and personality.

A number of investigators have now concluded that the
tendency to respond to the dental setting with tension and
pain appears to be chiefly the result of the way oral pain and
dentistry were presented in the home. Shoben and Borland
(115) proposed that parents who suffer traumatic experiences
involving the facial area, with dentists or physicians, become
emotionally sensitized and communicate fears to their
children. Forgione and Clark (54) subsequently argued that
the origins of dental fears were more complex. They
identified traumatic facial experiences, low pain tolerance,
and high trait anxiety, in addition to unfavorable dental
attitudes in the family, as factors related to the origins of
dental fears. Johnson and his associates (70,71) found that
mothers who reported high levels of anxiety in the dental
situation had children who exhibited more negative and
uncooperative behavior during tooth extractions and dental
examinations. Kleinknecht, Klepac and Alexander (73) also
implicate the role of vicarious arousal and classical
conditioning through exposure to the aversive reactions of
family and friends or through the mass media.

Abdominal pain. Recurrent abdominal pain, headaches and
limb pains during childhood frequently cannot be accounted for
by organic abnormalities, hence investigators have been led to
search for psychological causes (4,55,104,109). Studies of
children with recurrent abdominal pain were reported by Apley
(4), who collected comprehensive medical, personal and family
data for 1100 English school children. Children over the age
of three, who, within the previous year, had complained of at
least three episodes of pain severe enough to affect their
daily activities for a period longer than three months, were
contrasted with other children who did not exhibit this
pattern. One portion of the sample comprised 100 children
consecutively admitted for inpatient hospital care with
recurrent abdominal pain as the major symptom. A second group
of 1000 unselected school children provided the balance of the
sample, for the purposes of assessing the population incidence
of the complaint. It also permitted contrasts between
children complaining and not complaining of abdominal pain.

One hundred and eight (10.8%) of the children in the school
series satisfied the foregoing criteria for recurrent

abdominal pain, indicating that the complaint was relatively common. Medical histories of the families of the children complaining of abdominal pain indicated that their parents and siblings complained of the problem at an incidence 5.75 times greater than the control children's families. The member of the family most often reported to be affected was the mother, although two or three family members were affected in several families. The incidence of abdominal pain in relatives of the problematic children outside the immediate family (cousins, grandparents, uncles and aunts) was also several times higher.

Apley provided contrasts between cases in which an organic disorder clearly provide a reasonable basis for the abdominal pain and cases in which adequate organic pathology was not discovered after intensive investigations. Nearly half the children without verifiable organic disease had a positive family history of abdominal pain, whereas in children with organic disease the proportion was very low (1 in 8).

In discussing the pathogenesis of recurrent abdominal pain without adequate organic cause, Apley (4) described a number of mechanisms. Important psychological processes included: (1) the potential reinforcing effects of the social consequences of the pain complaint pattern, and (2) the impact of family interactions, as exemplified in the following, "Statistics do not give the whole story, but in a considerable proportion of my cases the children come from what I have called 'painful families' - practising doctors will recognize ruefully what this means. These are families with one or both parents suffering from recurrent pains and psychological problems, recurrent illnesses and pseudo-illnesses. With the background of a 'painful family' the child complaining of abdominal pains is most unlikely to grow up symptom-free (p. 95)." Parents in these families were often described as intensely preoccupied with their children's state of health and response to treatment.

Excessive attention to abdominal events was described as a critical antecedent to the development of recurrent pain. Apley (4) stated: "An 'awareness' of the abdomen may develop, may be reinforced or almost cultivated, in various ways. It can arise as a habit acquired from some other member of the family in which pain is commonplace or a dramatic abdominal accident has occurred. Alternatively, it may be precipitated by a transient disorder during which attention, associated with anxiety, was directed to the abdomen (p. 96)."

The observation was consistent with recent theoretical formulations of central pattern-generating, neural mechanisms that appear to be responsible for attacks of pain in the absence of injury or other adequate sensory input. The evidence indicates that neural substrates of the memories of earlier pain can be activated to produce pain in the absence of adequate noxious sensory input (99).

As a precaution, it should be emphasized that Apley found

the relative contributions of constitutional and social
influence determinants to be difficult to distinguish or
specify. Abdominal pain was associated frequently with
autonomic dysfunction, with this problem also recurring in
families. This suggested a role for genetic and
constitutional factors as determinants of the familial
consistencies in pain behaviour. Thus, the experiential
factors are as likely to operate in conjunction with
biological factors as alone.

Others have pursued contributions of familial experience to
the process whereby children learn to react with and to pain
(55,109). Oster (104) suggested that it was a tendency toward
exceptional pain proneness and not the more specific bodily
localization which showed a familial tendency. In the Apley
(4) studies, there was a tendency toward the same bodily locus
of pain as in other family members. In Oster's (104)
investigations, there was not as great a degree of agreement
in the specific complaints reported by children and their
parents.

Phantom limb pain. The literature on phantom limb pain
provided additional intriguing information as to the possible
role of modeling processes in the origins of patterns of pain
behavior. While virtually all amputees have phantom limb
experiences, in the form of some somaesthetic or kinesthetic
sensation (e.g., tingling, sweating, or itching), that is felt
as if it were as genuine as sensations in real limbs (96,105),
pain in the phantom limb is not nearly so frequent. Estimates
of its actual incidence among amputees differ, ranging from
between 2 and 10% (117), to 35% (96), depending upon the
criteria applied by the investigator. A critical determinant
of whether pain is likely to develop would appear to be the
patient's earlier experiences with pain. Phantom limb pain is
substantially more probable when pain has been suffered in the
limb for some time before amputation. In particular,
traumatic civilian accidents and battlefield injuries produce
little phantom pain if the limb is severed without warning, or
the individual had not regained consciousness subsequent to
the injury leading to its removal. If the injury or disease
process necessitating the amputation had been experienced as
painful, or intense pain had been experienced in the limb on
an earlier occasion, the phantom pain was likely to bear
considerable similarity to the earlier experience, insofar as
qualitative features of the pain were concerned.

In this case, past experience with pain, rather than social
models, appears to provide the basis for subsequent phantom
limb pain. However, evidence exists to suggest there are
interactions among past and present social experiences and
somatic sensory input (105). Emotional stress can precipitate
phantom limb pain (111) and accentuate the pain suffered by
paraplegics (99). Cases have been reported in which phantom
limb pain developed only after patients had interacted with

fellow amputees. Kolb et al. (75,76) observed that patients suffering phantom limb pain often had in their past histories important personal relationships with an individual who was an amputee. Fully 70% of individuals with painful phantom limbs had lived in close association with an amputee prior to their own loss (76).

Other pain. Past experience with others suffering various forms of acute and chronic pain have been implicated as determinants of the manner in which a variety of other pain states are conceptualized and expressed. Chapman (27) suggested that the patient who has observed a parent suffering from angina pectoris is likely to react differently to personally experienced attacks than other patients who have never observed cardiac pain behavior. There is evidence that reactions to heart attacks change over time. Patients suffering their first heart attack do not tend to be as anxious or demanding as on subsequent occasions (59). Vicarious learning would be expected to modify the nature of the reaction depending upon how serious the disease was for others important to the individual patient.

Surveys of patients with chronic low back pain have indicated that familial models for pain or other major disabilities were frequently available. In a questionnaire study of low back pain patients (60), 59% reported at least one close family member having suffered from either chronic low back pain or another debilitating physical disorder. These data are suggestive at best in the absence of data from control groups. Given a very high incidence of back distress in the general population, most people would be expected to have had some exposure to others with this problem (102). However, the observation that exposure to the symptoms and complaints of significant others may predispose the individual towards complaining of somatic problems when experiencing stress or minor injury deserves further study.

Common Interest Groups

Membership in certain groups of individuals with common identities or interests has also been associated with uniformities in pain behaviour. Some vocational, recreational, and social skills are executed better when high pain tolerance is displayed. Contact and endurance sports, heavy physical laboring, military service, and work in extreme climates frequently involve high risks of injury or pain. If the personal and social consequences of pain-induced performance deterioration are undesirable, one would expect efforts to control pain and persistence despite pain. The skills necessary to avoid, minimize, or tolerate pain may be acquired by members of these groups through observational learning.

Vicarious processes also may be involved when the pain-prone individual avoids high risk activities as a result of observing others suffering before attempting to participate personally. Ryan and Kovacic (114) found a relationship between willingness and ability to tolerate pain and the type of athletic activity in which individuals chose to participate. Their evidence suggested that appraisals of biological cues signalling anomalous activity were influenced by the example of significant others. Certain sensations became recognized as unacceptable, whereas others were accepted as normal.

Social Modeling in Pain Control Strategies

Traditional and innovative procedures presently used to achieve pain control, including analgesic medications, hypnoanalgesia, acupuncture, preparatory instructions, and other educational strategies, commonly include a variety of psychological influence techniques that are known to influence pain processes (117). Frequently they involve direct or symbolic exposure to other patients who have benefitted from the technique.

Modeling Components of Analgesic Intervention Strategies

Psychological and social influence procedures effective in reducing pain frequently incorporate modeling demonstrations to facilitate effectiveness of the procedure.

Hypnoanalgesia. One of the most dramatic and effective applications of hypnosis is in the production of analgesic effects (64). While evidence of these effects has been well-documented in reports of clinical investigations and experimental studies, the general public most frequently receives its confirmation of hypnotic benefits, including analgesia, during theatrical performances staged by professional entertainers. Meeker and Barber (91) described a series of tricks stage hypnotists use to dramatically demonstrate hypnotic phenomena to their audiences, including several illustrating the anaesthetic or analgesic effects of hypnotic states. Subsequent to an induction and appropriate suggestions of numbness and loss of feeling, the hypnotist could (1) ask to have the arm outstretched with the palm down and then pass a flame slowly back and forth beneath the hand, or (2) thrust a long needle or hatpin through the flesh of the hand or arm. An absence of reaction would be used to convince audiences that the hypnotic instructions induced analgesic states. However, Meeker and Barber (91) impress the reader with explanations that don't require the concept of an hypnotic state or an analgesic state. With respect to tolerating the flame, they note that heat can be tolerated readily if the flame is kept moving at a distance of about one

inch from the hand. A stage magician is quoted to account for
the pin through the flesh test: "The subject suffers very
little pain. Just as the needle pierces the skin, the
performer pinches the flesh, which practically deadens the
pain, with the exception of the needle point piercing the
outer skin. Just as soon as the first layer of skin is
broken, the pain ceases.... (91, p. 64)."

The persuasive character of this description, makes it
clear that the hypnotist intends the demonstration to have
telling effects on the audience. Among the possibilities
would be enhancement of the entertainment value of the
performance, enlisting audience cooperation by encouraging
favourable attitudes towards hypnosis, and fostering the
belief that audience members also were capable of enhanced
pain tolerance while under the influence of hypnotism. While
Barber and his colleagues reject the necessity of
conceptualizing the effects of an hypnotic induction in terms
of hypnotic states, or other altered states of consciousness,
they use similar dramatic demonstrations in attempts to
encourage audiences to use cognitive strategies to enhance
their personal capabilities (29,91).

In similar ways, professionals using hypnosis for
therapeutic purposes frequently symbolically model appropriate
hypnotic behavior by providing detailed examples in their
instructions of how the client should behave. Expectations
are usually elaborately described before clients are provided
with the suggestion that they can engage in an act, unless the
client is exceptionally cooperative. Hypnotists rarely
challenge clients to engage in dramatic behavior. When
analgesic effects are desirable this goal is only slowly
approximated. A great deal can be accomplished when the
hypnotist provides a model for how the client should behave,
either through exposure to others complying with suggestions
or through verbal description.

Acupuncture analgesia. Analyses of the dramatic successes
claimed for acupuncture in the relief of pain suggest that a
variety of social and psychological factors may be responsible
for its effects, beyond physiological factors described by
Eastern and Western writers (19,28,123,129). For example,
Chaves and Barber (28) attributed the effectiveness of
acupuncture to cultural conditioning, patient expectation,
adjunctive medication, pretreatment indoctrination,
distraction, and suggestion.

In the context of social modeling influences on pain,
descriptions of the methods used to prepare patients for
surgery with acupuncture analgesia are of special interest.
Acupuncture is rarely used without advanced preparation.
Capperauld (26) reported that acupuncture anaesthesia appeared
to work better in nonemergency situations in which patients
had several days preparation prior to surgery. Chaves and

Barber (28) observed that "The patient typically comes to the hospital two days before surgery and the surgeons explain to him exactly what they are going to do, they show him just how they will operate, and they explain to him what the acupuncturist will do and what effects the needles will have (p.15)."

In the areas of China where acupuncture is actively practised, children are instructed in its use with considerable description of both procedures and resultant beneficial effects. Wall (129) described a group of children who were copying acupuncture points and meridians onto an outline of the human body and practising pushing needles into stuffed socks. In some instances, children were provided with needles to practice insertion in themselves and others (26). Hsiao (65) reported that the Chinese explicitly used social modeling techniques "to build up confidence" by having new patients talk to those who had already gone through acupuncture anesthesia. Consequently, when acupuncture is chosen as an analgesic procedure, patients usually have had advance preparation, with a considerable amount of information conveyed through models.

Psychosocial programs for burn pain. Sensitive appreciation of the impact of the behavior of fellow patients with similar injuries on other patients' behavior was demonstrated in the development of a psychosocial treatment programme on an intensive burn care unit, as described by Fagerhaugh (52). In its intensity, severity, and persistence, burn pain can be one of the most frightful. Yet, on the nursing unit of interest, Fagerhaugh observed a striking infrequency of dramatic pain expression. Loud yelling, screaming, moaning and groaning, and constant requests for pain relief did not appear to be equal to patients' descriptions of pain. This relative absence of expressions of severe distress was attributed to the purposeful programming and organization of patients and staff members on the burn unit.

A variety of social interaction factors contributing to the success of staff in enabling patients to endure pain and to control its expression were described. Of particular interest, in the present context, were descriptions of observational learning opportunities, "The patients on a burn unit represent a group who are in various stages of the burn and pain trajectories, in open view of each other, and who spend a rather long period together in an enclosed space. These conditions give every patient a chance to rehearse and interpret his own illness and its pain trajectory and to compare his state to that of others. Through these activities he learns the norms and limits of pain expression and relief associated with the various phases of his illness: the probable duration of the various phases, the various methods of tolerating pain, and the complications that may alter his pain trajectory (52, p. 647)."

There occasionally were opportunities on this ward to examine the consequences of different kinds of exposure to others. For example, patients in early acute burn phases were normally relatively isolated through care in two-bed rooms. When limited bed space required immediate placement in a much larger ward, patients were described as learning about the temporal phases of pain earlier than otherwise would have been the case.

Other burn and chronic pain treatment programmes have reported the benefits of planned contacts between patients. Artz and Moncrief (5) stated, "Visual evidence of the likelihood of uneventful recovery is particularly encouraging in the early phase of hospitalization. Contact with patients who have had similar burns and are almost recovered is an important source of encouragement. Many patients are reassured by seeing photographs of other severely burned patients showing burned areas at the time of injury and after recovery (p. 284)." Swanson, Swenson, Maruta and Mcphee (121) found that two types of patients served as good social models on a chronic pain inpatient programme. These were the self-confident, independent patients who used treatment programmes effectively, and the highly suggestible patients who readily relinguished symptoms and identified strongly with staff members and programme goals. Other patients were reported to be attracted to them and to show unexpected progress as a result of this exposure. Ward settings clearly provide unique opportunities to control group interactions and to understand the complex social influences determining pain behavior.

Stress Inoculation for Experimental Pain. A pain tolerance training programme has been developed (92,124) that has proven successful in relieving tourniquet-induced ischemic pain and cold pressor pain in volunteer experimental subjects. The programme had a variety of components, including presentation of a conceptual framework for pain, discussing its relevance to the clients' personal experiences, instruction in a variety of behavioral and cognitive coping techniques, and rehearsal of the skills with feedback while the person in the process of training was subjected to a graded series of stress and pain-inducing conditions. The rehearsal phase used several imagery, role-playing and modeling techniques. They included having the trainer model effective use of the skills and having the subjects imagine themselves faltering, experiencing distress, and then coping with their inadequacies. The modeling influences were embedded within a complex array of techniques so that unique contributions of particular treatment components to the substantial overall pain-reducing effects were difficult to specify.

Treatment Programs Based on Modeling Therapies

Several treatment programmes have applied and evaluated modeling therapy techniques in the control of pain and related behavior problems.

Dental care. Melamed et al. (93) proposed that children's dental anxieties may be vicariously extinguished when a model is observed to be coping with the feared situation without experiencing adverse consequences. The sixteen children studied ranged in age from five to eleven years. None had prior direct dental experience. After an initial session providing a dental examination and the collection of psychometric and behavioral data, half the children viewed a thirteen minute film of an initially fearful but coping four year old experiencing a typical dental procedure with a friendly dentist. Consistent with principles describing conditions that facilitate therapeutic modeling effects (8), the model was initially fearful, but able to control the distress and subsequently discovered that there was nothing to fear. In addition, the model received reinforcement for cooperation in the form of verbal praise and a toy. The remaining children viewed a film involving a child engaged in activities unrelated to dentistry.

The modeling treatment had a substantial effect on several indices of emotional expression and cooperativeness throughout a subsequent dental treatment session that required the restoration of at least one carious tooth. On behavioral measures of disruptions, including crying, refusal to open the mouth, white knuckles, rigid posture, verbal complaints, and kicking, the group that had not received modeling treatment was markedly more disruptive than during the baseline assessment session and the treatment group was more cooperative. The group viewing the modeling film also was less anxious during dental treatment. The results clearly supported the use of modeling therapy, and suggested the potential preventive utility of this approach for children beginning a program of dental care.

Several other investigations have employed social modeling to modify and eliminate fearful behavior in dental settings (2,88,95,132). An innovative approach by Gordon, Terdal and Sterling (61) used a nine year old patient's nonanxious sister to demonstrate appropriate and cooperative behavior, while, at the same time, desensitizing the mother's ambivalence toward dental treatment by having her observe both daughters behaving in a relatively anxiety-free manner.

Surgery. Modeling has also been evaluated as a source of coping strategies and preparatory instruction for children about to be hospitalized for surgery. This potentially stressful and anxiety-producing experience frequently leads to behavior problems and a less than satisfactory response to surgery during postoperative recovery (32,82).

Melamed and Siegel (94) examined modeling treatments in a group of thirty children, ranging between 4 and 12 years of age. None had not been hospitalized prior to the occasion on which they were included in the study. The children were to undergo surgery for hernias, tonsillectomies and urinary tract problems.

Immediately prior to hospitalization, children in the modeling treatment group viewed a sixteen minute film depicting a seven year old boy in the course of hospitalization for corrective surgery of a hernia. A description of the film provided an understanding of the numerous events and experiences capable of influencing hospital adjustment. The film consisted of 15 episodes showing various events that the children were likely to encounter from the time of admission to the time of discharge. These included orientation to the hospital ward and medical personnel, having a blood test, exposure to standard hospital equipment, separation from the mother, and scenes in the operating and recovery rooms. There were explanations of the hospital procedures provided by the medical staff, and various scenes were narrated by the child, who described his feelings and the concerns he had at each stage of the hospital experience. Both the child's behavior and verbal remarks exemplified the behavior of a coping model, so that, while he exhibited some anxiety and apprehension, he overcame his initial fears. A second matched group of thirty children viewed an interesting film unrelated to hospitalization or surgery.

The films were evaluated for effects beyond those of procedures already used to reduce children's anxiety as standard routine in the hospital. These included a nurse's detailed explanation of what would happen on the day of surgery, what the child would observe and experience, and a visit by the surgeon or anesthesiologist who explained details of the operation, operating room and the method of anesthesia. Comprehensive measures were reported for subjective distress, behavior problems and physiological arousal (palmar sweat gland activity) prior to admission, the evening before surgery, and at follow-up 20 to 26 days after the child had been discharged from hospital.

The major findings were that the group viewing the peer-modeling hospitalization film displayed lower physiological arousal, fewer medical concerns and fewer anxiety-related behaviors on both the night prior to surgery and followup assessments. Children in the control group had substantially greater behavior problems during the 3 to 4 week posthospitalization period (e.g., bed-wetting, sleep disturbances, and tantrums). Contrary to expectations, the hospital's regular programme of nursing and medical staff's preparatory information and explanation was not associated with reductions in anxiety, suggesting to the authors that more preparation was needed than is ordinarily received once a child has been admitted to hospital. Carefully planned exposure to a model demonstrating coping skills satisfied this requirement.

Needle injections. The impact of realistic and nonrealistic filmed portrayals of children's affective reactions to needle injections was examined by Vernon (127) on children who were receiving preoperative injections prior to relatively minor operations (primarily tonsillectomies). The children ranged in age between 4 and 9 years. On the evening prior to hospital admission the children viewed in their own homes an 18 minute film depicting eight boys and eight girls enacting sick roles while receiving injections from a nurse. The children quietly lay on hospital beds. A nurse entered the room with a syringe and needle in a tray. She chatted briefly, positioned the child, gave the injection in the thigh, put on a bandaid and left. With this as the background, two films were prepared differing only in whether the children receiving injections "winced, said 'Ouch', and seemed to frown or pout, rather than remaining expressionless (p. 755)," or displayed no "apparent pain, fear, or emotional behavior (p. 755)." Two groups of 10 children viewed one of these films, while a third group saw neither film.

To measure the effectiveness of the films on clinical pain, trained observers rated the children on a global mood scale indicating how upset and frightened the children became prior to and during the delivery of preoperative medication by intramuscular injection. The findings indicated that the children who watched the models portraying realistic reactions to the injection were less distressed by the injections when administered to them than the children who had viewed unrealistic benign reactions, or those who were not provided with any advanced exposure. Viewing a model whose reaction to an injection was markedly less than normal expectations actually led to more distress when the observer was subjected to the needles than was displayed by either of the other two groups. In interpreting the adverse response, Vernon (127) suggested the model's unrealistic portrayal may have provoked distrust and anxiety over what would actually happen.

Several observations about how models could reduce or intensify pain reactions seemed appropriate (127). Modeling exposure would be most likely to reduce the pain and distress produced by noxious stimulation when accurate and realistic information is imparted about the probable experience of the viewer. If the viewer's expectations of pain prior to exposure to the model had been excessive, they would become more realistic. Alternatively, if the viewer erroneously anticipated a benign experience, the subsequent discrepancy between expectations and actual experience would be reduced. Modeled information could increase a viewer's subsequent pain and distress in some circumstances. When the model displays

strong tolerance and the message is credible, a condition
could arise in which the model leads to a striking
contradiction between expectations and actual experiences. In
addition, unbelievable messages could enhance distrust,
provoking added anxiety prior to and during the impact of
noxious stimulation. It would seem that the effects of
modeled information are the complex result of the credibility
of the model's role enactment, the viewer's expectations, and
the actual nature of the experience to be endured.

EXPERIMENTAL ANALYSES OF SOCIAL MODELING INFLUENCES ON PAIN

A great deal can be learned through systematic study of
modeling therapies and naturalistic observation in field and
clinical settings, but certain issues cannot be resolved
without difficulty because of practical and ethical reasons.
Laboratory research has provided an alternative approach to
examining the phenomena. The major advantage of laboratory
study is that variables that have potential or known effects
on pain can be subject to stringent control. When the source
of noxious stimulation is known, psychological and social
factors that may contribute to experiential and behavioural
pain responses can be carefully evaluated.

It is worth noting that the strong emphases of early
investigations of pain phenomena on sensory and physiological
processes led to deliberate attempts to exclude the operation
of psychological, social, and other contextual factors.
Consequently, these were rarely systematically studied.
Frequently, psychological variables were treated as nuisance
factors, or potential sources of measurement error, disguising
the investigator's understanding of the "real" pain the
individual was suffering. Experimental designs were invented
that would allow investigators to rule out explanations of
experimental effects based on psychological processes. The
use of placebo controls and double-blind designs in
evaluations of analgesic medications provide good
illustrations.

The Experimental Paradigm

The clinical and field observations make it clear that the
modeling influence process, whether intentional or
unintentional, is complex and can only be explained through
reference to a large number of variables. Before the
complexity could be explored in the laboratory, however, a
demonstration of the impact of modeling influences on pain was
needed. Craig and Weiss (45) examined the impact of exposure
to both tolerant and intolerant social models on verbal
reports of pain provoked by electrical stimulation. Volunteer
subjects described the discomfort and pain provoked by an
ascending series of shocks, while an experimental confederate

ostensibly undertook the identical task, but simulated
tolerance or intolerance proportional to the reports of the
subject. There was an impressive impact of the modeling roles
on both expressions of pain and willingness to accept currents
of increasing intensity. When the actor model was inactive,
the control group identified a mean current intensity of 6.3
mA (milliamperes) as painful. Subjects paired with an
intolerant model accepted only 2.50 mA before describing it as
painful, and exposure to a tolerant model led to reports of
pain at 8.65 mA. In addition to influencing pain reports, the
models also strongly inhibited or enhanced avoidance of the
shocks. Identifying the shocks as painful was the prearranged
signal to indicate an unwillingness to accept further shocks.
Several investigators have concluded that pain thresholds are
relatively stable and uninfluenced by psychological factors or
social constraints (57). Consequently, influencing this form
of pain expression represented a relatively severe test of
social modeling influences.

Subsequent studies examined the impact of models on clearly
painful levels of electric shock, ranging up to pain tolerance
levels, the intensities at which subjects were unwilling to
endure further increases in current intensity. In one
investigation (35), exposure to a tolerant model led to pain
tolerance at 9.93 mA, intolerant model exposure provoked
tolerance at 5.43 mA, and a control group unexposed to a model
endured 6.50 mA. The modeling influence strategy clearly
provided strong control over different forms of pain behaviour
in unselected volunteer subjects, and we concluded that the
experimental paradigm provided a basis for examining various
aspects of human pain behavior.

Enhancing Pain Reports

The early investigations had provided conceptual support
for clinical applications of modeling therapies designed to
reduce pain and inhibit pain behaviour, and also suggested
that modeling exposure could produce behaviour indicative of a
reduced capacity to tolerate noxious stimulation. The
reactions of pain to very low levels of stimulation roughly
paralleled expressions of distress and demands for treatment
in patients for whom there has been little or no evidence of
tissue pathology.

To study the acquisition of dispositions toward pain
proneness, using the modeling influence paradigm, two studies
(37,46) examined whether reports of pain could be elicited to
non-noxious electrical stimulation. In both studies a
constant, low-level, shock intensity, that usually leads to a
nonaversive experience commonly described as vibratory or
tingling, was delivered to subjects, while models described
the shock as progressively more uncomfortable, and ultimately
painful. In the combined studies, subjects exposed to the

intolerant model described the nonaversive shock as painful on 77% of the trials, whereas control groups characterized the shock as painful on but 3% of the trials. While physical trauma usually represents the source of pain behaviour, noxious stimulation is neither always necessary nor inevitably sufficient to evoke communications of pain or distress. Formulations of the origins of pain must consider the social context in which pain is reported.

Social Factors and Individual Differences

Several subsequent studies explored other social influence processes that may have contributed to the effectiveness of the modeling influence strategy, and personality characteristics that may have made subjects particularly prone or resistant to the model's example.

Pain communications were conceptualized as reflecting only one component of a network of events in which the individual in painful distress interacts continuously with others. For example, expressions of acute pain frequently lead to others' attempts at caretaking, which in turn can affect the frequency and nature of pain complaints. The complex nature of the modeling influence paradigm allowed analyses of various components of this reciprocal influence process, since participants interacted with each other over time.

In the early studies, communication networks between subjects and models were open insofar as information exchanges about the nature of the pain experience were concerned. Both participants were required to report reactions to the shocks. It became apparent that various features of the interaction process could be evaluated if communication channels were restricted. For example, requiring subjects to self-disclose their subjective experiences in the presence of a tolerant companion could have led to competitive feelings or tendencies to present oneself favourably. Subjects may have felt inferior to the model and resisted reporting distress despite considerable suffering.

A recent study (34) attempted to eliminate the effects of disclosing pain reactions to the peer companion by allowing subjects to make ratings of pain reactions without disclosure to the model. The study also allowed evaluation of the effects of the presence of a companion who was subjected to the same noxious experience as the subject but did not verbally report reactions. A recent investigation by Kleck et al. (72) had reported that the simple presence of an inactive observer attenuated reports of subjective distress, nonverbal expressive behaviour, and autonomic arousal to electric shocks. The results of the modeling study indicated that exposure to the tolerant model was a considerably more influential determinant of pain behaviour than the disclosure requirement, and the presence of a coactive companion had no apparent effect on pain. Removing the disclosure requirement only minimally affected pain ratings, whereas the tolerant model continued to exert a powerful effect, independent of whether or not disclosure was required. Exposure to the tolerant model led to a mean tolerance level of 15.23 mA, a substantially greater level of tolerance than was displayed in any earlier study in this series. While the self-disclosure requirement was minimally influential, other studies have successfully generated competitive motivation that inhibited expressions of pain. Lambert, Libman, and Poser (80), for example, found appealing to an individual's religious affiliation to be effective.

Other investigations have examined individual difference factors that could relate to the impact of models on pain behaviour. It is noteworthy that none of the laboratory investigations by Craig and his associates reviewed to this point had involved preselection of subjects on personality characteristics, suggesting that modeling influence strategies can have very general effects. However, it seemed likely that personality characteristics of models and subjects would affect the impact of modeling influences on pain behavior (cf. 29). There is a substantial social learning theory literature suggesting that interactions between characteristics of models and observers determine the extent to which their behaviours become matched (10).

In one investigation (35) determinants of feelings of control in settings involving noxious stimulation were examined. Feelings of loss of control frequently represent major distressing components of pain experiences. People who believe themselves unable to relieve or avoid pain or stress suffer more than those who perceive themselves to have control available (23,56). One source of perceived control could be long term dispositions to interpret situations as subject to personal influence. A wide range of behaviours has been found to be influenced by generalized, stable expectancies and personal beliefs about the ability to control situations (86,113). The present study examined the impact of individual differences in perceived control on pain behavior, and also whether this personality characteristic would influence the extent to which the model's pain behavior was matched.

The results indicated that perceived control was related to pain tolerance, with those believing themselves to have reasonably good personal control over reinforcement contingencies exhibiting somewhat greater tolerance than those believing themselves to have less control. This individual difference variable did not interact with the impact of the tolerant or intolerant modeling conditions. Consistent with earlier studies, the subjects displayed strong tendencies to match tolerant or intolerant models. In fact, the social influence variable was substantially more potent than the personality difference variable. This, in part, appeared

attributable to subjects' reports of beliefs that they
possessed considerable control over the model's ratings.   To
some extent, this was indeed the case.   The modeling influence
strategy provided for reciprocal control with the models
responsive to the subjects' behaviour, but biased in the
direction of tolerance or intolerance.   The study indicated
that it may be possible to provide feelings of control even
for those who generally don't consider themselves capable of
controlling external events.   We concluded that situational
factors were more important determinants of pain behaviour
than personality predispositions.

Public and Private Pain Behavior

While these investigations demonstrated an impressive
impact of exposure to social models on pain behaviour, they
did not provide direct measures of subjective experience.
Both formal and informal conceptions of pain usually emphasize
subjective distress as its most important qualitative
component (117).   Changes in overt, public behaviour are
important in their own right because they critically affect
reactions of others to the person in distress and the
self-perceiving behaviour of the suffering individual
(7,77,83), but overt verbal and nonverbal expressive behaviour
and subjective experiences can vary independently (42,72).
Depending upon the circumstances, an individual may be
provoked to considerable distress as a result of having been
subjected to noxious stimuli and either display evidence of
substantial discomfort, or stoical forbearance.   Self-report,
other expressive behaviours, and physiological processes, to
some extent, are all amenable to purposeful control and
dissimulation of evidence as to the nature of experiences,
depending upon situational demands.   While verbal reports of
pain represent the best available measure in clinical
practice, since they usually sensitively reflect tissue
pathology and analgesic medication (63), there are
circumstances in which this is not the case.   These are the
situations in which massive tissue damage is suffered with
minimal complaint, or there is considerable complaint without
apparent adequate organic pathology.

In several investigations, we have attempted to develop and
apply measures of less obvious, or private aspects of pain
behavior.   In these efforts to make private pain behaviour
public, multi-dimensional perspectives on pain have been
adopted.   A number of different frameworks have proven useful.
Sternbach's (117) description of interrelationships among
behavioral, subjective, and physiological components of pain
led to contrasts among self-reports, other overt behavior and
psychophysiological indices (41,42).   Sensory decision theory
(31,87) provided a rationale for differentiating between
sensory sensitivity to noxious stimulation and the effects of

biases in willingness to express discomfort (39,42,43). Magnitude estimation scaling procedures (34,38) were used to quantify the relationship between physical properties of noxious stimuli and the rate of perceived growth in the painful experience. Finally, distinctions between sensory-discriminative components of pain and affective-motivational qualities (17,100), and appropriate self-report measures of pain (97), led to investigations of the impact of models on different qualities of pain experience (76,48). While it seems unlikely that any single measure, or even group of measures, will entirely encompass as complex a process as pain, these distinctions were clearly important.

Psychophysiological Investigations

Measures of autonomic nervous system reactivity are not as subject to voluntary control as self-report, and reflect the biological processes mediating personal discomfort. The association between pain experience and physiological responses appears to reflect homeostatic mechanisms that are self-protective (20,21). The affective components of pain, in particular, appear to be closely associated with autonomic arousal, although the relationships are often complex (42,83). Sources of influence capable of inhibiting or enhancing painful distress would be expected to reduce or increase arousal in the autonomic nervous system. It should be noted, however, that while psychophysiological measures of autonomic activity have been used frequently to assess emotional arousal and distress (22), they are also responsive to non-affective stimuli (47,79,81), and caution is appropriate in interpreting their behavioural significance.

The impact of modeling on skin conductance and cardiovascular reactivity to electric shocks was recently examined (41). Groups of subjects exposed to tolerant and intolerant models differed substantially in the current intensities provoking pain thresholds, consistent with the models' role enactments, but they could not be differentiated on skin conductance or heart rate monitored during shock exposure. A subsequent study (42) used skin potential activity as an alternative electrodermal measure, because skin conductance measures appear to be overly sensitive to noxious stimulation and to exhibit early ceiling effects (125). Non-palmar skin potential and heart rate measures indicated that tolerant modeling exposure was associated with reductions in autonomic reactivity below that observed in a control group not exposed to a model (42). We concluded that, to the extent that these physiological variables reflected the biological substrates of the experience of pain, tolerant modeling exposure reduced fundamental affective qualities of the pain experience.

Sensory Decision Theory Analyses

Sensory decision theory, or signal detection theory as it traditionally has been known (30,31,87,106), also provided a rationale for conceptualizing the issue of whether verbal reports of pain are congruent with subjective experience. The major contribution of sensory decision theory has been the distinction between how well individuals detect or discriminate stimuli and their willingness to express discomfort in a given setting. A number of studies have now been completed applying this approach to the evaluation of the impact of social modeling influences on sensory-discriminative components of pain and verbal report response biases.

The initial study (39) examined the impact of tolerant and intolerant modeling on both shock-induced pain thresholds and sensory decision theory indices of sensory sensitivity. Consistent with earlier studies, the groups matched the tolerant and intolerant models in their reports of shock-elicited pain and willingness to accept strong current intensities. Sensory decision theory analyses of the data indicated that the impact of the intolerant model was to enhance differential sensitivity to the shocks. The groups exposed to this model displayed greater sensitivity to electrical stimulation than those exposed to the tolerant model, or the control group. Thus, the sensory component of the perception of electrical stimulation was influenced by the psychological influence strategy. Those exposed to the tolerant model showed no changes in sensitivity paralleling the reduced pain reports, hence this change appeared to be associated with a response criterion shift. The consequence of exposure to the tolerant model was reluctance to use the discomfort and pain labels at the low levels of stimulation delivered.

Because the electrical current intensities delivered during this study were at relatively low levels, increasing only to pain thresholds, and analgesic agents tend to be more effective at suprathreshold, strong levels of noxious stimulation, we sought to further evaluate tolerant modeling exposure at current intensities well above pain threshold (42), and increasing to tolerance levels (43). In both investigations, exposure to the model again produced substantial reductions in verbal reports of the amount of distress experienced. Sensory decision theory analyses of the data clearly indicated that the tolerant model reduced the extent to which subjects were discriminating differences between the noxious stimuli presented. Craig and Ward (43) also observed that the effects on verbal report and sensory discriminability persisted from the session during which there was modeling exposure to another session one week later when the model was inactive. Thus, the effects of exposure to the model were persistent, suggesting that training for pain tolerance may have durable, adaptive consequences.

The combined studies indicated that the social modeling influence strategy affected fundamental perceptual processing of noxious stimulation, beyond effects on willingness to complain of pain. Exposure to the intolerant model seemed to have its maximal effect on noxious stimuli at intensities representing the transition between the absence and presence of discomfort. When experience at this level was interpreted as reflecting distressing qualities through social influence, sensitivity seemed to be enhanced. People appeared to be trainable to be pain sensitive. On the other hand, exposure to the tolerant model reduced pain sensitivity, with the effects most apparent at strong levels of stimulation. The evidence of reduced physiological arousal and reduced sensory sensitivity when subjects were paired with the tolerant model suggested that the sensory information and affective arousal normally provoked by noxious stimulation were inhibited, thereby reducing available somatic cues to respond to as indicative of bodily pain. Similarly, low level somatic activity that would normally provide cues for anticipating more intense levels of distress would not be available. This would also be consistent with an interpretation that there was a change in attentional focus with the subjects reacting more to the social context and less to somatic cues.

Psychophysical Power Function Analyses

The magnitude estimation procedures used in several of the studies allowed the application of psychophysical power function analyses to describe the quantitative relationships between electric shock intensities and subjective judgments of physical intensity and discomfort (34,38). The scaling procedure is sensitive to the range of individual experience induced by noxious stimulation and potentially allows quantification of components of private pain behavior. Since early work by Stevens et al. (120), investigators consistently have reported that the perceived magnitude of experimentally-induced pain (Ψ) grows as a function of the physical value of the stimuli (ϕ) raised to a power (η), or $\Psi = \alpha\phi^\eta$ where α is the unit of scale. This has been the case with electric shock (49,51), cold pressor pain (62), and tourniquet induced ischemic pain (63,124). The power function has usually been interpreted as representing operating characteristics of the sensory receptors involved, with the exponent varying over different sensory modalities. However, various sources of information suggest that, at least in the case of shock-induced pain behaviour, the power function may reflect modulating roles of perceptual and cognitive factors. To the extent that the magnitude of the power exponent is subject to change as a result of variation in the social context, theoretical interpretations of its significance must include perceptual and cognitive processes in addition to sensory processes.

Craig et al. (38) found that the social modeling procedures changed the unit of scale and ideal estimates of the exponents of the power function, although the latter effect was not observed in conventional regression analyses and required range-derived estimates. In a subsequent investigation (34), in which the tolerant modeling effects were even more potent, insofar as verbal reports were concerned, regression analyses indicated direct effects of tolerant modeling on the exponent of the power function. The magnitude of the exponent was reduced indicating a slower rate of increase in perceived discomfort. Again, fundamental qualities of the shock-induced pain experience were changed as a result of influencing the individual's interpretation of the meaning of the experience.

The Language of Pain: Influencing Different Components

Multidimensional models of pain experience have led to attempts to characterize different diseases and pain disorders in terms of how they are represented on different qualitative dimensions (97). In clinical practice diagnosticians frequently rely on patients' descriptions of their symptoms. Agnew and Mersky (3) point out that there is a rich clinical literature describing the phenomonology of particular pains; for example, the burning pain of causalgia, the pressure and constriction of tension headaches, or the cramping qualities of visceral pain. Empirical evaluation of this clinical lore is only now becoming available (3,6,48). For example, Crockett, Prkachin and Craig (48) have identified dimensions of pain response whose extremes were represented to a greater or lesser degree among people experiencing clinical or experimentally induced pain.

The most generally accepted distinction between components of subjective reactions to noxious stimulation has been between sensory-discriminative and affective-motivational qualities (17,98). Sensory qualities concern the perception of physical properties of the painful event, including identification of its bodily location and distribution, time of onset, variation over time, and physical intensity. Affective-motivational qualities primarily concern emotional arousal, variations in affective tone, and motivational significance. Evidence exists indicating that people can restrict their reports to particular components of painful experiences and differentially report sensory and affective attributes (69,97).

A recent study (36) examined whether the social modeling influence paradigm would differentially influence reports of particular components of painful experiences. The social influence variable was expected to affect reports of affective discomfort more substantially than reports of physical

qualities of painful experiences. Complaints of distress
would appear to have a more important social functional value
than descriptions of the nonaffective qualities of experience.
The person in pain would be expected to be more sensitive to
the potential social consequences of talking about emotional
qualities than when describing sensory qualities. If this
were the case, clinicians could focus more heavily on reports
of sensory-discriminative qualities, since they would seem to
more directly reflect tissue damage. The investigation (36)
found that exposure to a tolerant model equally and
substantially influenced reports of both affective and sensory
qualities of shock induced pain. Reports of both components
of pain experiences seemed to be subject to the control of
social demands. This finding suggested that attempts to glean
information about a patient's disorder by ignoring or
suppressing affective material would not necessarily be an
effective strategy. Social biases appear to operate on
self-description of sensory experiences as well as affective
components. Further, because social factors indeed change
basic qualities of pain experiences, the effects observed
reflect changes in both public expressions of pain and
fundamental qualities of painful experience.

SUMMARY

Considerable evidence was reviewed on the immediate and
long-term effects of observing others experiencing pain. The
observational learning literature provided a perspective for
examining behavioral, cognitive and affective components of
reactions to the painful distress of others. Crosscultural
studies and investigations of the life histories of patients
suffering different kinds of clinical pain suggested that
parents, other family members, and individuals important to
the patient serve as models for the experience of pain and the
manner in which it is expressed. Modeling effects can be both
beneficial and maladaptive. Those components of conventional
and innovative treatment strategies involving live or symbolic
demonstrations of models coping with clinical or treatment
induced pain were described, as were several modeling therapy
programs specifically designed to control pain and related
behavior disorders. Finally, research studies of modeling
influences on pain were reviewed, including those indicating
that modeling intervention strategies affect not only
observable pain behavior, but also influence the processing of
sensory information and physiological responses to painful
stimulation.

REFERENCES

1.   Abel, G.G., Barlow, D.H., Blanchard, E.B., and Guild, D.
     (1977): Arch. Gen. Psychiatr., 34:895-903.

2. Adelson, R., and Goldfried, M.R. (1970): J. Dent. Child.,
    37:476-489.
3. Agnew, D.C., and Merskey, H. (1976): Pain, 2:73-81.
4. Apley, J. (1975): The Child with Abdominal Pains.
    Blackwell, Oxford.
5. Artz, C.P., and Moncrief, J.A. (1969): The Treatment of
    Burns. W.B. Saunders, Philadelphia.
6. Bailey, C.A., and Davidson, P.O. (1976): Pain, 2:73-81.
7. Bandler, R.J., Jr., Madaras, C.R., and Bem, D. (1978):
    J. Pers. Soc. Psychol., 9:205-209.
8. Bandura, A. (1969): Principles of Behavior Modification.
    Holt, Rinehart and Winston, New York.
9. Bandura, A. (1971): In: Psychological Modeling:
    Conflicting Theories, edited by A. Bandura, pp. 1-62.
    Aldine/Atherton, Chicago.
10. Bandura, A. (1977): Social Learning Theory. Prentice-
    Hall, Englewood Cliffs, N.J.
11. Bandura, A. (1977): Psychol. Rev., 84:191-215.
12. Bandura, A., and Menlove, F.L. (1968): J. Pers. Soc.
    Psychol., 8:99-108.
13. Bandura, A., and Rosenthal, R.L. (1966): J. Pers. Soc.
    Psychol., 3:54-62.
14. Barber, T.X. (1970): LSD, Marihuana, Yoga, and Hypnosis.
    Aldine, Chicago.
15. Baron, R.A. (1974): J. Pers. Soc. Psychol., 29:117-124.
16. Baron, R.A., and Byrne, D. (1977): Social Psychology.
    Allyn and Bacon, Boston.
17. Beecher, H.K. (1959): Measurement of Subjective Responses.
    Oxford University Press, Oxford.
18. Berger, S.M. (1962): Psychol. Rev., 69:450-466.
19. Berk, S.N., Moore, M.E., Resnick, J.H. (1977): J. Consult.
    Clin. Psychol., 45:612-619.
20. Bonica, J.J. (1953): The Management of Pain. Lea and
    Febiger, Philadelphia.
21. Bonica, J.J. (1977): Arch. Surg., 112:750-761.
22. Borkovec, T.D., Weerts, T.C., and Bernstein, D.A. (1977):
    In: Handbook of Behavioral Assessment, edited by
    A. Ciminero, K. Calhoun, and H.E. Adams, pp. 367-428.
    Wiley, New York.
23. Bowers, K.S. (1968): J. Consult. Clin. Psychol., 32:
    596-602.
24. Breuer, J., and Freud, S. (1956): Studies in Hysteria.
    Nervous and Mental Diseases Publishing Co., New York.
25. Buss, A.H., and Portnoy, N.W. (1967): J. Pers. Soc.
    Psychol., 6:106-108.
26. Capperauld, I. (1972): Surg. Gynecol. Obstet., 135:
    440-445.
27. Chapman, R.C. (1977): Proc. of Nat. Conf. Cardiac Pain,
    Health Sciences Inst., Princeton, N.J.
28. Chaves, J.F., and Barber, T.X. (1974): Psychoenerg Sys.,
    1:11-21.

29. Chaves, J.F., and Barber, T.X. (1974): J. Abnorm. Psychol., 83:356-363.
30. Clark, W.C. (1969): J. Abnorm. Psychol., 74:363-371.
31. Clark, W.C. (1974): Anesthesiology, 40:272-287.
32. Cohen, F., and Lazarus, R.S. (1973): Psychosom. Med., 35: 375-389.
33. Craig, K.D. (1968): J. Abnorm. Psychol., 73:513-520.
34. Craig, K.D. (1978): Can. J. Behav. Sci., 10 (in press).
35. Craig, K.D., and Best, J.A. (1977): Pain, 3:127-135.
36. Craig, K.D., Best, H., and Best, J.A. (1978): J. Consult. Clin. Psychol., 46 (in press).
37. Craig, K.D., Best, H., and Reith, G. (1973): Can. J. Behav. Sci., 6:169-177.
38. Craig, K.D., Best, H., and Ward, L.M. (1975): J. Abnorm. Psychol., 84:366-373.
39. Craig, K.D., and Coren, S. (1975): J. Psychosom. Res., 19:105-112.
40. Craig, K.D., and Lowery, J.J. (1969): J. Pers. Soc. Psychol., 11:381-387.
41. Craig, K.D., and Neidermayer, H. (1974): J. Pers. Soc. Psychol., 29:246-252.
42. Craig, K.D., and Prkachin, K.M. (1978): J. Pers. Soc. Psychol., 36 (in press).
43. Craig, K.D., and Ward, L.M. (1976): Social modeling influences on the discriminability of painful stimuli. Unpublished manuscript.
44. Craig, K.D., and Weinstein, M.S. (1965): Psychol. Rep., 17:955-963.
45. Craig, K.D., and Weiss, S.M. (1971): J. Pers. Soc. Psychol., 19:53-59.
46. Craig, K.D., and Weiss, S.M. (1972): Percept. Mot. Skills, 34:943-948.
47. Craig, K.D., and Wood, K. (1971): J. Exp. Res. Pers., 5:304-309.
48. Crockett, D.J., Prkachin, K.M., and Craig, K.D. (1977): Pain, 4:175-182.
49. Cross, D.V., Tursky, B., and Lodge, M. (1975): Percept. and Psychophysics, 18:9-14.
50. Davison, G.C. (1968): J. Abnorm. Psychol., 73:84-90.
51. Ekman, G., Frankenhauser, M., Levander, S., and Mellin, I. (1964): Scand. J. Psychol., 5:257-261.
52. Fagerhaugh, S.Y. (1974): Nurs. Outlook, 22:645-650.
53. Fordyce, W.E. (1976): Behavioral Methods for Chronic Pain and Illness. C.V. Mosby, St. Louis, Miss.
54. Forgione, A.G., and Clark, R.E. (1974): J. Dent. Res., 53:496-497.
55. Friedman, R. (1972): Clin. Pediatr., 11:331-333.
56. Geer, J.H., Davison, G.C., and Gatchel, B.I. (1970): J. Pers. Soc. Psychol., 16:731-738.
57. Gelfand, S. (1964): Canad. J. Psychol., 18:36-42.

58. Genest, M., and Turk, D.C. (1978): In: Behavioral Group Therapy, edited by D. Upper and S.M. Ross, Research Press, Champaign, Illinois (in press).
59. Gentry, W.D., and Haney, T. (1975): Heart Lung, 4:738-745.
60. Gentry, W.D., Shows, W.D., and Thomas, M. (1974): Psychosomatica, 15:174-177.
61. Gordon, D., Terdal, L., and Sterling, E. (1974): J. Dent. Child., 22:102-105.
62. Hilgard, E.R. (1967): Proc. Nat. Acad. Sci., 57:1581-1586.
63. Hilgard, E.R. (1969): Amer. Psychol., 24:103-113.
64. Hilgard, E.R., and Hilgard, J.R. (1975): Hypnosis in the Relief of Pain. William Kaufmann, Los Altos, Calif.
65. Hsiao, S. (1977): Amer. Psychol., 32:374-376.
66. Hygge, S. (1976): J. Pers. Soc. Psychol., 33:764-771.
67. Hygge, S., and Ohman, A. (1978): J. Pers. Soc. Psychol., 36:271-279.
68. Ireland, P., Sapira, J.O., and Templeton, B. (1967): Amer. J. Med., 43:579-592.
69. Johnson, J.E. (1973): J. Pers. Soc. Psychol., 27:261-275.
70. Johnson, R. (1971): Psychiatr. Med., 2:221-228.
71. Johnson, R., and Baldwin, D.C. (1968): J. Dent. Res., 47:801-805.
72. Kleck, R.E., Vaughan, R.C., Cartwright-Smith, J., Vaughan, K.B., Colby, C.Z., and Lanzetta, J.T. (1976): J. Pers. Soc. Psychol., 34:1211-1218.
73. Kleinknecht, R.A., Klepac, R.K., and Alexander, L.D. (1973): J. Amer. Dent. Assoc., 86:842-848.
74. Kleinknecht, R.A., Klepac, R.A., and Bernstein, D.A. (1976): Prof. Psychol., 7:585-592.
75. Kolb, L.C., Frank, L.M., and Watson, E.J. (1952): Proc. Staff Meet. Mayo Clin., 27:110-118.
76. Kolb, L.C. (1959): In: American Handbook of Psychiatry V., edited by I.S. Arieti, pp. 893-927. Basic Books, New York.
77. Kopel, S.A., and Arkowitz, H.S. (1974): J. Pers. Soc. Psychol., 29:677-686.
78. Krebs, D.L. (1975): J. Pers. Soc. Psychol., 32:1134-1146.
79. Lacey, J.I. (1967): In: Psychological Stress: Issues in Research, edited by M.H. Appley, and R. Trumbull, pp. 14-36. Appleton-Century-Crofts, New York.
80. Lambert, W.E., Libman, E., and Poser, E.G. (1960): J. Pers., 38:350-357.
81. Lang, P.J. (1971): In: Handbook of Psychotherapy and Behavior Change, edited by A.E. Bergin and S.L. Garfield, pp. 75-125. Wiley, New York.
82. Langer, E.J., Janis, I.L., and Wolfer, J.A. (1975): J. Exp. Soc. Psych., 11:155-165.
83. Lanzetta, J.T., Cartwright-Smith, J., and Kleck, R.E. (1976): J. Pers. Soc. Psychol., 33:354-370.
84. Lazarus, R.S., and Alfert, E. (1964): J. Abnorm. Soc. Psychol., 69:195-205.

85. Lazarus, R.S., Speisman, J.C., Mordkoff, A.M., and Davison, L.A. (1962): Psychol. Monog. 76 (Whole No. 533).

86. Lefcourt, H.M. (1972): In: Progress in Experimental Personality Research, Vol. 6, edited by B.A. Maher, pp. 1-39. Academic Press, New York.

87. Lloyd, M.A., and Appel, J.B. (1976): Psychosom Med., 38:79-94.

88. Machen, J., and Johnson, R. (1974): J. Dent. Res., 53:83-89.

89. Marlatt, G.A., and Perry, M.A. (1975): In: Helping People Change, edited by F.H. Kanfer and A.P. Goldstein, pp. 117-158. Pergamon, Elmsford, N.Y.

90. Mechanic, D. (1962): J. Chron. Dis., 15:189-194.

91. Meeker, W.B., and Barber, T.X. (1971): J. Abnorm. Psychol., 77:61-70.

92. Meichenbaum, D., and Turk, D. (1976): In: Behavioral Management of Anxiety Depression and Pain, edited by P.O. Davidson, pp. 1-34. Bruner/Mazel, New York.

93. Melamed, B.G., Hawes, R.R., Heiby, E., and Glick, J. (1975): J. Dent. Res., 54:797-801.

94. Melamed, B.G., and Siegel, L.J. (1975): J. Consult. Clin. Psychol., 43:511-521.

95. Melamed, B.G., Weinstein, D., Hawes, R., and Katin-Borland, M. (1975): J. Amer. Dent. Assoc., 90:822-826.

96. Melzack, R. (1973): The Puzzle of Pain. Penguin, Harmondsworth, Middlesex, England.

97. Melzack, R. (1975): Pain, 1:277-299.

98. Melzack, R., and Casey, K.L. (1968): In: The Skin Senses, edited by D.L. Kenshalo, pp. 423-443. Thomas, Springfield, Illinois.

99. Melzack, R., and Loeser, J.D. (1978): Pain, 4:195-210.

100. Melzack, R., and Torgerson, W.S. (1971): Anesthesiology, 34:50-59.

101. Merskey, H., and Spear, F.G. (1967): Pain: Psychological and Psychiatric Aspects. Bailliere, Tindall and Cassell, London.

102. Nachemson, A.L. (1976): Spine, 1:59-71.

103. Neufeld, R.W.J., and Davidson, P.O. (1971): J. Psychosom. Res., 15:329-335.

104. Oster, J. (1972): Pediatrics, 50:429-436.

105. Pasnau, R.O., and Pfefferbaum, B. (1976): Nurs. Clin. N. Amer., 11:679-685.

106. Pastore, R.E., and Scheirer, C.J. (1974): Psychol. Bull., 81:945-958.

107. Pilowsky, I. (1975): Aust. New Zeal. J. Psychiat., 9: 141-147.

108. Pilowsky, I., and Spence, N.D. (1976): Pain, 2:167-174.

109. Poznanski, E.O. (1976): Clin. Pediat., 15:1114-1119.

110. Rayner, J.F. (1976): In: Pain: New Perspectives in Therapy and Research, edited by M. Weisenberg and B. Tursky, pp. 93-112. Plenum Press, New York.

111. Riding, J. (1976): Anesthesia, 31:102-106.
112. Rosenthal, T.L. (1976): In: Progress in Behavior Modification. V. 2, edited by M. Hersen, R.M. Eisler, and P.M. Miller, pp. 53-97. Academic Press, New York.
113. Rotter, J.B. (1975): J. Consult. Clin. Psychol., 43: 56-57.
114. Ryan, E.D., and Kovacic, C.R. (1966): Percept. Mot. Skills, 22:383-390.
115. Shoben, E.J., and Borland, L. (1954): J. Clin, Psychol., 10:171-174.
116. Simpson, M.A. (1975): Can. Psychiatr. Assoc. J., 20: 429-437.
117. Sternbach, R.A. (1968): Pain: A Psychophysiological Analysis. Academic Press, New York.
118. Sternbach, R.A. (1974): Pain Patients: Traits and Treatment. Academic Press, New York.
119. Sternbach, R.A., and Tursky, B. (1965): Psychophysiology, 1:241-246.
120. Stevens, S.G., Carton, A.A., and Schickman, C.M. (1958): J. Exp. Psychol., 56:328-334.
121. Swanson, D.W., Swenson, W.M., Marata, T., and McPhee, M.C. (1976): Mayo Clin. Proc., 51:401-411.
122. Thomas, M.H., Horton, R.W., Lippincott, E.C., and Drabman, R.S. (1977): J. Pers. Soc. Psychol., 35:450-458.
123. Toomey, T.C., Ghia, J.N., Mao, W., and Gregg, J.M. (1977): Pain, 3:137-145.
124. Turk, O. (1977): A Coping Skills Training Approach for the Control of Experimentally Produced Pain. Doctoral Dissertation, University of Waterloo, Waterloo, Ontario.
125. Tursky, B. (1974): Psychophysiology, 11:95-112.
126. Tursky, B., and Sternbach, R.A. (1967): Psychophysiology, 4:67-74.
127. Vernon, D.T.A. (1974): J. Pers. Soc. Psychol., 29:794-799.
128. Trethowan, W.H., and Conlan, M.E. (1965): Brit. J. Psychiatr., 111:57-66.
129. Wall, P.D. (1974): New Sci., 3:31-34.
130. Weisenberg, M. (1977): Psychol. Bull., 84:1008-1044.
131. Weisenberg, M., Kreindler, M.L., Schachat, R., and Werboff, J. (1975): Psychosom. Med., 37:123-135.
132. White, W.C., Akers, J., Green, J., and Yates, D. (1974): J. Dent. Child., 30:106-110.
133. Wilfling, F.J., Klonoff, H., and Kokan, P. (1973): Clin. Orthop. Rel. Res., 90:153-160.
134. Zborowski, M. (1969): People in Pain. Jossey-Bass, San Francisco.

The Psychology of Pain, edited by R. A. Sternbach.
Raven Press, New York © 1978.

Pain and Personality

H. Merskey

*Department of Psychiatry, The University of Western Ontario, and Department of
Education and Research, London Psychiatric Hospital, London,
Ontario, Canada, N6A 4H1*

"It should not happen to you, all you that pass by. Look and
see if there is any pain like my pain which is done to me, with
which the Lord has afflicted me in the day of his fierce anger.
From above he has sent fire into my bones, he has made me deso-
late and faint all the day....." Lamentations (I,12)

A link between pain and the emotions was recognized both by
the Greeks and the ancient Hebrews. For Aristotle (3) pain was
one of the "passions of the soul" by which he appears to have
meant that it was both a sensation and an emotional state. In
the book of Lamentations by Jeremiah, mourning the destruction of
Jerusalem several centuries before Aristotle, we find a quotation
which clearly indicates that pain felt in the body was due to
emotional distress. The word he uses in the original unquestion-
ably means a pain located in part of the body, but curiously has
not always been given its literal translation. Devotees of
Handel's Messiah will recognize the expression "Is there any sorrow like unto my sorrow?", yet the original word is not sorrow
but specifically "pain". There may be more than one reason for
this mistranslation. One which we can easily recognize is the
tendency to equate pain with anguish. Pain, an experience which
we first of all associate with damage to the body, is readily
used for a symbol of suffering in general.

If we look a little longer at Jeremiah's words another aspect
is evident. The man who is in such an extreme state of pain because of the sack of Jerusalem has an experience like fire in the
bones and feels weary and faint all day. Take away the poetry,
speak of burning pains and chronic fatigue, and we have the picture of many patients who have pain for psychological reasons but
whose pain is associated with referral to the body. This serves
to emphasize the fact that when we speak of pain we mean an experience which is located in the soma. It may or may not have a
physical cause. Jeremiah's pain is described as entirely due to
emotions. But it is referred to the body, located in the bones.

The experience which is caused by the emotions and is itself an unpleasant affect, may thus in turn be a cause of further misery, at least in theory. Any such experience of pain, however, has to be distinguished from the purely metaphorical notion of pain: anguish, sorrow, misery, distress, etc. are not words which necessarily indicate any felt somatic disturbance. Mental pain is a different concept from pain and has to be kept separate. It might seem unnecessary to emphasize this point but confusion often arises when it is neglected.

PAIN AND MOOD

Enough has been said already to imply a strong relationship between pain and mood. More will be evident in other chapters also. Detailed reviews have been provided by Barber (5), Beecher (8) and Sternbach (59) and a further discussion by Merskey and Spear (45). Beecher (7) has particularly emphasized how the circumstances related to wounding affect the experience of pain. Those for whom pain has some advantage, like soldiers able to leave the battlefield, were shown by him to experience less pain for wounds of comparable size than civilians for whom the wounds from surgery were a wholly unwarranted interruption of their normal life. Anxiety is generally recognized as increasing pain, and so anything which diminishes anxiety can be expected to diminish pain, whilst, on the other hand, excitement or aggression may leave subjects oblivious of gross trauma. It is often remarked upon that football players and other sportsmen may be observed to suffer quite severe blows during a match or contest and yet do not appear to notice any pain until the match is over. Similar experiences are frequently reported in soldiers. In contrast with this, anxious patients, and those with a history of ready complaints to the doctor about somatic symptoms, frequently appear to have more pain than their physical circumstances seem to indicate. In general it can be said that high arousal reduces pain and moderate arousal enhances it. From this we can conclude that whilst some moods cause or promote pain others will abolish or alleviate it.

The evidence that mood alters pain is very varied. The commonest sources cited are the behaviour and experiences of men in battle and those of anxious patients, as already mentioned. In the first instance the prevailing mood reduces pain where it would otherwise be expected to be great. Thus in his famous study, Beecher showed that men wounded on the Anzio beachhead had far less requirement for analgesics than patients undergoing surgery in civilian life. The wounded soldiers were well able to appreciate a pin prick and other stimuli, but their concern with their wounds was not so great as that of the civilians, and hence their demand for relief of pain was less. The wounds which the soldiers had suffered, although obviously disadvantageous, also served to release them with honour from danger. There was no other benefit to the civilians in their surgery, except that it was necessary to restore them, if possible, to normality.

One of the problems with Beecher's study is that the types of trauma might be different in their ability to cause pain. Many of his military patients had wounds from high-speed missiles, and not all lesions that are suddenly produced cause pain. A colleague who broke a leg in a motor car accident related to me that his first feelings were of surprise that he could not stand on it. A boy of eight with a greenstick fracture of the radius brought it to attention because he could not extend his fingers normally. However Beecher (9) has shown that in different types of pathological events in civilians with acute or chronic pain the same degree of relief is produced by equivalent anesthetic agents. This is evidence against the objection just raised to Beecher's argument. He is supported further by a whole range of recurring anecdotal literature.

Beecher's study is not the only one to show how pain may be reduced in accordance with circumstances and expectations. Various placebo maneuvers and supportive and suggestive procedures also relieve pain. Placebos have repeatedly been shown to do this (8) and psychotherapy, psychoprophylaxis in childbirth, hypnosis, behavioural treatments and overt suggestion are regularly associated with reports that pain is lessened. Hypnosis both in this contest and in general is probably a form of suggestion and not any special trance state (5, 41). Egbert et al. (22) showed that demands for postoperative analgesia were halved in patients who had been given suitable preoperative encouragement compared with the control group. Jellinek (32) showed that 52 percent of patients with headache were relieved by placebos.

THE INCIDENCE OF PAIN

The frequency with which pain occurs gives some guide to the importance of factors in its causation. The fact that there are abundant psychiatric patients with pain does not necessarily mean that pain is most often a psychiatric problem. However, we find in surveys of the incidence of pain that it appears to be not only a majority symptom in psychiatric patients but also much associated with psychological illness in patients seen in more general medical practice. Sir Thomas Lewis (35) showed that 75 percent of patients with heart symptoms due to anxiety complained of pain. Interestingly, in the original report by Da Costa (18) on "Irritable Heart" the first patient described is a man who not only had the "Irritable Heart" but also had an aphonia due to supposed catarrhal laryngitis for a period of over eight months. It is plausible to suppose that that was a hysterical aphonia. Friedlander and Freyhoff (28) found precordial pain was a major symptom in 80 percent in their series of cases similar to those of Lewis. In medical clinics pains are common, affecting up to 97 percent of all patients (21). Gomez and Dally (29) found that no less than 84 percent of patients with abdominal pain in medical and surgical clinics were there for psychological reasons.

Devine and Merskey (20) found that 75 percent of those attending a gastrointestinal clinic had pain. Thirty-eight percent of those with pain and 40 percent of the remainder had a psychological disorder without associated evidence of organic disease. Klee et al. (33) showed that 61 percent of patients in a psychiatric outpatient clinic had pain, and Spear (57) observed that the incidence of pain was similarly high in psychiatric outpatients ranging from 53 percent with a spontaneous complaint of pain to 65.6 percent who admitted to pain on questioning at some time during medical/psychiatric observation. In general practice (4) 65 percent of patients with physical illness had pain. Patients with a psychiatric diagnosis, pain and no lesion constituted 17 percent of all those seen, and 59 percent of those with psychiatric diagnoses.

The lowest incidence of pain in a psychiatric series is 38 percent (19) and this refers to inpatients in a psychiatric hospital. In that study also the association of pain was greater with neurotic illness, less relatively with schizophrenia, and least with brain damage and transient situational disturbances. Pain is thus not quite so much associated with the most severe psychiatric illnesses as with intractable chronic personality problems and hysterical disorders, and it has an increased, although not overwhelming, association with anxiety and depression compared with other psychiatric disorders.

PSYCHIATRIC ILLNESS AND PAIN

Psychiatric illness has mainly been studied in relation to chronic pain that is of at least three months' duration. The largest series of psychiatric patients with pain is that of Walters (66) who reported on 430 with intractable pain. Anxiety and depression were the most frequent diagnoses although many had conversion symptoms in one form or another. In his view a hysterical conversion mechanism played a part in producing pain in these patients, but it was neither the sole nor usually the main factor in the origin of the pain. Previous to his work there had been much writing in the literature indicating that pain was related to repressed conflict, and especially resentment and aggression. Over 30 such reports were noted by Merskey and Spear (45), but there was no systematic study either of large numbers or in comparison with patients without pain. Engel (23, 24) had provided a series of cases, many with facial pain, studied in detail.

Merskey (40) reported on 100 patients with persistent pain and detectable physical causes for their illness compared with a control group who had persistent psychological illness and no pain. In that study most of the patients with pain had neurotic illness. A small number had endogenous depression, only two out of 100 had schizophrenia and the larger proportion had signs of anxiety or chronic hysterical traits. Some had well-defined conversion symptoms but a hypochondriacal personality type was more prominent. This pattern overlapped with the personality which had been described by Engel, to some extent, and by other authors. Some noticeable features in this hospital-based series were that the patients tended to be married and yet to be unsuccessful in their marriages, to come from large families, to be engaged in relatively unskilled or semi-skilled work and to seek many additional consultations. They emphasized bodily complaints in general and had an increased history of painful illness in the past. This was summed up by the writer (42) in the following description of the modal psychiatric patient with pain: "A married woman of the working or lower middle class, possibly once pretty and appealing, but never keen on sexual intercourse, now faded and complaining, with a history of repeated negative physical examinations and investigations, frank conversion symptoms in up to 50 percent of cases in addition to the pain and a sad tale of a hard life; together with depression which does not respond to antidepressant drugs." Such a description can only, of course, represent a pattern and that is only one amongst the actual clinical patterns which are to be found.

Similar patterns of findings appear however in the study of Pilling et al. (50) who used the Minnesota Multiphasic Personality Inventory (MMPI) on a series of psychiatric patients with pain as a presenting symptom. Compared with controls these patients had less depression and anxiety but much more hypochondriasis and more evidence of hysterical personality characteristics and a history of conversion symptoms. Some of them had a tendency to seek excessive operations and this trend was demonstrated as statistically significant by Spear (57) in his series.

Many of these last features of pain in association either with hysterical personality or conversion symptoms, intractable complaints persisting despite varied treatments, multiple investigations and repeated operations are parts of the stereotype nowadays of the chronic pain clinic patient, with or without a physical basis for the illness.

Another context in which pain is seen to be associated with hysteria has been elucidated by Guze (30) and his colleagues at St. Louis, Missouri. Ziegler et al. (73) originally reported 134 consecutive patients diagnosed as having conversion symptoms and found that pain was the primary complaint in 75 cases. Purtell et al. (53) in a series of 50 patients with hysteria found pain to be a common symptom (56 percent had back pain, 28 percent joint pains and 62 percent pains in the extremities). In later studies, Guze and his colleagues defined hysteria as a syndrome in which at least 25 symptoms from no less than 10 symptom complexes or systems appeared before the age of 30 (70). Pain was an extremely frequent symptom in this group and virtually never absent.

Epidemiological studies also suggest a link between pain and hysteria. In 1937-8 a Norwegian scientific expedition visited Tristan da Cunha and was able to record an epidemic of hysterical "spells" affecting many persons. In 1961 because of a volcanic eruption the islanders were evacuated to Hampshire in England.

Rawnsley and Loudon (54) noted a high incidence of headache amongst these patients, including headache of psychological origin. The latter was very significantly associated with a history of "spells" in the 1937-8 epidemic and with a marked tendency to seek extra medical consultations. This is significant evidence in support of the view that hysterical mechanisms are likely to be at work in the patients who consult frequently and develop pain for psychological reasons.

Occasional clinical instances show how pain may arise as a result of thought processes. For example, Freud (27) describes a man who was watching his anesthetized brother having an ankylosed hip straightened under an anesthetic. At the moment when the joint was straightened a loud crack was heard and the man felt a pain down the side of his leg. This is not necessarily pain due to a hysterical mechanism but it is hard to see it as anything but pain due to thought processes. The writer (41) has described a youth who had pains in most parts of his body and related them to an idea of a nail or a hammer against the back of his head, or a razor lying against his penis. The youth's view was that the thought of the nail or razor brought on his pain. Pain in any case has traditionally been associated with hysterical symptoms. Sydenham (1697) described the clavus or hysterical nail, i.e., a sensation of a nail giving rise to pain in the head.

There is thus much evidence of a relationship between pain and hysterical conversion symptoms, pain and thoughts and also pain and the hysterical personality. At this point it is worth indicating the distinction between conversion symptoms and the hysterical personality. Conversion symptoms are those which result from an emotional conflict, are not related to bodily disease directly and are ultimately in accordance with the patient's idea of loss of function in a part rather than with anatomy and physiology. If they affect the body they are called conversion symptoms. Comparable symptoms not affecting the body, such as hysterical loss of memory are known as dissociative symptoms. Both conversion and dissociative symptoms can be included under the one term of hysterical symptoms. Hysterical personality is an ancient concept which has been undergoing revision. Chodoff and Lyons (15) showed that hysterical conversion reactions do not occur solely by any means in patients with the characteristics of the hysterical personality. De Alarcon (2), however, from a review of the literature, has argued that it "may be safe to assume that probably all patients with symptoms of hysteria have some features of what we call hysterical personality." The stereotype of the hysterical personality referred to is characterized as showing evidence of histrionic, attention-seeking emotionally labile and manipulative traits, suggestibility and frigidity. De Alarcon (2) demonstrated that in 14 papers, including that of Chodoff and Lyons (15), such characteristics were repeatedly mentioned. Merskey and Trimble (47) have since shown that although conversion symptoms are not confined to patients with hysterical personality (as Ljungberg (36) had very fully demonstrated), they do occur significantly more often in association with the hysterical personality. It seems reasonable to conclude that when pain functions as a hysterical symptom, it is as likely to be associated with hysterical personality as are other conversion symptoms and this certainly reflects clinical experience.

A link between anxiety and depression and pain has been emphasized by other writers. A number of articles in the literature have suggested that pain may arise from these causes. Walters (66) finds it and in some instances so does Merskey (40). Bradley (13) reported a specific study of patients with pain and depression and there is no doubt that there is a subgroup of patients who have pain and depression whose pain recovers once their depression has been treated. One of the unresolved questions is how much pain is due to anxiety and depression in the population at large and how much it is due to hysterical mechanisms. The studies discussed so far have mainly been highly selected ones in patients with chronic pain. It is not unlikely that in a broader section of the population where hysterical mechanisms may be less prominent or less severe but pain no less frequent, anxiety and depression are more often a cause of pain than hysteria. There is no study as yet which tells us the answer on this point. One thing we do know is that not all tension headache is due to tension. Many headaches which are labelled for convenience as tension headache probably depend upon hysterical mechanisms but it is often too difficult to prove the latter point for an individual case and it is more acceptable to patients to phrase it in the former manner.

MASOCHISM

The idea that pain of psychological origin might serve a self-punishing function was developed by Schilder (55) and further expanded by Engel (23, 24) who summarised the work of other psychoanalysts. He stressed the frequency with which some patients sought out unnecessary operations and the fact that they sometimes tolerated pain of physical lesions with gusto. Other suffering, providing an alternative unhappy experience, could lead to the reduction of psychologically induced pain. Engel (23) considered that punitive or abusive parents were very important in the development of chronic pain with psychological causes. Blumer (10) subsequently described a large number of patients who demonstrated many of the same phenomena. No conclusive systematic study of these issues has been conducted except that in a recent investigation Merskey and Boyd (44) have found that amongst patients with pain those with no lesions (and probable psychiatric illness) had significantly more evidence of rejecting fathers, mothers with psychosomatic illness and mothers who were reported as punishing. There were significant trends for the patients with premorbid obsessional symptoms or personality traits or guilt feelings to have fathers lacking in warmth. Such findings need to be compared with those in psychiatric patients

without pain. Meanwhile it remains true that clinical case histories repeatedly seem to support Schilder's idea at least in a
broad sense, even if not in respect of the detailed psychodynamics which he postulated. Some very cogent, albeit extreme,
examples occur in the syndrome of so called "Hospital Addiction"
and are well described in such papers as that by Cramer et al.
(16).

PAIN CLINIC PATIENTS

A descriptive study of characteristics in pain clinic patients with chronic pain has been produced by Pilowsky and
Spence (51). From replies to a questionnaire the latter authors
provided a factor analytic description of 100 chronic patients.
Seven meaningful factors accounting for 63.3 percent of the variance were extracted and labelled as follows: general hypochondriacal factor, disease conviction factor, psychological versus
somatic factor, affective inhibition factor, affective disturbance factor, denial factor and irritability factor. Examining
the significance of these results the authors note that in terms
of the factors described, the patients show little phobic concern
about their pain though they are convinced that they do have some
sort of organic pathology (even where this has not been found)
and are preoccupied with their symptoms. Accordingly, the patients firmly reject any suggestion of their pain as a result of
psychological factors. It is worth remarking that this is not
true for many psychiatric patients with chronic pain who can be
said to show acceptance of the importance of psychological factors in causing their pain (12) although there is, of course a
large population to whom the findings of Pilowsky and Spence
certainly apply. A substantial proportion of the Pilowsky and
Spence patients admit that they have difficulty in expressing
their feelings, especially those of anger, to other people.
This is a tendency which the authors do not find to be common in
patients with psychomatic disorders at large - although the literature might be quoted against that view. Many also describe
themselves as being sad or anxious but presumably they would
explain this as being as a result of their pain.
The foregoing patients represent one end of the spectrum of
all patients with pain: those who are convinced that its presence is due to a physical cause even though none has been found.
This type of patient is typical of those who appear in pain
clinics. The yield from psychiatric treatment of these patients
is sadly poor. So is the yield from most other types of treatment. Fordyce (25, 26) and Sternbach (59) have emphasized the
approach by behavioural measures. There is no report of the successes of psychotherapy in any large number of patients. A few
attempts at treating such patients in groups have begun but there
is as yet no substantial literature on the subject. Reviews of
the effects of hypnosis do not suggest that this is any more val-

uable than other techniques (42). Biofeedback is still an unproven method in comparison with placebo (43). Where relevant
psychiatric illness can be diagnosed for which an adequate treatment is available, for example endogenous depression, the results
are as expected in such illnesses - namely good. Some individual
psychotherapy may work but in the chronic pain clinic patient it
is rarely of any benefit.

Many different treatments were tried simultaneously by Swanson
et al. (63) including a behaviour modification approach together
with group therapy, physical medicine treatments, transcutaneous
stimulation, biofeedback, relaxation techniques and involvement
of family members. Twenty-seven patients out of fifty were improved at the time of discharge. At three to six months follow-
up of 21 patients from the original group, 5 were back at work
and 15 were as well as or better than they had been on discharge.
A sustained 30% improvement rate and a 10% short term employment
rate is about as good as can be hoped for in this population but
is hardly attractive.

The main psychiatric function of pain clinics for such individuals is to reduce unreasonable expectations and to take many of
them off the plethora of conflicting drugs which they often
consume. Psychotherapy successes have occasionally been reported
and biofeedback is perhaps useful for chronic headache, although
still unproven as compared with relaxation or placebo. Cognitive
therapy and family therapy may be more appropriate techniques to
employ.

EFFECTS OF CHRONIC PAIN

Although it is obvious that pain from physical causes might
produce emotional change this consideration has been neglected in
the psychiatric and general literature on pain and is at the moment under some discussion. Weir Mitchell (48) described emotional changes in men suffering from painful nerve injuries. Of
one man he wrote "From being a man of gay and kindly temper,
known in his company as a good natured jester, he became morose
and melancholy and complained that reading gave him vertigo, and
that his memory of recent events was bad." Against this point of
view is the attitude that particular illnesses are due to the
basic personality of the individual. Wolff (67) reviewed the
literature on rheumatoid personality and concluded that the concept appeared to be unwarranted. Some common personality characteristics did appear such as neurotic response patterns, depression with over-concern with bodily functions, rigidity, dependency, emotional instability, low ego strength and feelings of
guilt. But these were not specific to rheumatoid arthritis,
could be observed in some other disease groups and are absent in
patients who have newly developed rheumatoid arthritis (Crown and
Crown (17)). The latter were not found to be particularly neurotic (17). Sternbach and Timmermans (60) have also produced evidence that the relief of chronic pain results in some ameliora-

tion of personality change. Woodforde and Merskey (69) found
that patients with pain of physical origin were actually more
anxious, more depressed and more subject to signs of neuroticism
than a comparison group of patients whose pain had no physical
cause and who were known to have psychiatric illness. The patients with physical illness had high L scores on the Eysenck
Personality Inventory. A rise in this scale has been shown by
others dealing with the physically ill including those in pain
(Morgenstern (49, 11), Jamison et al. (31)). Merskey and Boyd
(44), have further obtained evidence that, in a group of patients
similar to those reported by Woodforde and Merskey, there were
more indices of emotional disturbance and unfortunate childhood
experiences in those with pain and without organic lesions compared with those who did have both pain and an organic lesion.
We may interpret the results variously, but one plausible view is
that some physically ill patients saw themselves, correctly, as
having been persons who were well adjusted and emotionally
stable. Individuals who are aware of damage to their personalities and know that they have become subject to increasing anxiety
and depression may see the changes, not unreasonably, as due to
the chronic pain which they are suffering. Pilowsky and Spence
(51) do not appear to favour this view. They found, in the study
of illness behaviour in patients with chronic pain in a pain clinic, that the chronicity of the pain and the presence of organic
illness were not correlated with the particular personality
change. Rather the behaviour of the individual was in their view
related to pre-existing personality factors. The writer's preferences are for the simple view that chronic pain with physical
causes is a substantial factor in altering emotions and mood but
more evidence is needed on the subject. This does not mean that
Pilowsky and Spence are wholly wrong. Our own findings that patients who have psychological causes for pain have additional
indications of premorbid disturbance support part of their argument. However, both factors of premorbid personality and organic
lesion must be relevant and their significance will vary according to the different samples of patients studied. In the context of clear physical lesions, the balance of such evidence as
exists indicates that previously normal individuals do sustain
emotional and personality changes.

  Biological evidence of pain as a cause for irritability and
resentment can also be found. Ulrich et al. (64, 65) showed that
aggression frequently occurs in response to trauma. Rats given
electric shocks turn and bite their neighbours. Such aggression
is part of a fight or flight mechanism. We are accustomed to
think of pain as first and foremost intended to promote rest and
biological recuperation. But if pain occurs as a result of aggression against the individual, its significance may be to rouse
the affected organism to a suitable response. We might expect
that visceral pain would demand rest but that cutaneous pain
should in the first instance call for arousal and either active
fighting back or escape. If pain is experienced chronically and

referred to the skin it may well be the case that it causes chronic irritability and hostile arousal.

SOCIO-CULTURAL FACTORS AND PAIN

There are many reports about differences in individuals in response to noxious stimulation. Some of the characteristics which influence individual response are held to include work, sex and ethnic factors. All these, of course, play a part in determining personality responses and the willingness to feel pain from a given quantum of damaging stimulation. The literature was reviewed in 1968 by Wolff and Langley (68) and also by Merskey and Spear (45) and by Sternbach (58). Much of the experimental evidence is conflicting but certain findings emerge. We are dealing here not with actual complaints of pain but with the response to applied stimuli. So far as the evidence goes, it has been shown that workers in manual occupations tend to be less liable to complain of pain from a given amount of stimulation than do office workers (56). A number of differences between racial groups in respect to thresholds have been described but none of them has adequate consistent support (68). However, the report by Woodrow et al. (70) provides a massive investigation using a pressure test on the heel. This was undertaken with 41,119 patients who took an automated multi-phasic screening examination under the Kaiser Foundation Health Plan. Subjects were encouraged to tolerate the noxious stimulus as long as possible and a pain tolerance figure determined. The results showed very clearly that tolerance with this test decreased with age, men tolerated more pain than women, whites tolerated more pain than orientals and blacks occupied an intermediate position. Comparing their results with earlier work, the authors concluded that with increasing age tolerance to cutaneous noxious stimulation causing deep pain decreases. This finding is in harmony with the view just advanced that cutaneous pain causes more aggressive arousal than visceral pain since vigorous responses to aggression also diminish with age, whilst it is possible that in the age-range involved threats to health or life associated with deep pain may be more alarming than in the young. Socio-economic variables did not affect the results with their test.

Perhaps the most interesting studies are those which have taken up the hypothesis of Zborowski. This author found that major cultural differences determined attitudes toward pain (72). The author studied spontaneous pain qualitatively in 103 subjects (87 hospitalized patients and 16 of their healthy relatives or friends), but made his main comparisons between 26 "old Americans" i.e., white Anglo-Saxon Protestants, and 24 Italians and 31 Jews. He found that the hospital staff tended to uphold the "old American" tradition in which pain is reported and emotional responses are discouraged. The hospital staff members stated that Italians and Jews tended to overreact to pain, to be emotional about pain, and to complain excessively. Zborowski found that Italians sought immediate relief of pain whereas Jews also sought relief of pain but were skeptical or suspicious of the future and kept on complaining even after their pain had diminished. He concluded that Italians are present-oriented and demonstrate apprehension appropriately in the presence of pain. Jews are future-oriented and therefore present future-oriented anxiety when they are in pain. "Old Americans" resemble the Jews in being future-oriented but were more optimistic. They tended to withdraw socially while the Jews and Italians sought the social company of their relatives. Zborowski made the important points that similar reactions to pain (or as we would prefer to say noxious stimulation) by members of different ethnic or cultural groups do not necessarily reflect the same attitudes to pain, and the patterns of response may have different functions in various cultures.

Lambert, Libman and Poser (34), and Poser (52), were able to demonstrate that the responses in Roman Catholic and Jewish groups varied according to the apparent identity of the experimenter and the instructions given. Roman Catholic subjects produced similar responses to Jewish students when both had a Roman Catholic experimenter testing them. A Jewish experimenter only produced a significant change in the Jewish students, who then complained of pain sooner than under the other condition. It seems reasonable to suppose that cultural factors in terms of attitudinal variables, not only influenced behaviour but probably exerted a concommitant influence on pain perception. Cultural responses predispose an individual to evaluate some particular experience highly or less highly and it is also likely that he or she will have a somewhat altered subjective state. The well-known work of Bruner and Goodman (14), on the judgment of size is a fair indication of the way in which emotion colours responses, not only in regard to pain. Other work by Sternbach and Tursky (61), supports the conclusion that attitudinal differences account for psycho-physical and autonomic differences. These authors studied pain and skin potential responses to electric shock in 60 housewives. Some of them were Yankees, i.e., "old Americans" or Protestants of British descent, others were Irish or Italian Roman Catholics and still others orthodox or conservative Jews. The Yankees had the highest mean scores for acceptance of applied noxious stimuli, followed by Jews and then the Irish, with the Italians producing the lowest mean scores. There were no significant differences between the groups in stimulus magnitude estimation. The Yankees produced a significantly more rapid and greater decrease in skin potential than the other three groups. The Jewish housewives, being future-oriented, were not dismayed by the experimental pain and thus tended to resemble the Yankee and Irish groups whose attitudes towards pain were matter of fact.

The inherent problem in all of these studies is that the estimate of pain ultimately is a subjective one. It is not possible readily to compare one person's subjective estimate with another person's. The solution has been to utilise group differences to demonstrate the importance of culture and attitudes.

THE DESCRIPTION AND DEFINITION OF PAIN

It may seem surprising to turn now to the question of the definition of pain. But it is easier to consider the matter in the light of the data which we have been discussing than in the abstract and without an appreciation of the substantial impact of psychological factors on the production of pain. It should be clear enough at this point that many patients have pain for purely psychological reasons and that this is a common phenomenon. In clinical practice - and perhaps in the personal experience of the reader - it is often hard to tell from the description of the subjective experiences which we call pain whether or not the pain has a physical cause or a psychological one or both. The words patients use to describe pain are frequently identical (19, 46) whatever its cause, and although different words may be used for different types of pain all the words employed imply some physical change in the body. This is evident to anyone who consults the McGill Pain Questionnaire (38, 37). It is true that some distinctions can be made between groups of patients. Thus Agnew and Merskey (1), showed that sensory-thermal words such as burning, were more often used by patients with neurological lesions than by patients with pain and no lesions. Boyd and Merskey (12), found in psychiatric patients that throbbing pains tended to have a psychological cause whilst dull or aching pains tended to have physical causes. Sensory categories were the most common even amongst psychiatric patients (7) and this group tended to avoid evaluative words.

In an extension of the study with Agnew (1) by Merskey and Boyd (44), it was found that aching, aching plus stabbing pains, or aching plus throbbing pains were most often organic in origin, whilst throbbing or throbbing plus aching pains were predominant with patients with organic lesions. However there is considerable overlap and all groups of patients with pain share the view that it has physical characteristics. In fact, they routinely tend to describe it in terms of some disturbance to the tissues of the body and as something unpleasant.

Physicians find it hard to accept however, that pain can occur without relevant peripheral changes. Pain as a consequence of thought processes is a particularly difficult notion to accommodate. Perhaps this is because we believe we know a great deal about the physical mechanisms which promote pain both normally and when there is some pathological disturbance. We tend to think of pain as a change occurring in nerves and nerve pathways.

After the foregoing discussion, it should be evident nevertheless, that pain cannot be equated with mechanisms of the nervous system. Even if no patient ever had pain for Psychological reasons it would remain true that pain is a subjective experience. For this reason, it has to be defined in terms of psychology and not of physiology. If we do this consistently a plethora of problems melts away. For example, we do not have to give a physical explanation for pain when no physical cause is acceptable. If it is not conceptualized as a set of nervous impulses but rather as

a patient's experience, we do not have to call the patient a
liar if he has pain with no physical cause. If it is a psychological phenomenon, we can accept it as having psychological
causes. This does not mean that there are no physical correlates
to pain. It means instead that all pain has physical correlates
but sometimes they are brain events related to thoughts, sometimes they are pathophysiological brain discharges (as in central
pain) and sometimes they are brain events related to peripheral
changes.

We can still readily accept that the operational use of the
word pain is learned as a result of daily physical experiences.
As children we suffer knocks, bruises or other injuries and are
asked "Did it hurt? Is there a pain?" If we complain about the
injuries we are told that we are in pain. Thus we learn the use
of the word to describe unpleasant events located in the body and
characteristically of the type which are related to trauma.

To take account of these considerations the following definition of pain was drafted, "an unpleasant experience which we
primarily associate with tissue damage or describe in terms of
such damage or both", (39, 46).

I believe that it reconciles the somatic difficulties which
have bedevilled both the clinical treatment of patients and the
experimental investigation of the causes of pain. It further
excludes us from calling behaviour pain, or talking of reactions
as pain, but it allows us to consider all pain in terms of its
causes. Philosophically, this is a monistic solution.

REFERENCES

1. Agnew, D.C., and Merskey, H. (1976): Pain, 2:73-81.
2. Alarcon, R. De (1973): Psychiatr. Q., 47:258-275.
3. Aristotle. De Anima. (1931): Book II, chap. 2; Book III,
      chap. 1. (Trans. Smith, J.A. Ed. Ross, W.D.). Oxford:
      Clarendon Press.
4. Baker, J.W., and Merskey, H. (1967): J. Psychosom. Res.,
      10:383-387.
5. Barber, T.X. (1959): Psychol. Bull., 56:430-460.
6. Barber, T.X. (1969): Hypnosis: A Scientific Approach.
      Van Nostrand, New York.
7. Beecher, H.K. (1956): J. Amer. Med. Ass., 161:1609-1613.
8. Beecher, H.K. (1959): Measurement of Subjective Responses.
      Quantitative Effects of Drugs. New York: Oxford
      University Press.
9. Beecher, H.K. (1959): Science, 130:267-268.
10. Blumer, D. (1975): 'The Spine'. Vol. 2. Ed. Rothman,
      R.H., and Simeone, F.A. W.B. Saunders Co. Philadelphia.
11. Bond, M.R. (1971): Br. J. Psychiat., 119:671-678.
12. Boyd, D.B., and Merskey, H. (1978): Pain. (in press).
13. Bradley, J.J. (1963): Br. J. Psychiat., 109:741-745.
14. Bruner, J.S., and Goodman, C.C. (1974): J. Abnorm. Soc.
      Psychol., 13:33-44.

15. Chodoff, P., and Lyons, H. (1958): Amer. J. Psychiat., 114:734-740.
16. Cramer, B., Gershberg, M., and Stern, M. (1971): Arch. Gen. Psychiat., 24:573-578.
17. Crown, S., and Crown, J. (1973): J. Psychosom. Res., 17:189-196.
18. Da Costa, J.M. (1871): Amer. J. Med. Sci., 61:17-52.
19. Delaplaine, R., Ifabumuyi, O.I., Merskey, H., and Zarfas, J. (1977): Pain, 4:361-366.
20. Devine, R., and Merskey, H. (1965): J. Psychosom. Res., 9:311-316.
21. Douglas-Wilson, I. (1944): Brit. Med. J., 1:413-415.
22. Egbert, L.D., Battit, G.E., Welch, C.E., and Bartlett, M.K. (1964): New Engl. J. Med., 270:825-827.
23. Engel, G.L. (1951): Psychosom. Med., 13:375-396.
24. Engel, G.L. (1959): Amer. J. Med., 26:899-918.
25. Fordyce, W.E. (1974): Advances in Neurology. Ed. Bonica, J.J., Raven Press, New York. 4:415-422.
26. Fordyce, W.E., Fowler, R.S., Jr., Lehmann, J.F., De Lateur, B.J. (1968): J. Chron. Dis., 21:179-190.
27. Freud, S. (1893-1895): Studies in Hysteria. Complete Psychological Works. Standard ed., Vol. 2. London: Hogarth Press, 1955.
28. Friedlander, A., and Freyhoff, W.L. (1918): Arch. Intern. Med., 22:693-718.
29. Gomez, J., and Dally, P. (1977): Brit. Med. J., 1:1451-1453.
30. Guze, S.B. Seminars in Psychiatr., 2:392-402.
31. Jamison, K., Ferrer-Brechner, M.T., Brechner, V.L., and McCreary, C.P. (1976): Advances in Pain Res. and Therapy, Ed. Bonica, J.J. and Albe-Fessard, D. Raven Press, New York, 1:317-321.
32. Jellinek, E.M. (1946): Biomet. Bull., 2:87-91. Cit. Beecher, 1959.
33. Klee, G.D., Ozelis, S., Greenberg, I., and Gallant, L.J. (1959): Maryland State Med. J., 8:188-191.
34. Lambert, J.P., Libman, E., and Poser, E.G. (1960): J. Personal., 38:350-357.
35. Lewis, T. (1917): Report Upon Soldiers Returned as Cases of 'Disordered Action of the Heart' (D.A.H.) or 'Valvular Disease of the Heart' (V.D.H.). M.R.C. special report series No.8, London, H.M.S.O.
36. Ljungberg, L. (1957): Acta Psychiat. Scand., Suppl. 112.
37. Melzack, R. (1975): Pain, 1:277-299.
38. Melzack, R., and Torgerson, W.S. (1971): Anesthesiology, 34:50-59.
39. Merskey, H. (1964): An Investigation of Pain in Psychological Illness. D.M. Thesis, Oxford.
40. Merskey, H. (1965 b): J. Psychosom. Res., 9:291-298.
41. Merskey, H. (1968): Postgrad. Med. J., 44:297-306.
42. Merskey, H. (1971): Postgrad. Med. J., 47:572-580.

43. Merskey, H. (1977): Persistent Pain. Modern Methods of
     Treatment. Vol. I. Grune and Stratton, New York.
     Lipton, S., Academic Press, London.
44. Merskey, H., and Boyd, D.B. (1978): Pain (in press).
45. Merskey, H., and Spear, F.G. (1967): 'Pain: Psychological
     and Psychiatric Aspects'. Bailliere, Tindall and
     Cassell, London.
46. Merskey, H., and Spear, F.G. (1967): J. Psychosom. Res.
     11:59-67.
47. Merskey, H., and Trimble, M. (1978): Amer. J. Psychiat.
     (in press).
48. Mitchell, S.W. (1872): Injuries of Nerves and Their
     Consequences. Dover, New York, 1965.
49. Morgenstern, F.S. (1967): Chronic Pain. M.D. Thesis,
     Oxford.
50. Pilling, L.F., Brannick, T.L., and Swenson, W.M. (1967):
     Canad. Med. Ass. J., 97:387-394.
51. Pilowsky, I., and Spence, N.D. (1976): Pain, 2:61-71.
52. Poser, E.G. (1963): XVth. Internat. Congr. Psychol.,
     Wash., D.C.
53. Purtell, J.J., Robins, E., and Cohen, M.E. (1951): J.
     Amer. Med. Ass., 146:902-909.
54. Rawnsley, K., and Loudon, J.B. (1964): Brit. J. Psychiat.,
     110:830-839.
55. Schilder, P. (1931): Psychoanal. Rev., 18:1-22.
56. Sherman, E.D. (1943): Canad. Med. Ass. J., 48:437-441.
57. Spear, F.G. (1967): J. Psychosom. Res., 11:187-193.
58. Sternbach, R.A. (1968): 'Pain. A Psychophysiological
     Analysis'. Academic Press, New York.
59. Sternbach, R.A. (1974): Pain Patients. Traits and Treat-
     ment. Academic Press, New York.
60. Sternbach, R.A., and Timmermans, G. (1975): Pain, 1:177-
     181.
61. Sternbach, R.A., and Tursky, B. (1965): Psychophysiology,
     1:241-146.
62. Sydenham, T. (1697): Discourse Concerning Hysterical and
     Hypochondriacal Distempers. IN: Dr. Sydenham's Complete
     Method of Curing Almost All Diseases, and Description of
     Their Symptoms. To which are now added five discourses
     of the same author concerning the Pleurisy, Gout, Hysteri-
     cal Passion, Dropsy, and Rheumatism. 3rd. ed., Newman
     and Rich Parker, London, p.149.
63. Swanson, D.W., Floreen, A.C., and Swenson, W.M. (1976):
     Mayo Clin. Proc., 51:409-411.
64. Ulrich, R.E. (1966): Amer. Zoologist, 6:643-662.
65. Ulrich, R.E., Hutchinson, R.P., and Azrin, N.H. (1965):
     Psychol. Rec., 15:111-126.
66. Walters, A. (1961): Brain, 84:1-18.
67. Wolff, B.B. (1971): Bull. Rheum. Dis., 22:656-661.
68. Wolff, B.B., and Langley, F. (1968): Amer. Anthropol.,
     70:494-501.

69. Woodforde, J.M., and Merskey, H. (1972): <u>J. Psychosom. Res.</u> 16:167-172.
70. Woodrow, K.M., Friedman, G.D., Siegelaub, A.B., and Collen, M.F. (1967): <u>Psychosom. Med.</u>, 34:548-556.
71. Woodruff, R.A. (1968): <u>Brit. J. Psychiat.</u>, 114:1115-1119.
72. Zborowski, M. (1952): <u>J. Soc. Issues</u>, 8:16-30. Cit. Wolff and Langley, 1978.
73. Zeigler, F.J., Imboden, J.B., and Meyer, E. (1960): <u>Amer. J. Psychiat.</u>, 116:901-909.

The Psychology of Pain, edited by R. A. Sternbach.
Raven Press, New York © 1978.

Behavioural Measurement of Human Pain

B. Berthold Wolff

Pain Study Group, New York University Medical Center,
New York, New York 10016

INTRODUCTION

The measurement of pain has intrigued clinicians and researchers for centuries, but satisfactory quantification has as yet not
been entirely achieved. Major stumbling blocks are the lack both
of a generally accepted definition of pain (7;68;76) and of knowledge concerning the nature of the adequate stimulus for pain
(5;42;45). The latter problem has in recent years become less
of an enigma due to the development of sophisticated neurophysiological pain theories (79;90), associated with the realization
that the triggering mechanism for pain is dependent not upon some
static condition of the organism but upon a dynamic, ever-changing
state, continually influenced by a multitude of intrinsic and external stimuli impinging upon the organism. Therefore, it now
appears that the adequate (behavioural) stimulus for pain does not
have some kind of absolute or fixed value. In contrast, the problem of defining pain is still with us. While in recent years some
investigators have attempted to define pain (83;105), such definitions still lack general acceptance and applicability. Melzack
(76) points out that pain falls within the unique multidimensional
space of an individual and this implicitly makes a general definition difficult. Therefore, in discussing pain measurement the
obvious fact must be emphasized that it is not easy to measure
something if one is not sure what one is actually measuring. Fortunately, the use of operational definitions of pain has to some
extent permitted us to escape this dilemma, provided that it is
fully understood that such definitions are not all-encompassing

and generalizations are risky and not necessarily appropriate and require validation.

Pain measurement probably started with the classical experiments of Blix (9) in 1882 and Goldscheider (39) in 1884, who independently demonstrated the existence of specific pain spots in the skin, and thus permitted pain to be treated as a sensory modality. Schiff (99) in 1858 and Funke (37) in 1879, had previously suggested the existence of specific pain fibers, but the work of Blix and Goldscheider formalized the concept of pain as a specific sensory modality with its own receptors and nerve fibers. Actual psychophysical pain studies commenced with the laboratory pain-induction work of von Frey (131). While considerable anatomical, neurophysiological and surgical studies on pain were conducted during the end of the Nineteenth and beginning of the Twentieth centuries, relatively few psychophysical studies of human pain were published. It was not until the systematic investigations of pain by Hardy, Wolff and Goodell (41;42) at Cornell Medical College during the second quarter of this century that the era of modern pain measurement began. These investigators developed radiant heat stimulation into a psychophysical technique and studied the reactions to this heat stimulation under many diverse conditions.

Hardy, Wolff and Goodell (42, p.54) listed eight requirements for the laboratory measurement of human pain, as follows: ". . .

a) The measurable aspect of the stimulus should be closely associated with changes causing pain, i.e. with noxious stimulation.

b) The stimulus should be one for which, under the same conditions, reproducible quantitative measurements of the pain threshold are obtained.

c) The intensity of the stimulus should be controllable and measurable to a degree higher than the difference between two stimuli which evoke a just noticeable difference in pain sensation.

d) The stimulus should be one for which the ability of the subject to discriminate differences in pain intensity can be ascertained throughout the effective range of the stimulus, i.e. from threshold to "ceiling" pain.

e) The stimulus should cause minimal tissue damage at pain threshold and should be a minor hazard to the subject even at highest intensities.

f) The stimulus should be capable of evoking separately one of the qualities of pain--burning, pricking, aching.

g) The stimulus should be one which can be conveniently applied.

h) The stimulus should be one for which the perception and

identification of pain is clear cut, whether or not other sensations are evoked prior to, concomitant with or following the
pain.

We agree with six of these eight requirements, but differ with
item e and question item f. It is recommended that the stimulus,
even at levels well above threshold pain, should produce no or
only minimal tissue damage. Early pain experiments often involved a considerable amount of tissue damage (95), but such
laboratory procedures are no longer acceptable on ethical grounds.
Furthermore, it is now believed that tissue damage or injury is
not a sine qua non for pain. In regard to item f, it is not certain
just how many major types or "qualities" of pain exist and "burning, pricking and aching" may not be correct. There is evidence,
based on earlier work of Jarvik and Wolff (57) in our laboratory,
that there are two major types of pain--localized, sharp, well-
defined pain or diffuse, dull ache. In this context it is of interest to mention that noxious electrical stimulation is perhaps the
most widely used laboratory pain-induction technique. Yet the
electrically evoked response is one of discomfort rather than of
pain. Thus, it serves no useful purpose to limit the induced
sensations to three.

Beecher (7, p.14), in his discussion of the "ideal" method,
added four other requirements to those of Hardy et al, namely
". . .(i) The possibility of carrying our several to many repetitions of the stimulation even above the pain threshold value without interfering with subsequent determinations; (ii) Sensitivity so
that agents of low analgesic power can be detected; (iii) Differentiation among graded doses of analgesics through their power to
alter the effects of a standard pain stimulus; and (iv) Applicability
both to man and animals. . ."

The first of Beecher's additional requirements is very important
for systematic psychophysical studies. The statistical reliability
of a method depends on its repeatability. Furthermore, in psychophysical studies it is always advisable to make a series of
measurements and then calculate an average score in order to reduce variability. This requirement should apply equally well at
stimulus levels well above threshold pain as many modern methods
measure several such supra-threshold parameters, e.g. pain
tolerance.

Beecher's second and third points are desirable for their practical value. However, the third is based on a rather simplistic
assumption that the more potent the medication the greater the
relief of pain. This is not necessarily so. Beecher, of course,
was profoundly interested in human analgesic assays, and his
addition of these two requirements is thus not surprising. The

last of Beecher's requirements, namely applicability to both man and animals, is conceptually unnecessary.

Hardy, Wolff and Goodell at Cornell and Beecher at Harvard have played significant roles in the field of human pain measurement during the Mid-Century. Unfortunately, they were rivals and engaged in occasionally bitter controversy (3;43). Beecher is regarded as the Father of modern quantitative human analgesic assays with clinical pain. For many years, Beecher bitterly attacked and criticized the use of experimental pain, which he called "artificially contrived" (5). Beecher's attacks on experimental pain greatly hindered the progress of systematic laboratory pain studies during the Mid-Century as he was in an eminent scientific position and many investigators were influenced by him and refrained from pursuing such experimental projects. In turn, this tended to diminish the value researchers attached to the work of Hardy, Wolff and Goodell. It was, therefore, with considerable surprise that we heard Beecher (102) state in 1965 at the Twenty-Seventh Annual Meeting of the Committee of Drug Addiction and Narcotics (now the Committee on Problems of Drug Dependence) that he had changed his mind about experimental pain and that some techniques involving supra-threshold pain, such as the submaximum effort tourniquet pain method, may, after all, be of value. Consequently, from that time on it once again became "respectable" to study pain experimentally in man.

In recent years, there has been increased activity and interest in human pain research, utilizing both clinical and experimental pain. Many scientists have turned to experimental pain-induction methods to help them in their search for a better understanding of human pain and its control. Unfortunately, some have not been thoroughly versed in the rigorous requirements of good psychophysics and the complexity of human pain studies and, consequently, their results are often difficult to interpret and their conclusions have occasionally muddied rather than clarified the waters of our knowledge. Nevertheless, considerable progress has been made and we have now reached the point at which several pain response parameters have been identified and related to clinical pain phenomena. Such parameters can also evaluate the efficacy of various analgesic drugs and other pain-relieving therapeutic modalities.

HUMAN PAIN REACTIONS

Human pain behaviour may be categorized into voluntary and involuntary responses. All voluntary responses require consciousness and motor activity, whether verbal or non-verbal, and are under the individual's direct control. So-called "involuntary" exclamations, such as "Ouch, it hurts!" belong in this category. Involuntary responses are those not normally under direct conscious control of the individual, such as reflex reactions and autonomic nervous system activity, and are essentially nonverbal. However, such behaviour may under certain circumstances be learned and come under conscious control, such as in biofeedback.

Involuntary Evoked Responses

The search for objective and valid indices of human pain, especially in the hands of the experimental scientist, has frequently focused on involuntary, non-verbal evoked responses. These have usually centered on autonomic nervous system (ANS) reactions, such as heart rate, respiration rate, galvanic skin

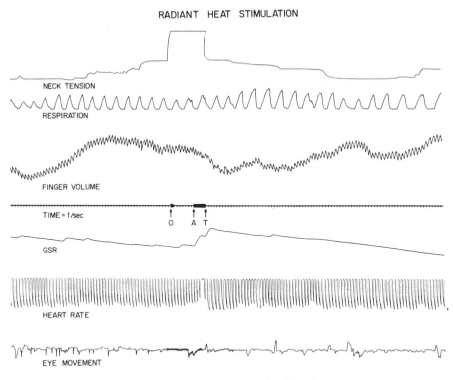

FIG. 1. 6-Channel polygraph record of ANS responses to radiant heat stimulation. 0= Onset of heat stimulation; A= Pain Threshold; T= Pain Tolerance.

reflex (GSR), muscle tension, etc. More recently, the development of computers has permitted the study of cortically evoked responses (CER). In the hands of a skilled technician it is relatively easy to demonstrate some kind of ANS response and/or CER to noxious stimuli. In the early days of our pain research, we used a 6-channel polygraph to record several types of ANS reactions to noxious stimulation. Fig. 1 shows a graph of radiant heat stimulation. It will be seen that there is a marked increase in heart rate, shallower respiration and significant GSR activity during the actual pain range. Ocular motion and digital plethysmography (finger volume) is less noticeable. Neck muscle tension (electromyography) changed throughout the stimulation period, whether below or during pain. It should also be noted that there tends to be a slight latency in response for most of these ANS parameters. However, as the noxious stimuli are repeatedly presented, one will find that gradually the ANS reactivity fades and eventually no response is obtained. Adaptation to stimulation has occurred. Furthermore, if by chance some extraneous stimulus, such as a sudden loud noise, should occur, one will again obtain an ANS response independently of the experimental stimulation. Therefore, it soon becomes apparent that these evoked ANS responses are non-specific and indicative of arousal rather than of pain. Consequently, ANS modalities are not suitable for human psychophysical pain measurement procedures, which require many repetitions of stimuli. Similarly, the CER does not seem to be pain-specific but more indicative of arousal.

Voluntary Pain Responses

There exists a host of voluntary pain responses under direct conscious control of the individual. In clinical pain states, verbal communication (i.e. complaints of pain), moaning, weeping and restlessness are common behaviour patterns. The individual in pain may use an additional variety of non-verbal motor behaviour, such as rubbing the sore site, favouring an injured limb, running to and fro, etc. In the laboratory, under experimental conditions, pain may be signalled by pushing a button, pressing a lever to reduce noxious stimulation, pressing a soft rubber ball connected to a kymograph to indicate degrees of pain, etc. However, similar to involuntary evoked responses, many of these response patterns are non-specific. While easily recognizable within the appropriate external milieu, such as the patient within the hospital, the injured soldier on the battlefield, or the hurt child with a bleeding knee, when taken out of context such behaviour patterns may not be identified as pain responses. The exception would appear to be the verbal report of pain. The statement "I am in pain" or "I hurt" conveys a specific message to the environment. This verbal communication is recognized by the observer as specifically indicative of the presence of pain. Unfortunately, like other verbal statements, it may not be true. We are, therefore, back at the problem of defining pain.

In our Society, the most common expression of pain is by verbal means. Szasz (126) distinguished three levels of symbolization according to a hierarchy of increasing complexity. The first is a signal to the individual that something is wrong--an intrapersonal communication. The second level is interpersonal--a cry for help, while the third is a more complex symbolic communication to others. The socio-cultural group in which we live also influences and modulates our pain behaviour (151;152). Anglo-Saxon influence emphasizes the "stiff upper lip," while Mediterranean cultures believe in freer expression. However, the simple verbal statement of pain is common and acceptable to both.

In clinical pain, the physician's best and most valid index of the presence of pain is the patient's verbal report. On physical examination, the patient may wince when a tender area is palpated, but the verbal description is, nevertheless, the most meaningful. Modern clinical trials of analgesic agents in humans are essentially based on measurement of the patients' "subjective" responses (7) and have yielded satisfactory scientific data. Melzack and Torgerson (78) used a selection of pain-descriptive adjectives categorized into sensory, affective and evaluative groups, to measure pain. This, in turn, led to the development of the McGill Pain Questionnaire (77). In the laboratory, operational definitions permit the use of specified words to indicate levels of pain. However, it is often argued that the verbal response is subject to distortion and manipulation and that non-verbal reactions may be more valid. Thus, interest has been shown in non-verbal responses, such as the visual analogue and graphic rating scales (55;100) for clinical pain, and button-pushing behaviour (44) for experimental pain. While it is correct that verbal responses may be falsified, the same applies to conscious non-verbal behaviour. A malingerer can as easily give false ratings non-verbally as verbally. On the other hand, verbal descriptions of different pain intensities may cause problems in understanding, especially in subjects with a limited education, and non-verbal methods, such as the visual analogue scale, may then be more valid. The point which is important is that in fact so-called "subjective" responses, be they verbal or non-verbal, are the best indices for pain measurement.

PSYCHOPHYSICAL METHODOLOGIES

Psychophysics is the study of stimulus and sensation in its broadest aspects, including sensory physics and psychosensory measurements. Psychophysics deals with the relationship between psychological or sensory quantities on the one hand and physical or stimulus quantities on the other (74). Joseph C. Stevens (109) divides the traditional questions posed by psychophysics into four categories. For a given sensory modality one may ask about ". . .(1) the smallest detectable energy (the measurement of sensitivity); (2) the smallest detectable change in energy (the measurement of resolving power); (3) the configurations of energy that produce an invariant sensory effect, such as a constant loudness or colour (the measurement of static invariances); (4) the way in which the magnitude of sensory effect depends functionally on the stimulus (the measurement of dynamic properties). . ."

In recent years, it has become customary to distinguish between the Classical or Old Psychophysics and the New Psychophysics. Classical Psychophysics focused on the measurement of the stimulus parameters as it held the view that it was meaningless to measure sensation directly. It thus used indirect means to measure sensation. In contrast, the New Psychophysics attempts to measure and quantify magnitudes of sensation directly.

Classical Psychophysics

Attempts to quantify sensation and perception in terms of stimulus parameters began about two centuries ago. However, Weber (133) is usually credited with the first quantitative statement, which ran as follows: "In comparing magnitudes it is not the arithmetical difference, but the ratio of the magnitudes, which we perceive"(150). This may be written mathematically as: $\delta S/S = W$, where S= stimulus intensity; δS= increment in stimulus intensity and W= a constant, sometimes called the Weber Fraction. Fechner (36), some years later, modified Weber's law as he recognized δS to be the Just Noticeable Difference (JND), sometimes called the DL for Difference Limen. Fechner believed that all JNDs were equal in subjective magnitude. He stated that: "The sensation is proportional to the logarithm of the stimulus" or "Equal stimulus ratios produce equal sensation intervals" or "As stimulus intensity increases geometrically, sensation intensity increases arithmetically." Fechner's logarithmic law may be written as:
Sensation= k log Stimulus.

Fechner's law produced much criticism throughout the years. A major objection is made to his assumption that all JNDs are equal in subjective magnitude. To quote James (56): "The many pounds which form the just perceptible addition to a hundredweight feel bigger when added than the few ounces which form the just perceptible addition to a pound." However, in spite of the recognition of flaws in the Weber and Fechner Laws, many psychophysicists still determine JNDs and use them on a practical basis in a variety of different measurement procedures. In particular, several classical psychophysical techniques are still in common use and will be briefly described. The emphasis of classical psychophysics is largely on the measurement of thresholds, both absolute threshold and difference threshold (i.e. JND). In so far that many pain researchers are interested in a pain threshold, some of these classical psychophysical techniques are of importance for pain studies.

Method of Limits

This method is known by several other names, such as the Method of Minimal Change, the Method of Serial Exploration or the Method of Just Noticeable Difference. Its application is for measurement of all thresholds, both absolute and difference, as well as points of subjective equality (PSE). This method is probably the best technique for obtaining thresholds. In order to measure the absolute threshold, the technique essentially consists of presenting ascending and descending series of stimuli to the subject. Ascending series are always started at a stimulus level well below the subject's threshold and then the stimulation is gradually increased until the subject first observes the stimulus. A descending series is commenced well above threshold level and gradually decreased until the subject reports the disappearance of the stimulus. Several each of these ascending and descending series are presented. The threshold may be computed in three different ways. (1) One may simply average (i.e. calculate the arithmetical mean) all ascending and descending thresholds. The standard deviation measures the individual's variability. (2) One may average each pair of successive ascending and descending trials to yield a threshold for each pair and then again average these thresholds. The obtained threshold is the same as before, but the standard deviation is smaller because the variation associated with separate ascending and descending series is reduced. (3) One may average all ascending thresholds to yield the mean ascending threshold and then separately average all descending thresholds to give the mean descending threshold. The final threshold is the average of these mean ascending and mean descending thresholds, and will again be the same as those calculated in the previously described fashion. However, the mean ascending and the mean descending thresholds are likely to be different due to "constant errors," such as set or anchoring effects. In an ascending series errors of habituation (set) are those where the subject tends to give the same reports, thus "over-shooting" the threshold. Errors of anticipation or expectation are the opposite, where the subject tends to expect a change and thus alters his report, i.e. it is premature. The purpose of alternating ascending and descending series is to balance out these errors(33). Fatigue, practice, distraction, reaction time and--for pain--emotional distress (50) may all influence the threshold.

To determine the JND, three instead of two response categories are used. On each trial two stimuli, a standard and a variable (comparison), are presented, and the subject judges if the variable stimulus is larger, equal or smaller than the standard. Ascending and descending series are used as before. Two points are measured in each series. In an ascending series these are the first "equal" and "larger," and in a descending series the first "equal" and "smaller." The upper and lower points are respectively averaged and the difference of the resultant means is called the Interval of Uncertainty, where equal judgements are most frequent. By definition, the JND= 1/2 Interval of Uncertainty. The PSE is defined as the mid-point of the Interval of Uncertainty, but due to "constant errors" it usually differs from the JND. Theoretically, the PSE is the point at which the variable stimulus is most likely to appear equal to the standard stimulus. It is the JND which must be added (or subtracted) to the standard stimulus for discrimination to occur.

There are several modifications of the Method of Limits when subjective or technical problems may interfere with presentation of complete ascending and descending series. Such modifications are particularly important for human pain experimentation. Sometimes, only ascending series of stimulus presentation may be employed, such as with the cold pressor method, which will be described later. The Stair-Case Method (28) is another modification, in which the direction is changed whenever the subject gives a response, i.e. each successive ascending (or descending) series starts at the threshold level of the previous series instead of well above or well below that level. This can save some time.

The standard psychophysical technique used by the New York University Pain Study Group for electrical stimulation (147) involves both the classical Method of Limits for pain threshold estimations and the Stair-Case Method for pain tolerance measures. The reason for this modification is that several response parameters are measured in a single trial (134) and at high stimulus magnitudes it would be both unethical and potentially hazardous to exceed the subject's tolerance levels.

Method of Constant Stimuli

This method is also known as the Frequency Method. It can be used to measure all thresholds, equality, equal intervals and equal ratios. The method is valuable for measuring stimuli which tend to lie in the transition zone between those that can usually be perceived and those that are rarely perceived. It consists essentially of presenting a fixed, constant stimulus and comparing it to several, usually from 5-7, comparison stimuli. These comparisons are selected to fall largely within the transition zone, but both the lowest and highest stimuli should almost always be discriminable by the subject. Usually at least twenty presentations per comparison stimulus are made, e.g. 100 trials for five comparison stimuli. Stimuli are presented randomly but balanced and the order of standard-comparison should also be counter-balanced. Responses are usually categorical, such as "Yes" and "No." There are several variations of this method, the two categories approach being the most common, but three categories, such as "Heavier," "Equal" and "Lighter," or single stimuli without the standard may also be used. A variety of statistical computations may be employed to determine the absolute threshold or JND, as well as the PSE and standard deviations, and the interested reader is referred to a textbook of psychophysics (33) for a detailed discussion of such mathematical calculations. An advantage of the Method of Constant Stimuli over the Method of Limits is that blank stimuli may be used.

This psychophysical technique is particularly useful for responses which are not easily measurable, but where the stimuli can be scaled. The obtained scores are the frequencies with which the subject applies the response categories to each comparison stimulus.

Method of Adjustment

This procedure is also known as the Method of Average Error or the Equation Method. Most commonly, this technique is used for measurement of the PSE. The subject manipulates a continuously variable comparison stimulus until it is equal to the standard stimulus. This procedure is repeated many times. It is a simple method and tends to have appeal for the subject as he himself is the manipulator. However, it is not applicable for stimulus modalities with discrete steps or intervals rather than a continuum.

New Psychophysics

The underlying view of the New Psychophysics is that one can make quantitative estimations of the magnitudes of one's sensory experiences. This is in contrast to Classical Psychophysics where the measurement of sensory magnitude is obtained indirectly by measuring some other variables or functions, such as stimulus intensities. The classical approach is often termed "indirect scaling." On the other hand, "direct scaling" procedures of sensory magnitudes are the basis of the New Psychophysics. While attempts at direct scaling involving ratios date to the late Nineteenth Century (80), a historical experiment in this area was published in 1930 by Richardson and Ross (96), involving estimation of loudness with respect to a standard tone. These investigators concluded that estimated loudness grows as a power function of sound pressure. This and other studies eventually led to S.S. Stevens' (115) statement of the Psychophysical Power Law and to the development of the Method of Magnitude Estimation (113;114). Stevens' Power Law (118) may be stated as follows: Equal stimulus ratios produce equal sensation ratios, i.e. $\Psi = k \, \Phi^\beta$, where Ψ represents the estimated psychological magnitude, Φ is the stimulus intensity, k is a constant, and β is the exponent.

Much work and many experiments have been done by Stevens (115;117;118;119;120) and other psychophysicists in checking the Power Law and to test its generality. It has been demonstrated that the Power Law appears to hold remarkably well for many different sensory modalities, such as loudness (110), taste (31), brightness (75) and weight lifting (32). Another approach which has been used extensively for validation and verification of the psychophysical power function is cross-modality matching (111; 112;116). This method involves the adjustment of stimuli along one sensory modality in order to match those along another sensory dimension, such as loudness versus brightness.

It would seem that while the psychophysical power law holds in general for most sensory modalities along most of the perceptual range, it may not be appropriate at low sensory levels at about the absolute threshold (108) deviating from linearity when plotted on log-log coordinates. It is also possible that the power law may not hold at high levels of sensory magnitude within the highly aversive and painful (i.e. pain tolerance) levels (121). Consequently, Stevens (118) has proposed a modification to correct for the absolute threshold, namely $\Psi = k (\Phi - \Phi_0)^n$, where Φ_0 is the stimulus intensity at absolute threshold. It is not within the scope of this Chapter to discuss in detail the many psychophysical studies focused on an evaluation of the power law, but the interested reader is referred to appropriate texts (e.g. 12;74).

The great importance of Stevens' Power Law in the field of pain is that nearly all psychophysical techniques for measuring clinical pain are based on methodologies derived from it, such as magnitude estimation and cross-modality matching.

Method of Magnitude Estimation

There are two forms of this method. The first presents a standard stimulus to the subject and defines the subjective value of that standard, say as "10." The subject then has to judge other variable stimuli in relation to the standard. A problem with this first form is that both the selection of the standard and the limitations of a "fixed" standard value may impose distortions in sensory judgements by introducing bias. The second and now more commonly used form is not to present a standard stimulus but to let the subject simply assign any value he wishes to the first variable stimulus and then judge all other variable stimuli in relation to the first. This reduces some of the bias. There are several ways of analyzing the data and plotting the power function, as described by Engen (34).

Cross-Modality Matching

This technique is perhaps more aptly termed a procedure rather than a formal psychophysical method. It essentially consists of having the subject match several standard stimuli along one sensory modality, e.g. brightness, by adjusting the value on a second sensory modality, e.g. loudness. The classical psychophysical Method of Adjustment can in fact be used for this purpose. The results of such cross-matching should demonstrate a linear equal sensation function when plotted along log-log coordinates with an exponent equal to the ratio of the exponents of the psychophysical functions for the two sensory modalities. The slope differs for the different sensory modalities.

Sensory Decision Theory

Sensory Decision Theory (SDT) or Signal Detection Theory is one of the three major spheres of psychophysics and the most recent. It was formally publicized by Swets et al (122;123;125) in

1961 with more recent reviews and discussions of the theory by
Green and Swets (40) and Swets (124). However, Swets credits
Peterson, Birdsall and Fox (93) and Van Meter and Middleton (129)
for developing SDT most fully. It started essentially as a technique to detect a weak signal above background noise and was
used in radar. It was then developed for use with humans as it
was realized that much of psychophysics deals with the detection
of signals (stimuli) above background noise (e.g. continuous
neural activity, interference, etc.). SDT makes two assumptions
about the sensory response. The first is that the sensory response that occurs in the presence of a given signal is variable,
the response being influenced by random noise. The second is
that the sensory response is an unidimensional variable. SDT
also separates the subject's bias--the Likelihood-Ratio Criterion
--from the purely sensory aspects of the signal. The relative
operating-characteristic (ROC) curves of subjects are similar to
theoretical curves based on a Gaussian distribution. These
curves can be characterized by a single parameter, termed "d',"
which is the sensory discriminatory function and defined as the
difference between the means of the signal-plus-noise and
noise-alone distributions, divided by the standard deviation of
the noise distribution. The slope of the curve at any point equals
the value of the Likelihood-Ratio Criterion.

Fundamentally, SDT allows the separation of the subject's response bias or criterion for giving a response from the purely
sensory aspects of the stimulus, and thus differs from classical
psychophysics which can only provide a single measure of
threshold, which includes both the sensory and judgemental components of the response. It utilizes a "YES" or "NO" response
dichotomy of signal present or absent, and each response may be
a "hit" or a "miss." An implicit assumption of SDT is that there
exists no absolute sensory threshold and that, therefore, classical psychophysics errs in its attempts to measure such sensory
thresholds.

In view of the theoretical concepts of SDT it has been grouped
separately from "Old" and "New" Psychophysics. However, it
has not replaced "New" Psychophysics or Direct Scaling. In
fact, some contemporary psychophysicists show very little interest in SDT. There is still much controversy among theoretical
orientations in the field of psychophysics and for some SDT plays
a very minor role.

SDT, however, has had important effects on contemporary pain
research. It was introduced to the field of pain in 1969 by Clark
(21). It excited many pain investigators as they believed that
SDT now provided them with a technique for separating the purely

sensory characteristics of the pain response from the individual's attitudinal and judgemental components of the pain response. However, it has also led to considerable confusion as some pain researchers mistakenly consider the response bias to include all kinds of psychological characteristics, such as emotional varia- bles, etc. Furthermore, it has also had a kind of band wagon effect on pain research, and many investigators consider that SDT is the only correct approach to psychophysical pain studies.

This decade has seen an emergence of experimental pain stu- dies in which SDT has been used. A review of the literature (70;98) indicates that nearly all published human studies in this area were chiefly carried out by four groups of investigators, namely Clark et al (22-26) at Columbia; Chapman et al (14-18) at Seattle; Craig et al (29) in Vancouver, and Bloedel et al (10) in Minneapolis. Furthermore, nearly every published experiment used one of two noxious stimulation techniques, either radiant heat (10;15;17;21;23;24;26;35) or electrical stimulation (18;29;44). The noxious stimulation was modulated by a variety of factors, such as drugs (17), placebo (21), age (24;44), suggestion (23), modelling (29), acupuncture (14;26) and (therapeutic) electrical stimulation(10). In addition to the traditional parametric analysis of the data, non-parametric methods have also been used (10;48). These data have been summarized in tables by Lloyd and Appel (70) and Rollman (98). While the results are somewhat confusing, in general, "psychological" modulators tended to change the criterion without altering d', while "physical" modulators, such as drugs and acupuncture tended to change d' alone or together with the criterion.

The enthusiastic reception of SDT into pain research has recent- ly been tempered by a serious critique of Rollman (98) in which he questions if, indeed, SDT is applicable to human pain research. Rollman essentially raises two major issues, involving conceptual and methodological considerations. The latter consist of criticism that SDT pain investigators have not used a sufficient number of stimulus presentations, that the subjects have not been carefully trained, that there are problems in deriving the optimum number of rating categories, and, fourthly, that usually only one pair of stimuli, signal or blank, instead of many variable stimuli are presented. However, Rollman concedes that these methodological deficiencies can be overcome by improved techniques. Much more important is the fundamental criticism that SDT is inappro- priate for high stimulus intensity experiments, such as pain stu- dies, and that d' under such conditions reflects discrimination but not sensory sensitivity. Rollman concluded that SDT mea- sures discrimination but not pain. In a reply, Chapman (13) dismisses much of Rollman's criticisms as irrelevant or based on misunderstanding of SDT. In particular he rebuts the alleged charge that SDT pain researchers are attempting to separate sensory and emotional components of pain. He also rejects the criticism that SDT is inappropriate for high intensity stimulation, citing dental pulp studies in which (non-painful) detection is very close to pain. (The latter is actually a weak answer, as recent research clearly demonstrates the existence of a range of non-painful sensation during electrical tooth pulp stimulation before pain threshold is reached (87;88).

It is considered that Rollman does in fact raise an important issue concerning the actual meaning of d'. This problem is also raised tangentially in another, much more favorable, review (70). Is d' really a measure of pure sensation? Originally, SDT was developed as a technique for detecting weak stimuli from a relatively strong background noise. Furthermore, it was assumed that the background noise is constantly changing. Thus detection became a function of both the intensity of the signal (i.e. a stronger signal is more easily detectable than a weaker one) and the observer's criterion, dependent to a large extent on the payoff. In contrast, in human pain studies conducted in the laboratory under controlled experimental conditions the magnitude of the noxious stimulus at pain threshold value is usually quite large in comparison to the background noise. More important, contemporary pain researchers have begun to be more interested in supra-threshold pain than in pain threshold responses (e.g. pain tolerance). Under such conditions the noxious stimulation is quite intense. Consequently, the healthy subject under the experimental conditions invariably detects the stimulus and the pain response becomes a judgemental and not a sensory response. Manipulating the independent variable may produce changes in the supra-pain threshold responses, but it would appear that such changes are judgemental and not sensory. Background noise is really quite unimportant under such conditions. Therefore, we are concerned that in such supra-threshold pain studies it is not at all clear what d' actually measures. It is unlikely to be a purely sensory component. Is it possible, that, contrary to the basic assumptions, SDT under such conditions measures two components of the total "psychological" spectrum (e.g. attitude, affect, criterion, etc.) rather than both a sensory and a bias component? This is an area which requires much more investigation and careful exploration.

Finally, it should be stated that in the field of pain it was not the SDT investigators who first attempted to differentiate the sensory from the judgemental components. Chapman and Jones

(19) in 1944 and later Gelfand (38) in 1964 suggested that the experimental pain threshold measured the physiological (sensory) components of the pain response whereas the pain tolerance measured the psychological components. This hypothesis intrigued us, and we conducted several studies to explore this further. On the basis of our studies we concluded that, while both threshold and tolerance had sensory and psychological components, the experimental pain threshold was more highly loaded with sensory than with psychological variables, whereas the pain tolerance had proportionally higher loadings of psychological than of physiological (sensory) components (140;148). Clark (23) has challenged this view, using SDT analysis. Nevertheless, it is of considerable interest that current human analgesic assays with experimental pain still support this view (144).

CLINICAL PAIN

The behavioural measurement of clinical pain was made possible by the development of direct scaling methods--the New Psychophysics. Classical psychophysics, by its emphasis on the stimulus rather than the sensation, offered relatively little to clinical pain measurement. In clinical pain, the exact stimulus is usually not known, or if known, not easily manipulated so that the experimenter does not have direct control. It was probably no accident that allowed Beecher (2;6;7) to introduce measurement techniques of clinical pain for human analgesic assays by utilizing the patient's subjective responses. Beecher and S. S. Stevens were both together at Harvard and the latter's development of direct scaling techniques, especially magnitude estimation, influenced the former. In any event, Beecher's approach was to use magnitude estimation by having the patient rate his clinical pain along a (subjective) numerical (verbal) scale. Beecher is regarded as the Father of modern clinical analgesic assays and he worked with or trained many of the leading clinical pharmacologists, such as Lasagna, Keats and Houde, who, in turn, have trained the current "generation" of clinical investigators. Yet, all this covers only approximately a quarter of a century.

Beecher's contribution to pain measurement and analgesic evaluations was not simply restricted to evolving a methodological approach involving magnitude estimation, but also in stating two essential requirements for clinical analgesic assays, namely the use of (a) the double-blind procedure, and (b) a placebo control. These two requirements seem so obvious and commonplace to the contemporary investigator, but only two decades ago most clinical trials lacked these controls. The double-blind condition requires that neither the patient (or subject) nor the physician (or experimenter) know which of the possible treatments (or drugs) is being used. Placebo corresponds to blanks in psychophysics and used to be defined (incorrectly) as an inert treatment. However, since placebos do exert an analgesic effect it is more correctly defined as a treatment which mimics the qualities and characteristics of the active treatment except for the variable under study, i.e. the actual analgesic properties. It is not easy to find such a placebo and more often than not the placebo differs from the active treatment in several attributes. In oral analgesic studies, lactose is frequently chosen as the placebo, while in parenteral studies saline is often employed. However, like the contemporary clinical investigator, modern patients have also become more sophisticated and are not that easily "fooled," e.g. saline is a poor placebo for morphine.

Subjective clinical pain measurements are most commonly applied to human analgesic assays and the standard procedure is to use patients with acute rather than chronic pain, such as post-operative or post-partum pain. A nurse, trained in the methodology of clinical analgesic trials, and called the nurse-observer, has the patient rate his pain, utilizing a 4- or 5-points scale, such as no pain, mild pain, moderate pain, severe pain and excruciating pain. The drug is then given under double-blind conditions and the nurse-observer returns hourly and has the patient re-evaluate his pain level. Commonly, a patient is only included if his original starting pain is at least moderate or severe, and the hourly changes in pain recorded as the pain relief scores, i.e. successive pain scores are subtracted from the starting pain score. Placebo is used as control and graded doses of the active medication are given (6;51-54;59;61;65-67;85). It is of interest to comment that the patient's subjective pain ratings are not linear (as known from magnitude estimation), yet the data is treated statistically as being linear.

The use of a verbal rating scale for pain is, of course, not restricted to pharmacological studies. It has been observed that the subjective verbal ratings of pain tend to yield limited categories, the average patient usually has difficulties if more than five categories (i.e. four pain and one no pain) are used. In part, this is due to semantic rather than scaling problems, e.g. what is the difference between mild and slight and moderate pain? Yet, there also seem to be inherent scaling problems. Some time ago, the author in an unpublished exploratory study stimulated the backs of healthy volunteers with 20 graded radiant heat intensities ranging from no pain to severe pain (based on each individual's earlier control response). The subjects were requested to rate the pain intensities. The average number of discriminations (i.e. intensity levels) was only seven, and ranged from five to eleven. In an interesting paper, Miller (84) commented upon the "magical" number seven in psychophysics. He observed that most investigators tend to use seven plus or minus two categories for psychophysical discriminations. Thus, he suggested, somewhat humourously, that indeed seven may be a magical number. However, more scientifically, he proposed that human sensory information processing has limits placed upon it, and that about seven categories are as many as can be effectively analyzed (discriminated). Similarly, in pain it would appear that relatively few discriminatory categories are available and that more lead to confusion. This contradicts Hardy, Wolff and Goodell's Dol Scale of 21 steps (42).

Recently, the visual analogue scale has been employed increasingly with pain estimations (55), although such scales had been used previously for rating illness-well being (27). A visual analogue scale is a straight line, either horizontal or vertical, the ends of which are fixed by a statement of the extreme limits of the sensation to be measured, e.g. No Pain and Excruciating Pain. A graphic rating scale is simply a visual analogue scale, which, in addition to the defined fixed end-points, also has descriptive terms placed at specified intervals along its length, e.g. mild, moderate and severe. The visual analogue scale has been compared with the graphic rating scale (100) and with the more traditional verbal rating scale (92;149), and with the pressure algometer and an audiometric scaling method (149). While most types of these scales tend to demonstrate high interscale correlations, the audiometric correlations were lower but statistically significant, while there were no correlations between the pain threshold, measured by the pressure algometer, and the other subjective scales. In general, the visual analogue scale emerges as superior to the other subjective scales by its apparent greater sensitivity to changes in pain following analgesic treatment. The success of the visual analogue scale in Britain has stimulated interest in the United States of America where it is now used by several investigators and additional reliability and validity studies should become available soon.

Yet another approach to the quantitative measurement of clinical pain is provided by the McGill Pain Questionnaire (77;78). The Questionnaire consists of 102 words descriptive of pain, divided into three major categories of sensory, affective and evaluative. The patient's choice of words is analyzed in three different ways, consisting of (a) a pain rating index, which is based on numerical values assigned to the chosen words; (b) the

number of words chosen; and (c) the present pain intensity on a
1-5 points intensity scale. The Questionnaire is said to be
sensitive to changes in pain following different analgesic treatment methods. A number of investigators are currently studying
the use and validity of the McGill Pain Questionnaire and pertinent results should become available in the near future.

In some pilot trials with chronic pain and chronic arthritis
patients, we have found that many of the words are too difficult
for the "average" patient, especially those without college education, and the applicability of the Questionnaire thus becomes
rather restrictive. It, therefore, is of interest to see what future
data will indicate in terms of the Questionnaire's validity with
patients of low socio-economic background and from non-English
speaking sub-cultures.

Finally, cross-modal measurement methods should be mentioned.
Strictly speaking, the visual analogue scale and the graphic
rating scale are both such cross-modal approaches, as the
patient's pain is transformed to another, visual, modality. However, more traditionally, experimental pain-induction techniques
have been used and the patient has to equate his subjective pain
intensity to the magnitude of the applied noxious stimulus (i.e.
find the PSE) (60). This approach, however, has not been too
successful for clinical pain measurements for two reasons. First-
ly, most clinical pain tends to be more severe than that measured
by an experimentally induced pain threshold. Yet, in the past,
many pain investigators have been wary of applying greater stimulus intensities to patients in pain in the fear of possibly causing
some tissue damage. The pain threshold, itself, is not a good
measure of clinical pain (149). Secondly, it is a nuisance and
inconvenient to drag apparatus to a patient's bedside, unless it
is a simple device, such as the pressure algometer. Therefore,
the use of non-traumatic and easily administered self-rating
scales, such as the visual analogue scale, are probably the best
cross-modal approach to clinical pain measurement.

EXPERIMENTAL PAIN

Modern, systematic experimental pain studies in man commenced with the meticulous investigations of Hardy, Wolff and
Goodell (41,42) at Cornell, but floundered with the strong
attacks of Beecher (3; 5) upon them, as discussed earlier in this
Chapter. Beecher's (102) eventual change of mind in turn made
such studies more acceptable. In recent years, human experimental pain studies have again flourished, in part due to an

increased public interest in pain, in part due to the application of SDT, and in part due to some interesting and important findings relating experimental pain to clinical pain.

The major criticisms of experimental pain have been that (a) there is no significant psychological involvement and implication for the subject, so that there is no real "suffering," which is in sharp contrast to clinical pain; (b) the duration of experimental pain--seconds, minutes, perhaps a couple of hours--is much shorter than clinical pain, which may last many years; and (c) the intensity of experimental pain is usually much less than the severity of clinical pain. These criticisms are well-founded. While it is technically possible to manipulate experimental pain to yield somewhat similar patterns of "suffering," anxiety, duration and intensity as in clinical pain, such manipulations are, fortunately, both unethical and probably illegal. However, let us look at the advantages of experimental pain, which are based chiefly on the experimenter's precise control of the stimulus and the laboratory conditions, combined with careful recording of the subject's response behaviour. This is not possible in clinical pain. Furthermore, if it can be established that there is some direct or indirect relationship between experimentally-induced and clinical pain then there would be ample justification for laboratory pain studies. Such relationships will, in fact, be discussed later in this Chapter. The reader is also reminded of both Hardy, Wolff and Goodell's (42) and Beecher's (7) requirement for a laboratory pain-induction method, which were listed at the beginning of this Chapter.

Pain Response Parameters

There are five pain response parameters which are or have been in common use in experimental pain studies. These are the pain threshold, the JND, the pain tolerance, the pain sensitivity range and the drug request point. In addition, there is a non-painful response, the detection threshold, which is simply the point at which any kind of sensation along the sensory continuum under study is first perceived. The detection threshold is particularly useful in experiments involving electrical stimulation as it serves as a check that the equipment is working satisfactorily and the subject is responding properly.

In addition to these five pain response parameters, recent work has isolated a specific pain factor, which is based on some of these (primary) pain response parameters and may thus be considered a second order variable. This pain factor will be discussed in greater detail later in this Chapter.

The reader interested in reviewing the literature in this area is warned to beware of semantic difficulties. Different names have been applied to a given pain response parameter by different investigators, and, worse, the same name has been used by different experimenters for different parameters (135). We have attempted to introduce uniformity of labelling these pain response parameters for many years, and gradually, many investigators are beginning to apply common terms. The names used in this Chapter are those which we consider the most suitable and which are receiving a growing number of supporters.

Pain Threshold

The pain threshold is that point at which the subject just begins to feel pain in an ascending trial or at which pain just disappears in a descending trial. Alternately, it may be defined as that point at which pain is just perceived 50% of the time. It is usually measured in terms of stimulus parameters. Psychophysically, the pain threshold is thus an absolute sensory threshold.

The experimental pain threshold has been subjected to much criticism. SDT questions its very existence (122) while Beecher (5) questioned its purpose and relevance for clinical pain. In the past, many studies tried to relate the pain threshold to clinical pain, usually without much success (73). In experimental human analgesic assays, the pain threshold's sensitivity or reactivity to analgesic drugs is equivocal (101;103;104;146). Some investigators have claimed that the pain threshold is highly unreliable, fluctuating both within and between experimental sessions (89;97;132), while others consider it to be a highly reliable (i.e. test-retest) measure (20;91;141). What then is the status of the pain threshold now?

Conceptually and statistically one has to examine both the reliability and validity of the pain threshold. Reliability refers to the (intrasubject) consistency of repeated measures under the same experimental conditions both within and between experimental sessions. It is usually expressed in terms of test-retest reliability coefficients, ranging from 1.0 for perfect reliability to 0.0 for no reliability. In view of the relative crudity of behavioural pain measures, we recommend a fairly lenient, rule of thumb, approach. It is suggested that split-half or within session reliability coefficients of 0.6 or above are acceptable, 0.8 or above are very good and those above 0.9 are excellent. For between sessions with intervals of a week or more, reliability coefficients are acceptable at somewhat lower values, provided statistical significance is maintained.

Reliability is dependent upon the pain-induction method and the experimental procedure and consequently varies between methods or for different procedures with the same method. It is considered that the controversy about the reliability of the pain threshold is largely due to the selection of poor pain-induction methods or to faulty stimulation procedures, such as lack of familiarity with rigorous psychophysical techniques, or both. If possible, it is advisable to administer several trials within an experimental session and to calculate the mean score rather than present only a single trial as this increases reliability. In our laboratory, all pain-induction methods (except for the cold pressor) are presented at least five times per subject per experimental condition and the score from the first trial excluded and the mean score calculated from the remaining trials. Rejection of the first score is based on our observations over many years of testing that the first presentation usually yields the largest deviation from the mean score. Therefore, exclusion of this first trial score considerably reduces the variability of the mean score, based upon the remaining trials. Furthermore, each research assistant receives intensive training in stimulus application and experimental behaviour vis-a-vis a subject and has to "pass" a test with a senior staff member acting as a difficult subject before being allowed to participate in data collection and experimentation. Consequently, the New York University Pain Group consistently obtains very high reliability coefficients with most of its standard pain-induction methods. Immediate test-retest reliability coefficients for the pain threshold were found to be 0.96 for intramuscular hypertonic saline stimulation (0.79 between sessions after a median time interval of two weeks) (143); 0.96 for intramuscular hypotonic saline stimulation and 0.92 for radiant heat stimulation (141). In recent years, we tend to obtain coefficients of 0.95 and above for cutaneous electrical stimulation (and 0.85 to 0.90 for between sessions trials), based on a series of many different studies involving a total of over 500 healthy subjects. Cold pressor reliabilities tend to be lower. Clark and Bindra (20) have published immediate retest reliabilities of 0.81 for electrical, 0.91 for mechanical (pressure), and 0.88 for radiant heat. Merskey and Spear (82) obtained a reliability coefficient of 0.65 for the pressure algometer (a different mechanical method from that used by Clark and Bindra). These are just a few examples of published data in this area which have been selected because they specifically focused on the reliability of the pain threshold.

On the basis of the above cited data and our experience, we believe that there is a hierarchy of retest reliabilities for four of the most commonly used pain-induction methods, which places cutaneous electrical stimulation at the top, followed by radiant heat, pressure algometer and the cold pressor method. It must be emphasized, however, that when the experimental conditions or stimulation procedures are altered, that the test-retest correlations are no longer reliability scores and may decrease. Instructions (8;140;148), anxiety (132;139), drugs (145), diurnal variation (97) and other variables may all influence the pain threshold.

The next point concerns the validity of the pain threshold. Validity refers to the problem whether or not the variable being studied actually measures what it is supposed to measure. In other words, does the pain threshold measure pain? In a very restricted sense, using operational definitions and the subjective response, the experimental pain threshold does in fact measure pain as presumably the subject responds to the noxious stimulation when first perceiving pain. However, in a broader sense, has the pain threshold any meaningful relationship to pain in general? There are three approaches to this question, consisting of (a) comparing different pain thresholds across various sensory modalities; (b) directly comparing the pain threshold with clinical pain; and (c) indirectly, by testing the pain threshold's reactivity (sensitivity) to an analgesic treatment known to have efficacy for clinical pain.

Cross-modal pain threshold studies indicate very large differences in correlation. Wolff and Jarvik (142) obtained correlations ranging from a low of 0.13 (no correlation) to a high of 0.53 (significant) for four pain-induction methods, consisting of radiant heat, cold pressor, intramuscular hypertonic and hypotonic stimulation. Clark and Bindra (20) found the pain threshold correlations to vary from 0.58 to 0.77 for three methods, including radiant heat, electrical and mechanical stimulation. Davidson and McDougall (30) observed pain threshold correlations from a low of 0.0 (completely unrelated) to a high of 0.49 for four methods, namely electrical, cold pressor, radiant heat and pressure algometer. Lynn and Perl (71) found correlations from 0.10 to 0.52 with three methods, involving pin prick, pinch threshold and heat (thermode). These examples suffice to show that cross-modal studies of the experimental pain threshold are at best equivocal and hardly support, but also do not necessarily negate, the validity of the experimental pain threshold as a measure of pain.

Direct comparisons of the experimental pain threshold with clinical pain have not been too fruitful (149). Generally speaking, in so far that the experimental pain threshold is by definition a minimal measure of pain, conceptually it would really not be necessary for it to be significantly correlated with clinical pain, which is supra-threshold pain even at moderate severity. Thus, the experimental pain threshold inherently is probably a relatively poor index of clinical pain.

The effects of analgesic drugs on the experimental pain threshold have yielded ambiguous results. Years ago, Beecher (7) already criticized this response parameter as unrelated to clinical pain. Kutscher and Kutscher (64) in a review of 90 papers on the radiant heat method concluded that it was an equivocal technique for human analgesic assays if one uses the pain threshold. Incidentally, however, the radiant heat method is one of the two most common techniques for measuring analgesia in animals, where it is known as the tail-flick method. Our own work with human analgesic assays has suggested that the experimental pain threshold is less reactive or sensitive to commonly used analgesics than other pain response parameters (144;146;147). However, some of our current analgesic studies suggest that perhaps, after all, the experimental pain threshold may be of some value for mild oral analgesics, such as aspirin (138). We are now investigating this possibility more thoroughly.

Finally, some years ago, Wolff and Jarvik (141) stated two hypotheses: (a) Pain thresholds induced by different noxious stimuli impinging upon different tissues or body loci will be significantly correlated if the resultant subjective pain sensations are qualitatively similar; and (b) Pain thresholds elicited by different noxious stimuli impinging upon the same body locus or tissue will be significantly correlated irrespective of the subjective quality of the induced pain. The first hypothesis was supported in a later study (142), but the second hypothesis was questioned. The recent work of Lynn and Perl (71) also questions the role of the body locus, but, unfortunately, failed to investigate the effects of the subjective sensations.

Difference Limen (JND)

The JND or Difference Limen or Difference Threshold is the stimulus interval or distance between two stimulus points which can just be discriminated. According to the Weber-Fechner Law, this interval increases logarithmically with stimulus magnitude. The JND is based upon classical psychophysics and with the introduction of direct scaling methods has become of little interest to pain researchers. However, historically, it is of importance to mention that Hardy, Wolff and Goodell (42) developed a pain scale, which they called the Dol-Scale, which is based upon JNDs. The Dol-Scale was derived from their meticulous studies with radiant heat during which they stimulated the entire

body surface. The Dol-Scale consists of 21 steps or JNDs from
no pain through pain threshold to pain tolerance. Hardy et al
defined 1 dol= 2 JNDs. The range of pain spans 10 dols (or 20
JNDs) while the odd number reflects the 0 point of no pain. It
has already been mentioned before that the "average" subject
usually yields about seven categories of pain and rarely exceeds
eleven with five being the optimal for clincal pain estimations.
Consequently, the Dol-Scale is rarely used these days.

Pain Tolerance

The pain tolerance is essentially the upper threshold of experimental pain. It is that point at which the individual terminates
noxious stimulation. It is the highest level of supra-threshold
experimental pain, i.e. pain used in the laboratory, but it must
not be confused with severe or excruciating clinical pain, which,
probably is of greater subjective intensity. It has already been
mentioned that this is a parameter which has only come to the
fore in relatively recent years. Hardy's et al work with radiant
heat focused almost exclusively on the pain threshold, except
for the Dol-Scale studies which, in a limited manner, included
pain tolerance. Chapman and Jones (19) compared different pain-
induction methods, but restricted their work to the pain threshold
and supra-threshold pain reactions but not pain tolerance. Therefore, some of the earliest systematic experimental work with pain
tolerance seemed to have been done by Clark and Bindra (20) and
somewhat later by Wolff and Jarvik (141). In the last fifteen
years, pain tolerance has been used in several studies by different investigators, but there still appears to be a reluctance by
some workers in the field to use pain tolerance levels in experimental work. In our opinion, appropriate selection of the pain-
induction method to avoid potential tissue damage together with
the fact that the subject is in control of stimulation make the use
of such high pain levels ethical.

The reliability of the pain tolerance tends to be high. Clark
and Bindra (20) obtained reliability coefficients of 0.91 for electrical, 0.86 for mechanical, and 0.85 for radiant heat, while we
obtained a coefficient of 0.93 for the latter (141). Merskey and
Spear (82) found the pressure algometer tolerance to have a reliability of 0.81. However, the pain tolerance is very sensitive to
manipulation (140).

Cross-modal comparisons of different pain tolerance levels
yield ambiguous data. While Clark and Bindra (20) found relatively high correlations, ranging from 0.65 to 0.78 for electrical,
mechanical and radiant heat stimulation, Davidson and McDougall

(30) obtained very low correlations, varying from 0.08 to 0.32 for four methods, consisting of electrical, cold pressor, radiant heat and pressure algometer stimulation. Therefore, the validity of the pain tolerance as a measure of pain is equivocal when cross-modal experimental pain data is used. However, clinical comparisons appear much more fruitful (60) than for the pain threshold. It is in human analgesic assays that pain tolerance comes to the fore as a valid measure of pain. In many studies in our laboratory we have demonstrated that the pain tolerance is very sensitive to the analgesic effects of moderate and potent analgesics, such as propoxyphene, codeine, morphine, etc. (138;144; 145;147), and these findings are supported by those of Smith et al (101;103;104).

It was indicated earlier in this Chapter that the pain tolerance may have proportionally much higher loadings of psychological than physiological factors, while the opposite seems to hold for the pain threshold (19;38;141). Consequently, one would expect the pain tolerance to be easily modulated by such psychological variables.

Pain Sensitivity Range

The pain sensitivity range (PSR) is simply the arithmetical difference between the pain tolerance and the pain threshold, i.e. Pain Tolerance – Pain Threshold = PSR. We became interested in this variable when we were looking for a relatively stable measure of pain not easily changed by extraneous or intrinsic factors. The pain tolerance initially appeared to be such a measure, but its reactivity to other variables made us look for another parameter. While the PSR is somewhat more stable than the pain tolerance, it also can be influenced by external factors, such as drugs. Centrally acting analgesics, such as narcotics, have a more profound effect on the PSR than peripherally acting drugs, such as aspirin (147). However, the importance of the PSR was revealed in a factor analytic study in which we isolated a specific pain factor, which will be discussed shortly.

Drug Request Point

Several investigators in the past have used a response of this nature to signal the subject's desire for a pain-relieving drug. We define the drug request point as that point at which the subject would like to take a mild pain-killing medication, such as aspirin, were he to experience a similar pain to the experimentally-induced pain in a real life situation. The reason for using this pain response parameter, which lies between the pain threshold and pain tolerance, is the wish to have a parameter which is particularly sensitive to analgesic drugs. Our studies (138;144) show that the drug request point is a pain response parameter with reactivity to a broad spectrum of pain-relieving drugs from mild, oral medications, such as aspirin, through moderate drugs like propoxyphene, to the more potent narcotics. It thus fills a practical need, although it probably has no great theoretical significance.

Laboratory Pain-Induction Methods

Potentially, there are probably as many different ways to induce pain experimentally as there are pain researchers to think up such methods. Fortunately, a number of such methods have become "standard" techniques, used by many investigators, thus allowing systematic studies and comparisons. For purely practical purposes we like to divide laboratory pain-induction methods into three categories depending on the site of the stimulus application, namely, (a) cutaneous for superficial stimuli or for intradermal or subcutaneous stimulation; (b) deep somatic for stimulation of the deeper tissues, such as striated muscles; and (c) visceral for stimulation of internal organs and smooth muscles. In view of ethical considerations, visceral stimulation techniques, such as swallowing a balloon which is then inflated (19) or intraperitoneal stimulation with various chemicals (58), tend to be frowned upon and are no longer used routinely. Deep somatic pain-induction methods are more common, especially those involving mechanical pressure, while cutaneous techniques are the most common, in particular superficial stimulation. Detailed discussions and reviews of many different experimental pain-induction methods have been provided by Hardy et al (42), Beecher (7) and by Wolff (137) and in this Chapter only brief summaries of a few more commonly used methods will be presented.

Thermal Methods

Radiant heat method. It is most appropriate to list the radiant heat method first as it was used so extensively by Hardy et al (41;42). The traditional Hardy-Wolff-Goodell apparatus consists of two components, a dolorimeter which controls the electrical output and contains a timer and variac, and a projection lamp, which contains a high intensity bulb housed in a gun-like casing with a multiple lens system focusing the light and heat on an aperture, 2 cm in diameter. The exact radiant heat flux at the aperture, expressed in $mcal/sec/cm^2$, is controlled by the dolorimeter. The aperture is placed against the blackened skin surface and stimulation is either applied traditionally by 3 sec exposures of different heat intensities, i.e. fixed time, variable heat intensity, or by the single-trial technique (134) with a constant radiant heat flux and time in sec as the dependent variable. The latter technique permits the measurements of pain threshold, drug request point and pain tolerance in one trial, while the traditional approach requires many stimulus applications for single measures of these variables. The heat may be applied to the forehead, volar surfaces of the forearms or the back, while hairy skin surfaces are less suitable. Contemporary investigators frequently use more modern equipment for radiant heat stimulation.

A recent development by Mor and Carmon (86) uses a laser to produce the radiant heat. However, at present it is not clear how safe this technique is for human experimentation. We personally know of several pain researchers who have been badly blistered by this laser method.

Cold pressor method. This method, together with electrical stimulation, are perhaps the most widely used pain-induction methods at present. The cold pressor method was first published by Hines and Brown (47) as a technique for measuring vasomotor reactions. In our laboratory, we standardize the skin temperature of the hand by immersion in a warm water bath maintained at body temperature ($37^{\circ}C$) for 2 min and then plunging the hand into an ice water bath saturated with ice chippings and essentially at $0^{\circ}C$. Subjective verbal responses of "PAIN" (i.e. pain threshold) and "STOP" (i.e. pain tolerance) are used. Hilgard et al (46;130) use a modification with several different cold water temperatures.

We have observed the cold pressor method to be less reliable than some of the other methods, as we only take one measurement per condition as it takes some time for the circulation to be restored to normal after immersion. In contrast, it appears to be one of the most valid methods for measuring pain, such as in human analgesic evaluations (144). Consequently, this is a good example where excellent validity outweighs reliability considerations.

Electrical Methods

All kinds of electrical stimulation for pain induction have been used in the past. Electrical stimulation is a very convenient technique, easily controllable, although it does have several very complex parameters. It can be applied at all tissue levels, from superficial cutaneous to deep somatic and visceral. The main requirement is that the subject is electrically isolated for safety. Constant current stimulators are preferred to constant voltage units. The most commonly used body loci are the fingers, hand, forearms and the healthy tooth pulp. We also use intramuscular stimulation of the gluteus medius muscle. There are many publications dealing with electrical stimulation and the interested reader is referred to Wolff (137) for a more thorough discussion. However, it should be mentioned again that electrical stimulation is very reliable and seems reasonably valid. It produces a sensation which is rather unique and often called "discomfort" rather than "pain," although it can become very aversive.

Chemical Methods

Cantharidin blister method. This procedure (1; 62) is largely used in England and consists of applying a cantharidin plaster to the skin of the volar surface of the forearm for 4-6 hr during the evening before the day of the experiment. A blister develops overnight after the plaster is removed. On the next day, the fluid is aspirated and the raised epidermis cut away. Small volumes of various chemicals are then dropped on the exposed and very sensitive skin. Each chemical stimulus is washed away with sterile isotonic saline before stimulating again.

Tourniquet ischemic method. This method was introduced by Smith and Beecher (101-104) as the answer to experimental pain threshold techniques. They labelled it the sub-maximum effort tourniquet technique, modified from an earlier method described by Lewis et al (69). Essentially it consists of draining the arm of venous blood, constricting the blood flow by means of a tourniquet wrapped around the upper arm and having the subject perform several types of exercises with the hand. Some modifications were added by Sternbach (106).

Smith et al have claimed that this tourniquet method is a good and valid instrument for analgesic assays, and superior to other experimental pain-induction methods. However, some other investigators (11;132) have seriously questioned the reliability and validity of this tourniquet ischemia method.

In our laboratory, we experimented with the tourniquet method and various modifications of it for two years and concluded that it was quite unreliable for human psychophysical pain measurements. We found it to be inferior in comparison to the other experimental pain-induction methods used commonly by us. Chief points of our criticisms were that the tourniquet itself often produced discomfort more severe than the ischemic pain; frequently, fatigue prevented the onset of "real" pain; it required anywhere from 8-25 min to reach pain threshold; within sessions replications were not possible; and data could not be replicated in another session.

We have been puzzled why this tourniquet method is still being used when there exist several much simpler and significantly more reliable experimental methods. It is suggested that part of the answer may lie in Beecher's tremendous prestige and influence. Beecher (102) introduced this technique as the answer to the "inadequate" old-fashioned pain threshold methods and his halo may still surround it. This explanation is supported in part by a recent paper (107) in which the tourniquet method failed to be a valid tool for analgesic discriminations. Yet, in spite of and in opposition to the actual obtained results, the investigators, nevertheless, spuriously concluded that the tourniquet method is useful.

Mechanical Methods

Pressure algometer. Keele (63) has described a spring-loaded gauge with a plunger which is applied to the skin over a bony surface and increased pressure applied gradually. This he termed the pressure algometer, which has been used extensively in Britain (81;82) and to a lesser extent in the United States (72). In our laboratory we prefer to apply the pressure algometer to the thumb knuckles and the medial surface of the ankles.

Sphygmomanometer cuff. Hollander (49) attached a metal grater inside a sphygmomanometer cuff and placed it around the upper arm of the subject and gradually inflated it to induce pressure pain. Poser (94) used a modification, sewing 94 pointed projections inside the cuff. This technique is not very satisfactory and tends to leave marks on the skin lasting several days. However, some investigators still seem to use it.

PAIN ENDURANCE

In our search for better experimental measures of pain, we decided to apply the statistical technique of factor analysis to a large matrix of correlations obtained from many experimental and clinical pain variables as well as several personality and cognitive measures. Specifically, in a three years longitudinal study with chronic arthritis patients, who were undergoing corrective or reconstructive orthopaedic surgery on an arthritic joint (fusions being excluded) each patient was admitted pre-operatively for five days to a special research ward and given a large variety of experimental and clinical tests and procedures. These included three cutaneous (electrical, cold pressor and radiant heat) and two deep somatic (electrical and hypertonic saline) pain-induction methods, and the pain thresholds, pain tolerance levels and PSRs measured. Pre- and post-operative subjective self-ratings of clinical pain as well as clinical observations by three experienced physicians were also included. Following surgery, the patient had to start exercising the operated joint within 24 hr in order to maximize range of motion, participating in an intensive physical exercise regimen. Initially, this tended to be very painful and post-operative outcome was largely dependent upon such active patient participation. The use of potent analgesic drugs was contra-indicated as they tended to interfere with the patient's physical exercise program. Each patient was evaluated six months post-operatively in terms of post-operative success or failure, which largely depended upon the patient's ability to tolerate the clinical pain during joint motion. The various clinical and experimental measures, collected blindly, were factor analyzed and a factor, which seemed to be pain-specific, was isolated. This factor was most highly loaded with PSRs from the various experimental pain-induction methods, and was the only pre-operative factor which was significantly correlated with the 6-months post-operative clinical ratings (136). Therefore, Wolff labelled this factor "pain endurance."

Recently, Timmermans and Sternbach (127) carried out a second factor analytic study based on back pain patients, and used many clinical, experimental pain as well as psychological variables. These investigators also were able to isolate a pain-specific factor, which appears to resemble the pain endurance factor previously obtained by Wolff. A more sophisticated statistical analysis (canonical correlation analysis) by Timmermans and Sternbach (128) confirmed their earlier findings.

Therefore, in view of these two separate and independent studies carried out by different investigators in different laboratories with different patient populations, there is strong evidence that there exists a specific pain factor which seems to be aptly named pain endurance. It seems to be a measure of a patient's ability to tolerate pain. This experimental approach appears to have provided a direct link between experimental and clinical pain.

Recent work in our laboratory related to both the above discussed factor analyses and human analgesic assays have suggested the following hypothesis (138): Directly measurable experimental pain response parameters, such as pain threshold, drug request point and pain tolerance, appear to be measures readily influenced by intrinsic and extrinsic variables, such as drugs. Therefore, they tend to be parameters suitable for evaluation of modulators of pain, such as analgesics and other pain-relieving treatments. In contrast, they are relatively poor predictors of a given individual's reaction to and tolerance of pain. On the other hand, indirect and second-order variables, such as the PSR and the pain endurance factor, are more stable characteristics of an individual and as such more suitable for prediction of the individual's ability to tolerate pain.

SUMMARY AND CONCLUSIONS

This Chapter has provided a summary of psychophysical methodologies and problems encountered in the behavioural measurement of human pain. It was indicated that originally the introduction of SDT to pain research appeared most promising. However, it has not supplanted direct scaling and some classical psychophysical techniques and questions are now being raised as to its actual suitability for human pain measurement. This is an important area for further investigations.

One of the more exciting developments in recent years has been the application of the visual analogue scale to pain measurement. It is a direct scaling technique and, like verbal rating scales, has been found to have great validity. The possibility that the visual analogue scale is more sensitive and has greater discriminability than some of the other scaling methods has interesting implications. Can it be that the optimal 4-5 pain categories based on verbal self-ratings are limited by the crudity of such subjective scales or does it mean that the visual analogue discriminates changes in pain following treatment more readily?

Important progress has been made in the area of experimental human analgesic assays. The stage has now been reached where it is possible to screen analgesics in man successfully with experimental pain. These laboratory procedures tend to be faster and more economical than the traditional clinical trials with patients in pain. We have also observed that the simpler the experimental pain-induction method the better it seems to work for such pharmacological assays.

The isolation of a specific pain factor also holds considerable promise for a better understanding of the behavioural mechanisms of pain. Insofar that the pain endurance factor is a second-order variable, there are some practical problems in using it as a potential predictor of a given individual's tolerance to pain. However, such techniques can easily be developed.

Finally, the area of psychophysical measurement of human pain responses is yielding exciting and important data which will greatly assist our understanding of behavioural pain mechanisms.

Experimental results are no longer isolated from "real" pain problems and will eventually contribute to objective evaluation and prediction of the individual's pain behaviour.

ACKNOWLEDGEMENT

The studies and work reported in this Chapter were in part supported by Grant No.: GM-20228 from the National Institute of General Medical Sciences; Grant No.: DA-01679 from the National Institute on Drug Abuse; and Grant No.: DE-04095 from the National Institute of Dental Research; United States Department of Health, Education, and Welfare. I would also like to thank the staff of the New York University Pain Study Group for their advice and assistance with this Chapter.

REFERENCES

1. Armstrong, D., Dry, R.M.L., Keele, C.A. and Markham, J.W. (1951): J. Physiol., 115:59-61P.
2. Beecher, H.K. (1952): Science, 116:157-162.
3. Beecher, H.K. (1953): Science, 117:166-167.
4. Beecher, H.K. (1956): J.A.M.A., 161:1609-1613.
5. Beecher, H.K. (1956): J. Chron. Dis., 4:11-21.
6. Beecher, H.K. (1957): Pharm. Rev., 9:59-209.
7. Beecher, H.K. (1959): Measurement of Subjective Responses. Oxford University Press, New York.
8. Blitz, B., and Dinnerstein, A.J. (1968): J. Abnorm. Psychol., 73:276-280.
9. Blix, M. (1884): Z. Biol., 20:141-160.
10. Bloedel, J.R., McCreery, D.B., and Erickson, D.L. (1976) In Advances in Pain Research and Therapy, I, edited by J.J. Bonica and D. Albe-Fessard, pp. 433-437. Raven Press, New York.
11. Bloomfield, S.S., and Hurwitz, H.N. (1970): J. Clin. Pharmacol., 10:361-369.
12. Cain, W.S., and Marks, L.E. (1971): Stimulus and Sensation: Readings in Sensory Psychology, Little, Brown and Co., Boston.
13. Chapman, C.R. (1977): Pain, 3:295-305.
14. Chapman, C.R., Chen, A.C., and Bonica, J.J. (1977): Pain, 3:213-227.
15. Chapman, C.R., and Feather, B.W. (1973): Psychosom. Med., 35:330-340.
16. Chapman, C.R., Gehrig, J.D. and Wilson, M.E. (1975): Science, 189:65.

17. Chapman, C.R., Murphy, T.M. and Butler, S.H. (1973): Science, 179:1246-1248.
18. Chapman, C.R., Wilson, M.E. and Gehrig, J.D. (1976): Pain, 2:265-283.
19. Chapman, W.P. and Jones, C.M. (1944): J. Clin. Invest., 23:81-91.
20. Clark, J.W. and Bindra, D. (1956): Canad. J. Psychol., 10:69-76.
21. Clark, W.C. (1969): J. Abnorm. Psychol., 74:363-371.
22. Clark, W.C. (1974): Anesthesiology, 40:272-287.
23. Clark, W.C. and Goodman, J.S. (1974): J. Abnorm. Psychol., 83:364-372.
24. Clark, W.C. and Mehl, L. (1971): J. Abnorm.Psychol., 78:202-212.
25. Clark, W.C. and Mehl, L. (1973) J. Abnorm. Psychol., 97:148-153.
26. Clark, W.C. and Yang, J.C. (1974): Science, 184: 1096-1098.
27. Clarke, P.R.F. and Spear, F.G. (1964): Bull. Br. Psychol. Soc., 17:18A.
28. Cornsweet, T.N. (1962): Am. J. Psychol., 75:485-491.
29. Craig, K.D. and Coren, S. (1975): J. Psychosom. Res., 19:105-112.
30. Davidson, P.O. and McDougall, C.E.A. (1969): J. Psychosom. Res., 13:83-89.
31. Ekman, G. and Åkesson, C. (1965): Scand. J. Psychol., 6:241-253.
32. Ekman, G., Hosman, B., Lindman, R., Ljungberg, L. and Akesson, C.A. (1968), Percept. Mot.Skills, 26:815-823.
33. Engen T. (1971): In: Woodworth & Schlosberg's Experimental Psychology, edited by J.W. Kling and L.A. Riggs, pp. 11-46. Holt, Rinehart & Winston, New York.
34. Engen, T. (1971): In: Woodworth & Schlosberg's Experimental Psychology, edited by J.W. Kling & L.A. Riggs, pp. 47-86. Holt, Rinehart & Winston, New York.
35. Feather, B.W., Chapman, C.R., and Fisher, S.B. (1972): Psychosom. Med., 34:290-294.
36. Fechner, G.T. (1860): Elemente der Psychophysik. Breitkopf & Härtel, Leipzig.
37. Funke, O. (1879): In: Handbuch der Physiologie der Sinnesorgane. 3:297.
38. Gelfand, Sidney (1964), Canad. J. Psychol., 18:36-42.
39. Goldscheider, A. (1884), Mschr. Prakt. Derm.,3: 283-303.
40. Green, D.M. and Swets, J.A. (1966), Signal Detection Theory and Psychophysics. Wiley, New York.

41. Hardy, J.D., Wolff, H.G., and Goodell, H. (1940). *J. Clin. Invest.*, 19:649-657.

42. Hardy, J.D., Wolff, H.G. and Goodell, H. (1952), *Pain Sensations and Reactions*, Williams and Wilkins, Baltimore.

43. Hardy, J.D., Wolff, H.G., and Goodell, H. (1953), *Science*, 117:164-165.

44. Harkins, S.W. and Chapman, C.R. (1976), *Pain*, 2:253-264.

45. Hebb, D.O. (1949), *The Organization of Behavior*, John Wiley and Sons, New York.

46. Hilgard, E.R., Ruch, J.C., Lange, A.F., Lenox, J.R., Morgan, A.H., and Sachs, L.B. (1974): *Am. J. Psychol.*, 87:17-31.

47. Hines, E.A. and Brown, G.E. (1932): *Proceedings, Staff Meetings of the Mayo Clinic*, 7:332-335.

48. Hodos, W. (1970): *Psychol. Bull.*, 74:351-356.

49. Hollander, Edward (1939): *J. Lab. Clin. Med.*, 24:537-538.

50. Horland, A.A., and Wolff, B.B. (1973): *J. Abn. Psychol.*, 81:39-45.

51. Houde, R.W. and Wallenstein, S.L. (1953): *Drug Addic. & Narc. Bull.*, Appendix F: 660-682.

52. Houde, R. W., Wallenstein, S.L., and Beaver, W.T. (1965): In: *Analgetics*, edited by G. de Stevens, pp. 75-122. Academic Press, New York.

53. Houde, R.W., Wallenstein, S.L., and Beaver, W.T. (1966): In: *Clinical Pharmacology, International Encyclopedia of Pharmacology and Therapeutics*, Section 6, Vol. 1, edited by L. Lasagna, pp. 59-97. Bergamon Press, London.

54. Houde, R.W., Wallenstein, S.L., and Rogers, A. (1960): *Clin. Pharmacol. Therap.*, 1:163-174.

55. Huskisson, E.C. (1974): *Lancet*, 2:1127-1131.

56. James, W. (1892): *Psychology: Briefer Course*. Holt, New York.

57. Jarvik, M.E., and Wolff, B.B. (1962): *J. Appl. Physiol.*, 17:841-843.

58. Kantor, T.G., Jarvik, M.E., and Wolff, B.B. (1967): *Proc. Soc. Exptl. Biol. Med.*, 126:505-507.

59. Kantor, T.G., Sunshine, A., Laska, E., Meisner, M. and Hopper, M. (1966): *Clin. Pharm. Therap.*, 7:447-456.

60. Kast, E.C. (1962), *The Journal of New Drugs*, 2:344-351.

61. Keats, A.S., Beecher, H.K., and Mosteller, F.C. (1950): J. Appl. Physiol., 3:35-44.
62. Keele, A., and Armstrong, D. (1964): Substances Producing Pain and Itch. Edward Arnold, London.
63. Keele, K.D. (1954): Lancet, i:636-639.
64. Kutscher, A.H., and Kutscher, H.W. (1957): Int. Rec. Med., 170:202-222 and 228-230.
65. Lasagna, L. (1955): J. Chron. Dis., 1:353-367.
66. Lasagna, L. (1960): Ann. N.Y. Acad. Sci., 86:28-37.
67. Laska, E., Kantor, T., and Sunshine, A. (1966): In: International Encyclopedia of Pharmacology and Therapeutics, Section 6, Vol. I, edited by L. Lasagna, pp. 115-132. Pergamon Press, Oxford.
68. Lewis, T. (1942): Pain. Macmillan, New York.
69. Lewis, T., Pickering, G.W., and Rothschild, P. (1929-1930): Heart, 15:359-383.
70. Lloyd, M.A., and Appel, J.B. (1976): Psychosom. Med., 38:79-94.
71. Lynn, E.C., and Perl, E. (1977): Pain, 3:353-365.
72. McCarty, D.J., Gatter, R.A., and Phelps, P. (1965): Arth. & Rheum., 8:551-559.
73. McKenna, A.E. (1958): J. Appl. Physiol., 13:449-456.
74. Marks, L.E. (1974): Sensory Processes: The New Psychophysics. Academic Press, New York.
75. Marks, L.E., and Stevens, J.C. (1966): Perception and Psychophysics, 1:17-24,
76. Melzack, R. (1973): The Puzzle of Pain. Penguin Books, Harmondsworth.
77. Melzack, R. (1975): Pain, 1:277-299.
78. Melzack, R., and Torgerson, W.S. (1971): Anesthesiology, 34:50.
79. Melzack, R., and Wall, P.D. (1965): Science, 150:971-979.
80. Merkel, J. (1888): Philosophische Studien, 4:541-594.
81. Merskey, H., Gillis, A., and Marszalek, K.S. (1962): J. Ment. Sci., 108:347-355.
82. Merskey, H., and Spear, F.G. (1964): British Journal of Social and Clinical Psychology, 3:130-136.
83. Merskey, H., and Spear, F.G. (1967): Pain: Psychological and Psychiatric Aspects. Bailliere, Tindall & Cassell, London.
84. Miller, G.A. (1956): Psychol. Rev., 63:81-97.
85. Modell, W., and Houde, R.W. (1958): J.A.M.A. 167:2190-2198.

86. Mor, J., and Carmon, A. (1975): Pain, 1:233-237.

87. Mumford, J.M. (1976): Toothache and Orofacial Pain. Churchill Livingstone, Edinburgh.

88. Mumford, J.M., and Bowsher, D. (1976): Pain, 2:223-243.

89. Neisser, U. (1959): J. Appl. Physiol., 14:368-372.

90. Noordenbos, W. (1959): Pain, Elsever Publishing Co., Amsterdam.

91. Notermans, S.L.H. (1966): Neurology, 16:1071-1086.

92. Ohnhaus, E.E., and Adler, R. (1975): Pain, 1:379-384.

93. Peterson, W.W., Birdsall, T.G., and Fox, W.F. (1954): Trans. Professional Group on Information Theory, PGIT-4: 171-212.

94. Poser, Ernest G. (1962): American Journal of Psychology, 75:304-305.

95. Rhode, H. (1921): Arch. F. Expermient. Pathol. U. Pharmakol., 91:173-217.

96. Richardson, L.F., and Ross, J.S. (1930): J. Gen. Psychol. 3:288-306.

97. Rogers, E.J., and Vilkin, B. (1978): J. Clin. Psychiat., 39:431-438.

98. Rollman, G.B. (1977): Pain, 3:187-211.

99. Schiff, J.M. (1858): Lehrbuch der Physiologie, 1:228.

100. Scott, J. and Huskisson, E.C. (1976): Pain, 2:175-184.

101. Smith, G.M., and Beecher, H.K. (1969), 10:213-216.

102. Smith, G.M., Egbert, L.D., Markowitz, R., and Beecher, H.K. (1965), Proceedings, Committee on Drug Addiction and Narcotics, 27th Meeting, Appendix 13, 4201-4211.

103. Smith, G.M., Egbert, L.D., Markowitz, R.A., Mosteller, F., and Beecher, H.K. (1966): J. Pharmac. Exp. Ther., 154:324-332.

104. Smith, G.M., Lowenstein, E., Hubbard, J.H., and Beecher, H.K. (1968): J. Pharmac. Exp. Ther., 163:468-474.

105. Sternbach, R.A. (1968): Pain--A Psychophysiological Analysis. Academic Press, New York.

106. Sternbach, R.A. (1974): Pain Patients: Traits and Treatments. Academic Press, New York.

107. Sternbach, R.A., Deems, L.M., Timmermans, G., and Huey, L.Y. (1977): Pain, 3:105-110.

108. Stevens, J.C. (1967): Percept. and Psychophysics, 2:451-454.

109. Stevens, J.C. (1971): In: Stimulus and Sensation: Readings in Sensory Psychology, Little, Brown and Co., Boston.

110. Stevens, J.C. (1964): J. Accous. Soc. Am., 36:2210-2213.

111. Stevens, J.C., Mack, J.D., and Stevens, S.S. (1960): J. Exp. Psychol., 59:60-67.
112. Stevens, J.C., and Marks, L.E.(1965): Proc. Nat. Acad. Sci., 54:407-411.
113. Stevens, S.S. (1936): Psychol. Rev., 43:405-416.
114. Stevens, S.S. (1956): Am. J. Psychol., 49:1-25.
115. Stevens, S.S. (1957): Psychol. Rev., 64:153-181.
116. Stevens, S.S. (1959): J. Exp. Psychol., 57:201-209.
117. Stevens, S.S. (1960): Scan. J. Psychol., 1:27-35.
118. Stevens, S.S. (1961): Science, 133:80-86.
119. Stevens, S.S. (1970): Science, 170:1043-1050.
120. Stevens, S.S. (1971): Psychol. Rev., 78:426-450.
121. Sullivan, R.A. (1968): Proc., 76th Ann. Conv. Am. Psychol. Assoc., 115-116.
122. Swets, J.A. (1961): Science, 134:168-177.
123. Swets. J.A. (1961): Psychometrika, 26:49-63.
124. Swets, J.A. (1973): Science, 182:990-1000.
125. Swets, J.A., (1961): Psychol. Rev., 68:301-340.
126. Szasz, T.S. (1957): Pain and Pleasure. Basic Books, New York.
127. Timmermans, G. and Sternbach, R.A. (1974): Science, 184:806-808.
128. Timmermans, G. and Sternbach, R.A. (1976): In: Advances in Pain Research and Therapy, I., edited by J.J. Bonica and D. Albe-Fessard, pp.307-310. Raven Press, New York.
129. Van Meter, D., and Middleton, D. (1954): Trans. Professional Group on Information Theory, PGIT-4, 119-145.
130. Voevodsky, J, Cooper, L.M., Morgan, A.H., and Hilgard, E.R. (1967): Am. J. Psychol., 80:124-128.
131. Von Frey, M. (1894): Ber. U. D. Verhandl. D. K. Sächs. Ges. D. Wiss. Z. Leipzig, Math.-Phys. Kl., 46:185-196, and 288-296.
132. Von Graffenried, B., Adler, R., Abt, K., Nüesch, E., and Spiegel, R. (1978): Pain, 4:253-263.
133. Weber, E.H. (1846): Handwörterbuch der Physiologie, 3: 481-588.
134. Wertheimer, M. (1952): Am. J. Psychol., 65:297-298.
135. Wolff, B.B. (1964): Canad. J. Psychol., 18:249-253.
136. Wolff, B.B. (1971): J. Abnorm. Psychol., 78:292-298.
137. Wolff, B.B. (1977): Acupuncture and Electro-Therap. Res. Int. J., 2: 271-305.
138. Wolff, B.B. (1977): Clin. Pharm. and Therap., 21:123.
139. Wolff, B.B., Cohen, P. and Greene, C.T. (1976): In: Advances in Pain Research and Therapy, Vol. I., edited by J. J. Bonica, and D. Albe-Fessard, pp. 327-333. Raven Press, New York.

140. Wolff, B.B., and Horland, A.A. (1967): J. Abnorm. Psychol., 72:402-407.
141. Wolff, B.B., and Jarvik, M.E. (1963): Canad. J. Psychol. 17:37-44.
142. Wolff, B.B., and Jarvik, M.E. (1964): Am. J. Psychol., 77:589-599.
143. Wolff, B. B. and Jarvik, M.(1965): Clin. Sci., 28:43-56.
144. Wolff, B.B., Kantor, T.G., and Cohen, P. (1976): Advances in Pain Research and Therapy, Vol. I, edited by J. J. Bonica and D. Albe-Fessard, pp. 363-367. Raven Press, New York.
145. Wolff, B.B., Kantor, T.G., Jarvik, M.E., and Laska, E. (1966): Clin. Pharmac. Therap., 7:224-238.
146. Wolff, B.B., Kantor, T.G., Jarvik, M.E., and Laska, E. (1966): Clin. Pharmac. Therap., 7:323-331.
147. Wolff, B.B., Kantor, T.G.., Jarvik, M.E., and Laska, E. (1969): Clin. Pharmac. Therap., 10:217-228.
148. Wolff, B.B., Krasnegor, N.A., and Farr, R.S. (1965): Perceptual and Motor Skills, 21:675-683.
149. Woodforde, J.M., and Merskey, H. (1972): J. Psychosom. Res., 16:173-178.
150. Woodworth, R.S. (1950): Experimental Psychology. Methuen and Co., London.
151. Zborowski, M. (1952): J. Soc. Issues, 8:16-30.
152. Zborowski, M. (1969): People in Pain. Jossey-Bass, San Francisco.

The Psychology of Pain, edited by R. A. Sternbach.
Raven Press, New York © 1978.

Pain: The Perception of Noxious Events

C. Richard Chapman

*Departments of Anesthesiology, Psychiatry and Behavioral Sciences, and Psychology,
University of Washington, Seattle, Washington 98195*

INTRODUCTION

Pain is an unpleasant, subjective experience that occurs when tissues are damaged or stressed. A major problem in contemporary medical practice, it has eluded attempts to prevent or control its occurrence in a variety of settings. In recent decades, chronic pain has emerged as a syndrome of epidemic proportions (10), and pain problems are foremost in the difficulties faced by physicians managing cancer patients and burn trauma victims. That pain control persists as one of the great problem areas of contemporary medicine after more than a century of research in this field suggests that the nature of the human pain experience has been poorly understood by investigators.

Historically, there has been substantial ambiguity about whether pain belongs to the domain of sensory physiology or to that of perceptual psychology. Fundamentally, this is simply a question of which explanatory scheme is best suited for dealing with the subjective experience that we call pain. For many years the physiological/anatomical model dominated thinking, and pain was conceptualized as a straightforward sensory process that informed the brain about tissue damage. Early theorists, sometimes termed specificists, believed that certain receptors detected tissue damage and generated sensory messages that traveled pain-specific pathways in the spinal cord to a pain center in the brain. While it is now known that each receptor structure has its own adequate stimulus and that pain-generating receptors transmit impulses that follow certain pathways in the spinal cord and thalamus, the pain experience is recognized to be a much more complex phenomenon. Contemporary theorists stress that pain involves emotional arousal, motivational drive, and cognition in addition to sensory information transmission.

While pain can be studied by the sensory physiologist at the peripheral and central levels, it may also be studied by the psychologist as a form of perception; that is, at the level of phenomenal sequences of subjective experience. The task of perceptual psychology as a broad field is to discover and refine

the irregularities and lawful connections that determine the
central coding and experiencing of sensory messages. In the area
of pain, the mandate of the perceptual psychologist is to explore
those phenomenal and sensory impressions characterized by
aversive feeling states generally associated with tissue injury
or·disease, and to elucidate the central coding and organization
processes that determine such experiences.

The purpose of this chapter is to review the concept of
perception as a domain of psychological inquiry and to develop
our understanding of pain within this framework. The narrative
will describe the peripheral and central physiological mechanisms,
central attentional processes, and central organizational
mechanisms of perception that determine the pain experience,
integrating the concepts and hypotheses put forth with clinical
observations. This will begin with a concrete overview of the
peripheral neurophysiology of pain, but it will necessarily
become increasingly abstract as the central processes are
considered. This progression reflects the state of knowledge and
theory in the field at present. Finally, the issues of measurement in the perceptual psychology of pain will be considered,
and Sensory Decision Theory methods will be described and reviewed.

PERIPHERAL MECHANISMS

Fundamental Concepts

The sensory physiology subserving the pain experience is the
most intensively studied aspect of the pain process. The
putative existence of injury-specific receptors has been a major
issue among sensory physiologists, and this issue continues to
evolve and survive inspite of compelling data supporting the
basic premise of the specifists. Pain pathways in the spinal
cord and pain relay areas in the thalamus have also attracted
much interest among physiologists. The descriptions that follow
are broad overviews of these research areas. These overviews
incorporate physiological findings that reflect the interests and
interpretations of the perceptual psychologist.

Receptors Classes: In the broadest sense, perception is the
process by which human consciousness becomes aware of the environment in which it exists. This environment may be conveniently
divided into two components: the somatic and the external. Constellations of information about the latter come to the brain
from highly refined sense organs at the periphery of the nervous
system such as the eye, ear, nose, tongue, and a host of cutaneous
receptors. Similarly, a variety of receptor organs provide the
brain with information about the body's movement, posture, the
condition of the viscera and muscles, and its general health.
Sherrington defined sensory organs that generate information
about the external environment as exteroceptors, while those that
convey input from the internal organs were called interoceptors.
Structures that provide information about muscle tension, posture,

and equilibrium were termed proprioceptors. In light of contemporary physiology it seems useful to expand and modify
Sherrington's classical distinction. For the purpose of this
chapter, exteroceptors will be defined as those sensory organs
that provide information about the surrounding physical environment, while interoceptors will be construed as those receptors
whose function is to provide information about body tissues; the
internal environment is defined as all body tissues, and not just
viscera alone. The concept of proprioceptors will remain
unaltered.

The expanded definition of interoceptors allows us to think
of these structures as existing in skin, dental pulp, cornea, and
mucous membrane as well as in viscera. In cutaneous tissues they
co-exist with receptors that primarily serve as exteroceptors,
and some skin receptor organs may serve a dual purpose. For
example, receptors that normally provide information about objects
or energy sources in the environment that damage skin may change
their function when pathology occurs (e.g. sunburn) so that they
generate signals about tissue stress or disease.

Receptor Organs for Noxious Stimulation

Sensory end organs that are activated by tissue damage or
stress are termed nociceptors, which indicates that they fire in
response to noxious stimulation. Nociceptors convert noxious
stimulation into a barrage of sensory impulses, and this afferent
barrage is the basic building block of the pain experience.

Cutaneous Tissues: Nociceptors of various kinds are found in the
skin, blood vessels, fascia, subcutaneous tissue, periosteum,
and viscera in addition to other structures. They are activated
by mechanical injury, chemical irritation, ischemia, thermal
energy, certain kinds of electrical stimulation, or other noxious
events that threaten the integrity of tissue. It is now known
on the basis of research on cat and monkey that nerve endings of
certain subgroups of the small unmyelinated C fibers and the
larger thinly myelinated A-delta fibers function as cutaneous
nociceptors. High threshold damaging stimuli provoke 10-25% of
the A-delta fiber population into activity. These fibers generate
a fast, bright pain sensation that is well localized by the
perceiver. With repetitive stimulation this pain decreases. In
contrast, 50-80% of the slow conducting unmyelinated C fibers
respond to noxious stimulation, generating a diffuse nagging and
particularly unpleasant sensation that is poorly localized. This
pain increases in intensity with recurrent stimulation. Both of
these fiber types have their cell bodies located in the posterior
root ganglia and they enter the posterior horn of the spinal cord
with termination in laminae I, IV, and V.

Deep Tissues: Muscles, joints, and tendons are innervated with
nociceptors similar to those in skin, although the adequate
stimuli for these end organs differ somewhat. Deep pain endings

are excited by ischemia, prolonged muscle contraction, or rhythmic contraction, mechanical force, or chemical irritation. Sustained contraction in skeletal musculature is responsible for a large proportion of common aches and pains including tension headache.

Viscera: Pain originating in the viscera is less well understood and these organs are sparsely innervated (64). It is sometimes asserted that the viscera are relatively insensitive because they can be cut, crushed, or burned in the operating room without pain. However, the adequate stimuli for these structures are not these forms of tissue damage, but rather distension, spasm, ischemia, and chemical irritation. Viewed within the context of their own environment, visceral organs are highly sensitive.

While somatic nerves mediate cutaneous pain, visceral sensations are conducted in sympathetic neural pathways for the most part. Nerves serving the viscera generally follow an artery to the abdominal aorta where they enter the splanchnic nerve without synapse. They then course through the sympathetic chain, and reach the spinal nerve. In addition to these pathways, some visceral pain originates in organs that are served by the pelvic and vagus nerves. Certain structures are innervated principally by the thoracic, upper lumbar spinal, and phrenic nerves, which are somatic rather than autonomic.

Teeth: Yet another body structure that commonly gives rise to pain and that has attracted much attention among pain researchers is dental tissue. While it has not been widely recognized as such, the tooth is a highly developed sensory organ. In lower animals such as rodents that gnaw environmental objects, teeth serve an important function in the interaction of the organism with the environment. Broadly speaking, the receptor mechanisms associated with the teeth may be divided into two classes: intradental and periodontal. In man, periodontal receptors play an important role in biting and chewing, but intradental receptors appear to generate pain sensations almost exclusively. It is common knowledge that a sensation of pain can be evoked from the human tooth when it is stimulated by pathologic change, dental drilling, variation in temperature, or electrical shock. Intradental receptors are similar to those observed in other tissues, consisting of both myelinated and unmyelinated fibers of differing diameters.

The tooth is unique in that it contains a very high density of nerve fibers at the pulp, which is encapsulated in hard tissue. The greatest concentration of nerve endings intradentally is in the pulp horns. Some nerve fibers actually course through the dentine and predentine of the tooth, but evidence currently available suggests that these nerves do not mediate pain. Application of either local anesthetic or protein precipitant to exposed dentine fails to block pain, and this indicates that pain is probably mediated entirely within the dental pulp (2). While

not all fibers in the pulp are sensory in function, dental
stimulation consistently results in pain (3). It is generally
assumed that pain of dental origin is mediated by A-delta fibers
and C-fibers.

Periodontal receptors are concerned with movement of the teeth
in the socket and respond to the influence of such movement on the
periodontal ligament. These are probably more often activated than
the intradental receptors, since even very light touch can excite
them. Almost certainly, there are high threshold pain-generating
endings in periodontal tissues which become activated with disease
or trauma and give rise to pain.

Transmission Pathways

In the posterior horn of the spinal cord, the A-delta and C
fibers synapse with neurons that transmit nociceptive impulses
to various parts of the neuraxis. Some travel to the anterior
horn and synapse with motor neurons, while others passing to the
anterior horn stimulate preganglionic neurons of the sympathetic
or parasympathetic nervous systems. The impulses that follow
these pathways are responsible for the motor and autonomic
reflexes associated with tissue injury.

Two Ascending Pathways: The afferent barrage that eventually
results in the conscious experience of pain ascends to the
thalamus via two different systems: the neospinothalamic tract
and the paleospinothalamic tract. A distinction that was made
earlier in the discussion of peripheral nerve fibers, that of
fast and slow conducting fibers, is roughly evident in the
spinothalamic tract as well. The spinothalamic tract is composed
of long fibers that make direct connection with the ventrolateral
and posterior thalamus where they synapse with fibers that project
to primary somatosensory cortex. Thus, this system conveys most
nociceptive impulses quite rapidly. It is generally considered
to be responsible for the delivery of discriminative information
about the site, intensity, and duration of damaging stimuli:
e.g., it gives rise to the perception of sharp, well localized
pain.

The older paleospinothalamic tract is composed of long and
short fibers that project to the reticular formation, the medulla,
the lateral pons, the midbrain, the periaqueductal gray, the
hypothalamus, and the medial intralaminar thalamic nuclei. Some
of these fibers contact neurons that connect with the limbic
forebrain structures while others connect with diffuse projections
to many other parts of the brain. Because of the multiple
synapses within this system, impulses conveyed by it are much
slower in reaching higher centers. This system is generally
assumed to be responsible for the perception of poorly localized,
dull, aching and burning pain, although conclusive evidence for
this is lacking.

Two Functions of Nociception

Warning and Reminding Systems: Current knowledge of anatomical
pathways, physiological evidence involving nerve conduction
times, and subjective descriptions of pain sensations all suggest
that there are two subsystems of pain signals with roughly two
different functions. The first which involves A-delta fibers is
a warning system that provides immediate information about the
presence of injury, the extent of injury, and its location. The
second, which utilizes C-fibers acts as a reminding system. By
generating slow, diffuse, particularly unpleasant, nagging pain,
the second system repeatedly reminds the brain that injury has
occurred and hence that normal activity should be restricted and
the injury should be given more attention. In terms of the
expanded definitions of Sherrington's concepts described previously, warning system nociceptors would be considered exteroceptors since they provide information about harmful environmental
events. Reminding system nociceptors would be construed as
interoceptors because they signal tissue distress or pathology.

First and Second Pain: The classical distinction between first
and second pain mirrors this distinction in function. Both forms
of pain are generated by sudden traumatic injury. First pain is
characterized by precise localization of injury, a bright quality,
and a sharp, well defined sensation. In contrast, second pain,
which occurs just after the first pain disappears, is vague,
poorly localized, and persistent. Mumford and Bowsher (56) and
Price et al. (60) have recently reviewed this distinction and
noted that the dual uniqueness of first and second pain is now
generally accepted. Most investigators hold that, at the time of
injury, pain is first mediated by A-delta fibers and later by C
fibers. Subjectively, with cutaneous injury, this corresponds to
a bright, well localized flash of pain followed by a poorly
localized but particularly disagreeable burning or aching. Price
et al. have shown that first pain shows adaptation with repetitive
noxious electrical skin stimulation while second pain shows a
summation phenomenon that results in the sensation seeming more
intense and the area of painful skin seems to be larger.

The Nature of Noxious Sensory Messages

While the distinction between the two types of fibers is
useful, it must be remembered that most natural pain experiences
involve the stimulation of multiple fiber populations. Both
A-delta and C fibers are activated during injury along with a
variety of other sensory end organs that are not necessarily
nociceptive in function. Thus, naturally occurring pain experiences are the result of a barrage of sensory impulses that
reflect a constellation of information from multiple receptor
populations, both interoceptive and exteroceptive in nature.

From the historical perspective, there is some question about the relationship of the activity of nociceptors to the energy of the stimulus source that provokes them. This question is not only academic but also of direct clinical relevance, since subjective pain intensity in patients is very poorly correlated with the degree of injury, the extent of tissue damage, or the number of receptors affected.

Stimulus Energy Versus Information Processing Hypotheses: Traditionally, sensory physiologists assumed that receptor structures were sensitive to stimulus energy, and that their function was one of transducing the amount of energy encountered into neural signals. In contrast, as Garner (34) has recently emphasized, contemporary theorists hold that it is not stimulus energy that is processed by receptor organs such as the eye, ear, or skin but rather the information contained in the stimulus. Since a single injury stimulus usually excites a configuration of nociceptors and other end organs, it is potentially a rich source of information. The crucial concept is that injury involves an entire receptive field and that response entails a large number of cells acting in unison. It is because cells react in unison to natural injury stimuli that information transmission rather than energy transduction occurs. A stimulus may result in a barrage of impulses from the receptive field that conveys several classes of information, particularly if the stimulus itself has several properties that can vary. That is, a stimulus may be said to have several attributes, dimensions, or distinctive features and it may represent a different level or value on each dimension. Visually, a bird flying through the air has attributes of movement, shape or contour, color, and distance. The retinal receptive field is able to process all of this information. Similarly, a nociceptive barrage originating at the skin may have multiple dimensions of information. It may be bright or dull, intense or mild, well-localized or diffuse, deep or superficial, or possibly novel or familiar. Pain generally results from the information generated in a relatively large interoceptive or exteroceptive receptive field, and it may involve a complex rather than a simple sensory message.

ATTENTION

Information Filtering

Perception depends on the constant monitoring of the multiple barrages of impulses from the many intero-, proprio-, and exteroceptors and the filtering of this input to select for awareness that information which is relevant and useful, excluding that which is of secondary importance or which carries no new information. This process of selection and integration of sensory input from the external and internal environment is the process

of attention. It is sometimes described as the process of
focussing the perceiver's sensory and cognitive abilities on
certain configurations of input from internal or external sources
or on internally generated imagery or thought patterns.

At the most fundamental level, attention involves the filtering of relevant signals from the sensory noise created by the
constant barrage of input from the many sense organs. At a
higher level, it involves the integration of information across
sensory modalities to permit the organization of meaningful forms
of experience. When a victim suffers injury, attentional processes
select the information from the nociceptors as being important on
the basis of its novelty and information content while sensory
messages from other somatic modalities are pushed into the
background. A multiple modality receptor orientation occurs as
the victim looks at and touches the wound, perhaps moving the
injured limb to generate kinesthetic input as well. There is an
attempt to gain new information about the noxious stimulus from
as many sensory modalties as possible. A characteristic of pain
and the other aversive senses (itch, vertigo, etc.) is that these
modalities often demonstrate a unique ability to captivate attention. Aversive interoceptive sensory input intrudes like an alarm
bell into normal waking consciousness, interrupting and disturbing
the ongoing activity and mental pre-occupation of the perceiver.

Filtering Mechanisms: Recent literature indicates that there are
physiological mechanisms that inhibit the barrage of nociceptive
sensory input (9). These include peripheral adaptation mechanisms,
brain stem inhibitory circuits (55), and higher central processes.
Such mechanisms are particularly valuable in times of intense
external stress when survival depends on the ability of the perceiver to concentrate completely on the surrounding physical or
social environment. Activation of these mechanisms ensures that
there will be no distracting competition for attention from the
nociceptive system.

The best studied of the pain inhibitory systems is that
described by Liebeskind in another chapter of this volume. An
area of gray matter surrounding the sylvian aqueduct appears to
play a major role in control of pain. It is responsive not only
to direct electrical stimulation but also to a variety of chemical
substances, including certain peptides that are endogenously
produced, and are bound to specialized receptors. Narcotic drugs,
which share certain characteristics with these endogenic peptides,
also bind to the receptors that activate neurons in the periaqueductal gray area. Activation of this area of the brain leads to
a change in the firing rate of the cells, and this in turn stimu-
lates a structure immediately below the area of the sylvian aqueduct called the dorsal raphé magnus. Long axons from neurons in
the dorsal raphé magnus descend to various levels of the spinal
cord, and in the dorsal horn their activity inhibits the transmission of nociceptive impulses from the periphery.

In spite of the rapid development of research in pain inhibitory processes, understanding of the function of this pain inhib-

itory system is still incomplete. A survey of the literature
suggests, however, that this auto-analgesia system is responsive
to a wide variety of stress experiences that the perceiver may
encounter and that its function is to protect the information
processing centers of the brain from competing nociceptive input
during times of danger when complete concentration on the environment is necessary for survival.

Vigilance: Perceivers sometimes show a readiness to select out
and respond to a certain kind of weak or infrequent stimulus from
the external or internal environment. This predisposition to
attend to certain classes of events is commonly termed vigilance
(52). The term was first introduced in the psychological literature by Mackworth (52). Because it is often a product of a learning process, the occurrence of vigilance reflects the effects of
past experience on present perception. It may result from
straightforward instructions to "pay attention" to particular
events, or it may develop as a perceptual habit because of selective reinforcement for identifying certain kinds of stimuli in the
past. Fordyce (32) has described the effects of reinforcement on
pain behavior elsewhere, and this need not be detailed here. It
is important to note, however, that some individuals develop perceptual habits of vigilance for somatic distress signals, in particular, pain sensations. In extreme instances, this behavior is
associated with the patient's belief that he has a horrible
disease that doctors either cannot identify or are afraid to tell
him about. In other cases, a patient may have a phobia about
catching a serious disease. In both instances, the patients are
suffering from well defined syndromes of hypochondriasis (58, 59).
In other cases, the problem is less obvious and patients often
succeed in obtaining needless exploratory surgery or drugs. Convinced that a noxious signal from, for example, the abdomen must
mean something bad, the patient keeps a constant vigil for the
dreaded sensation and reports every twinge to his doctors, often
with some exaggeration in order to be sure that the doctor does
not underestimate the problem.

Current theory about the origin of chronic pain holds that
the hypervigilant pain patient develops his perceptual habits
because family members have reinforced pain complaints by giving
attention, concern and special favors in response to announce-
ments that he has experienced pain (32, 65). Pain complaints
have profound impacts on the patient's social environment, and
in some instances, they may be directly linked to financial
reward. Clinical experience shows that the automobile accident
victim who must await trial to gain a handsome payoff from litigation is likely to make every effort to preserve his pain symptoms
in spite of nature's tendency to heal. In such cases, the secondary gains associated with pain are enough to make the patient
somatically hypervigilant.

The foregoing considerations illustrate some of the ways in
which beliefs, attitudes, and expectancies control the perception
of painful events. The pain experience is very much determined

by cognitive factors at both the level of selective attention and
in higher organizational processes. Unless the stimulus source
is clear and the stimulus is intense, noxious sensory input is
characterized by substantial uncertainty. When uncertainty
exists, the impulse barrage is susceptible to classification
at several different levels of information processing. Such
classification may reduce it to a trivial pain experience, lead
to an experience that is not pain but some vaguely similar
sensation (e.g. tightness, cramping), or it may amplify the
sensory signal and associate it with great threat.

Arousal and Emotion: The purpose of attention is obvious--it makes
possible efficient and effective interaction of the perceiver with
his environment. Diseases of attention processes, such as infan-
tile autism, provide dramatic examples of the importance of attentional mechanisms. Perhaps less obvious is the link between
attentional focus and arousal or emotion. Efficiency of performance depends on emotional arousal and activation of the organism.
The autonomic nervous system, the endocrine system, and the
central nervous system all contribute to the responsiveness of
the perceiver and the relationship of arousal to performance is
generally accepted to be an inverted U-shaped function (33).

Stimulus Property Versus Perceptual Disruption Hypotheses: Many
early theorists held that a pleasant stimulus should be expected
to evoke arousal patterns associated with pleasure while noxious
stimuli would be predicted to provoke arousal characterized by
displeasure and fear. However, the literature does not support
this hypothesis (53). Arousal appears to be a function of
interruption of attention, the surprise of stimulation, novelty
of the stimulus, as well as incongruity and uncertainty about the
meaning of the stimulus. There is reduction in arousal when the
perceiver finds a means of coping with the conflicts in attentional focus generated by these variables. Often the resolution of
conflict is a matter of acquiring new information so that the
perceiver can reorganize his perception and come to an understanding of his situation.
   The hypothesis that the association of pain with anxiety
(emotional arousal) is due to the disrupting effects of a sudden
nociceptive sensory barrage on attention rather than to an intrinsic
reflexive response within the limbic system or autonomic nervous
system is not widely held among pain theorists. Nonetheless, this
concept provides a basis for explaining the dramatic differences in
response to injury that so often puzzle health care professionals.
It suggests that pain problems can be effectively managed in some
settings by properly preparing patients in advance for expected
encounters with pain sensations. Such preparation prevents uncertainty and surprise when noxious events are experienced and perceptual disruption is minimized. The instructions given Chinese
patients before acupuncture analgesia surgery and the intraoperative

coaching almost certainly play a role in the success of the acupuncture treatment (1).

The ability of many parturients to undergo labor and delivery gracefully and without significant suffering after attending classes in natural childbirth also illustrates this principle (61, 67). The sensations and the sequences of events experienced are well known and can be taught in detail, together with coping skills, to the patient. The result of such preparation is that the novelty and uncertainty inherent in the situation is reduced to a minimum. The configurations of sensory information from muscle contraction and tissue stress or damage are not altered by the educational process, but prophylaxis has occurred inasmuch as these signals no longer generate intense aversive emotional arousal.

There is substantial literature on the control of anxiety during recovery from surgery (11, 28, 57). Psychological preparation, the provision of information, and familiarity with the environment can markedly reduce both the severity of postoperative anxiety and pain as well as the time of convalescence. One explanation for the benefits of psychological preparation is that it allows the patient to maximize his coping skills, and it reduces the surprise and uncertainty associated with both the procedures and the sensations.

The perceptual disruption hypothesis also accounts for the ubiquitous observation (65) that patients with chronic pain have relatively low anxiety levels. When pain has persisted for months or years, the experience has become devoid of novelty, surprise, and uncertainty. In many cases, the pain becomes the center of attentional focus around which everything else in the patient's life is organized. A stark contrast may be observed in most patients with persistent pain who have been given a diagnosis of cancer. Any change in the pain or the appearance of pain in a new area of the body may generate intense emotional arousal, because it may signal metastatic progression of the disease.

In some instances, recurrent bouts of pain may reliably trigger emotional arousal even though the experience is all too familiar to the patient. This occurs when the pain may signal an acute life threatening event. Many heart disease patients with angina pectoris repeatedly experience high anxiety with each successive onset of retrosternal pain because such pain may herald a fatal heart attack. In this case the uncertainty about survival associated with the pain generates anxiety (12).

CENTRAL PROCESSING

Central perceptual organization processes cannot be discussed in detail apart from consideration of the numerous theories of perception. Historically, the field has been characterized by both the parallel and successive development of numerous theories of perceptual processes. Nevertheless, all perceptual theories have a great deal in common and are not as different in basic concept as one might suppose. Recently, Avant and Helson (6) noted, "That various approaches to perception have much in common is a sign of the maturity and the scientific character of the theories, for the more advanced a science is, the more do the pieces it studies hang together."

The following discussion is an attempt to present the most basic constructs from theory on central organizational processes that repeatedly appear in the various theoretical frameworks, and to relate them to pain. In most instances, the concepts are developed in the least technical language, although any of several different sets of descriptive terms taken from different theories might have sufficed. The concept of figure-ground derived from Gestalt Psychology, for example, could also be described in terms of signal-noise (Signal Detection Theory) or information-uncertainty (Information Theory). An excellent review of the various perceptual theories has been provided by Avant and Helson (6) and the evolution of thinking in this field has been recounted by Wertheimer (69).

Figure-Ground Phenomena

Perceptual Field: During normal waking behavior the perceiver is actively scanning his perceptual field. The field consists of 1) the immediate external physical and social environment, 2) the immediate internal somatic environment, and 3) imagination processes that involve, in addition to imagery, both memory and expectancies. Only information that is relevant is of interest to the perceiver. This relevancy is determined in three ways. It includes:

1. That which meets some immediate personal need. Such needs may be basic such as hunger and thirst, and relief from boredom, or the needs may be psychological, such as dependency or affiliational needs, or they may even be social needs such as status recognition. Fundamentally, the perceiver is interested in that which is of immediate value in negotiating with the physical and social environment.

2. That which will help achieve a future goal. This is an abstract process, but the perceiver is concerned with environmental objects, social contacts, or even somatic symptoms that will be of use in attaining some goal in the future. For example, if a patient is contemplating litigation or hoping to get compensation for on-the-job injury, any kind of physical symptom suddenly becomes very important to him.

3. That which warns of or indicates the presence of threat or harm. This involves not only environmental warning

signals but also any of the warning signal systems in the somatic environment such as pain, nausea, itch, or vertigo.

There is a continual fluid change inherent in the scanning process, although focus of perception may remain relatively fixed for long periods on a highly complex exteroceptive stimulus sequence such as television, a movie, a musical piece, or during intense physical activity such as participation in an athletic event. The emergence of one configuration of sensory messages and the concomitant receding of others into the background is termed the figure-ground phenomenon.

Perceptual Units: Gestalt psychologists contended that perceptual experience consisted of a series of highly organized configuration units, called Gestalten, each of which was characterized by a figure-ground structure. Moment-to-moment experience was thought to involve scanning processes that led to a blending of one Gestalt into another. Because the concept of organization extended beyond perception and into all aspects of psychology, the configurationists conceived of each gestalt unit as a part of a larger organized Gestalt of meaning and mental function. Certain disorders of fluid figure-ground functioning are well known as syndromes of psychopathology: e.g., obsessive-compulsive behavior, thought rumination, phobia, and hypochondriasis. Such pathologic states occur when perceptual organization is limited by habit to certain rigid structures.

As mentioned previously, nociceptive sensory input and other aversive sensations in the body often have the ability to dominate the perceptual field, particularly if they are characterized by surprise, novelty, or uncertainty. Typically, perforation of a duodenal ulcer results in an intense pain that emerges as figure with everything else in the patient's surroundings being forced into the background. In contrast, however, a tension headache may gradually and insidiously develop, emerging from the background to dominate perceptual processess only when it has become exceedingly intense. In many instances, common headaches reach only a light or moderate intensity and are generally ignored by the perceiver while he is active. Notice is taken of the presence of pain only when the individual has a few moments in a quiet environment.

Hypnosis and Figure-Ground Transition: There are certain psychological mechanisms that may be employed to control the figure-ground transitions associated with the experience of pain. Hypnotic suggestion is a form of social control of the perceiver's figure-ground functioning so that the process becomes rigidly exclusive of perceptual organizations in which pain is the figure. This kind of control can be achieved only in certain suggestible individuals (43) and it works reliably only in limited circumstances. Barber (8) extensively reviewed both clinical and experimental evidence of hypnotic analgesia and concluded that the "pain experience is at times reduced but is rarely, if ever, abolished (8, p. 328). While hypnosis can be used to control the pain of surgery when minor procedures are carried out and in cases where nature provides for muscular relaxation (for example, caesarian section), these procedures do not work well where profound muscular relaxation is necessary (50).

Hypnosis can be used in the management of chronic pain states and for pain associated with terminal disease since it provides a technique for the re-interpretation of the pain experience, time distortion, control of emotional response, or displacement of pain (43), but it is rarely, if ever, successful in the direct abolition of chronic pain.

It seems clear from a number of studies and reviews of the literature that hypnosis does not involve an actual loss in sensory function (8, 42, 44, 48). Blood pressure remains elevated during testing under hypnotic analgesia as it does during the normal experience of pain and this suggests that the patient is undergoing nociceptive stimulation at some level of awareness. Hypnotic subjects engaging in automatic writings or other dissociative procedures while undergoing a cold pressor test may assert verbally that they are comfortable while they write "it hurts" with the dissociated hand. This "hidden pain" phenomenon (43) suggests that there is a rigid figure-ground limitation imposed on the hypnotic subject so that pain is experienced only in the background of the perceptual field and never as the figure.

The distinction between overt and covert pain experiences made by Hilgard and Hilgard (43) parallels the figure-ground concept. In describing subjects from a cold pressor test experiment, who demonstrated both overt and covert pain during hypnotic analgesia, these authors commented that "the hidden pain was sensory pain of high intensity, but unaccompanied by suffering. After amnesia for the covert report was lifted, subjects commonly remembered what their covert reports were, but could not remember actually feeling the pain reported in that way" (43, p. 172). Thus, it seems useful to describe or interpret the phenomenon of hidden pain during hypnotic analgesia as a background pain that has been barred by the hypnotist from emerging into the foreground.

When the pain cannot emerge as the figure, it apparently does not provoke the emotional and aversive responses that one normally observes with patients in pain. The matter was nicely stated by one of the subjects in the experiment reported by Hilgard and Hilgard (43) "...when you are hypnotized, there are certain questions that just aren't answered, and you just don't probe them in your mind. I think you are aware that the pain exists, but it is not appropriate to deal with it just then." This observation is consistent with the previously presented hypothesis that pain normally generates arousal because of its disruptive effects on perception rather than because emotion is an intrinsic quality or component of the pain experience.

Perceptual Stability

A fundamental theme of all perceptual theories is that all perceptual experience tends toward stable organization. That is, sensory messages conveying information from the surrounding sources of stimulation are organized together with imagery and thought into a phenomenal whole or a configuration of sensory experience. The tendency to maintain stable patterns in perception ensures that potentially distorting or destructive influences in the environment will not break up perceptual continuity and thus compromise the safety or well-being of the perceiver. Licklider and Miller (51) studied the perception of human speech. They observed that peak clipping of the voice signal to as much as 94% of its original amplitude resulted in only a decline of 5% in the intelligibility of monosyllabic words. Many other examples of stability in visual and auditory modalities are available in introductory psychology texts. This tendency to perceive objects and events as stable, even when the energy delivered to receptor structures is severely altered, is called constancy. The constancy principle is responsible for protecting the integrity of perceptual configurations, or wholes, once they are experienced.

Perceptual Wholes: To perceive and react to wholes, or Gestalten, is more natural, easier, and occurs earlier than the perception of parts. Thus in visual experience, for example, one finds it easier to review an entire face as a pattern or configuration that is meaningful than to search and assemble all of the visual "parts" that make up the experience of the human face. By forcing the details of objects, events, imaginations, and somatic sensation into wholes, the perceiver is able to classify and categorize his experiences. He can accurately identify novelty, incongruity, threat, etc., so long as he can dismiss most of the things in the perceptual field as familiar or old. With stimuli forced into meaningful configurations, the perceiver can develop efficient strategies for dealing with a complex perceptual field.

How are perceptual wholes formed? In some cases, the parts of the stimulus array naturally go together to form certain configurations. In other cases, the past experiences of the perceiver determine on the basis of learning, the organization that will occur. In still other circumstances, the needs of the perceiver will lead him to organize ambiguous sensations into a meaningful whole that is relevant to the need.

Once perceptual wholes have been formed, they resist change. The strength of a whole depends on the redundancy of the information it contains. When the parts of the whole are highly redundant, the whole can be predicted from any part while poor or weak configurations are not predictable from any part (34). Good patterns or wholes are associated with fewer alternative configurations than are poor wholes and hence they are more unique.

<u>Closure and Perseverating Pain</u>:   Pattern perception research in
the exteroceptive modalities has repeatedly demonstrated that the
removal of certain parts from a strong whole does not necessarily
destroy it or necessitate perceptual restructuring. If a visual
circle is partly obliterated so that it becomes a continuous
curved line of dots, it will still be perceived as a circle. This
phenomenon is termed closure. Just how this tendency to maintain
stability of form affects the perceiving of interoceptive signals
is not developed in the literature.

Certain chronic pain syndromes seem to be problems of perception that are related to excessive stability of perceptual organi-
ization. At the University of Washington, referral pain clinic
patients who have had pain for many years are given a thorough
diagnostic testing. It is common for such patients to suffer with
pain that defies explanation on an organic basis. As part of the
diagnostic procedure, the patients receive a series of nerve blocks,
each with a different anesthetic agent or a saline placebo. Epi-
dural blocks of the spinal cord are often used, since this procedure leaves the patient insensitive to sensory impulses originating
below the neurologic segment where the block is given. The duration of anesthetic effect can be accurately predicted for each of
the drugs used. Interestingly, a significant number of patients
maintain their complaints of pain even when they have received a
spinal block that leaves them numb to pinprick or needle insertion
in the affected area. Thus, a patient who comes to the clinic
with an abdominal pain of ten years duration may complain that
the pain persists even when the block has made him completely numb
below the nipple line. Such phenomena can occur, according to the
organizational stability hypothesis, because nociceptive signals
are only a small part of the complex stimulus configuration that
the patient refers to when he complains of pain. If that part is
removed, closure occurs and the stimulus configuration is perceived as being unchanged. Other elements that frequently contribute to the complex stimulus constellations that give rise to
complaining and health care utilization in chronic pain patients
are loneliness, insomnia, a sense of helplessness and hopelessness,
and anger (13, 65).

<u>Body Integrity and Perceptual Reorganization</u>: When injury suddenly
occurs under normal conditions and a barrage of nociceptive input
is generated, ongoing perceptual configurations of body integrity
are broken down and a state of tension exists until a new perceptual whole is formed. As in other forms of perception, this may
require the addition of new information obtained through other
sense modalities such as vision, hearing, kinesthesia, etc. By
looking, posturing, and touching, the victim gains more information
about the injury, and this permits the restructuring of perception
so that the injury event is translated from confusion and surprise
into a meaningful, albeit unpleasant, configuration of experience.
Occasionally constancy, the tendency toward maintaining stability,
may be so strong that experience is reorganized into a sort of

compromise configuration that does not veridically represent the environment, and an illusion is created. This process is easily demonstrated and well investigated in the field of vision, but almost nothing is known about the way in which individuals organize perceptual experience that is dominated by pain.

The perceptual reorganization hypothesis has been used to explain the occurrence of phantom limb pain (31, 54), a peculiar syndrome that occasionally appears in patients who have suffered the loss of a limb due to trauma or surgical amputation. It is common for most amputees to briefly experience sensations that suggest that the limb is still present. After surgery, some still believe that they have the limb until they observe the stump (29). Initially, the illusory limb seems to be identical in size and shape to the original, but with the passage of time it tends to shrink and it usually disappears. In a small percentage of patients, the phantom part persists and becomes excruciatingly painful, and sometimes the phantom hand or foot seems to be contorted into a bizzare position. Finneson (31) has suggested that the patient possesses a persisting concept of total body image, and that he tends to perceive his body, like other objects, as a complete unit. For the amputee, the perceptual organization of bodily integrity is so stable that it resists change even though visual and proprioceptive information necessitate perceptual reorganization. Pain in the phantom limb could be interpreted as a symptom of the tension created by the incongruity of the new information with the old perceptual whole.

Figure-Ground Among Perceptual Units

Influence of Context: Gestalt psychologists were the first to emphasize the unique importance of organizational factors in perception. Indeed, for them such factors determined all aspects of behavior. In specifying Gestalten as segregated configurations of perceptual experience, they conceptualized each unit of perception as an organized figure-ground phenomenon that takes place against the background of a broader perceptual and cognitive organization. Each Gestalt must necessarily depend to some extent on the perceptual context in which it occurs and on the internal norms for perception that have developed with a lifetime of learning experiences.

The way in which past experience and stimulus context affect perception is crucial to an understanding of pain. Cultural differences in response to injury and intra-individual differences in pain behavior in varying social contexts are among the most fascinating curiosities in the area of pain research. Common clinical observations support the assertion that pain differs as the context changes. It is often noted, for example, that pain is less noticeable in physically active patients, that pain problems seem most intense at night and that masking stimulation such as white noise or superficial electrical stimulation can relieve the annoyance of a painful condition.

Adaptation Level: Adaptation Level Theory was developed by Helson
(41) to account for the influence of context on the perception of
objects. Because persisting pain is primarily interoceptive
rather than exteroceptive, the model does not fit smoothly when
it is extended to nociception. Nonetheless, the principles which
it encompasses are of value for pain research.

Helson (41) asserted that the judgment of a stimulus depended
on a process termed adaptation level (AL) that is a product of
three factors: the focal stimulus, the background or contextual
stimuli and residual stimuli (those factors not accounted for by
focus or background, such as reflectance). The AL was construed
as the weighted log mean of the three factors. The model accounts
for the common observation that a given stimulus is perceived
differently by people with different backgrounds of prior experience and by the same individual in two different contexts. Both
context effects and anchor effects have been demonstrated in a
variety of perceptual modalities. The latter refers to the biases
in judgment induced by a stimulus that serves as a standard for
other test stimuli.

A potential problem is foreseeable for the application of AL
methods to pain research. Pain results from activation of both
warning system structures (first pain) and reminder system structures (second pain), as described previously. While the former
perceptual experiences may well conform to the AL model, the
latter probably do not. Price et al. (60) recently compared and
contrasted first pain and second pain phenomena. Repetition of
noxious heat stimulation in human subjects led to disappearance of
first pain but second pain appeared to summate, even when the
stimulation location of the contact thermode was changed. Since
an increase in intensity and expanded localization may occur when
second pain is repeatedly evoked, this sense modality differs
significantly from the exteroceptive senses for which the AL model
was developed. Because most pathologic pain problems involve
primarily second pain, strict application of AL constructs may be
only partly successful in accounting for pain phenomena.

Illusions and Context

Illusions and Metastability: Study of perceptual illusions suggests
that background and context can actually distort the perception of
stimuli. For example, small objects feel much heavier than larger
objects with the same weight when they are presented together.
Gregory (37) describes how a large can and a small can of equal
weight will seem different to a perceiver lifting each of them.
The small can will feel up to fifty percent heavier. In this case,
the visual input alters the weight judgment that normally involves
both pressure and muscle senses. He states, " I believe all systematic distortion illusions are essentially similar to this
size-weight illusion."

Gregory (37) goes on to present and describe a series of
visual illusions in which the perceived size or shape of an object

is systematically distorted by the visual background against which it appears. For example, two rectangles identical in size look distinctly unequal if they are superimposed on a photograph of converging railroad tracks. By varying the background, it can be shown that perspective creates visual distortions. In concluding his article, Gregory notes that such illusions of distortion should be expected to arise in any effective perceptual system because they occur as imperfect solutions to the problems faced by a data handling system dealing with ambiguous sources of information. The extent to which sensory background alters veridical perception of tissue damage has never been systematically explored.

Illusions and Metastability: Many well known illusions seem unrelated to background. Geldard (35) emphasized that the experience of illusion is very general and that it intervenes on all agents of perception, and in all sense modalities. He stated, "The frequency with which illusion is upon us is not ordinarily appreciated. Indeed, one cannot go far into the study of human perception without making the important discovery that illusion, not veridicality, is the rule. All sense channels are normally subject to illusion, both with respect to time and space" (35, p. 16). In describing a cutaneous movement illusion created by applying several vibration sources to the skin (possibly another example of sensory summation), Geldard introduced the concept of perceptual metastability which refers to the tendency of a sense modality to systematically distort reality in its representation of the environment. He contended that certain cutaneous senses, such as touch, show less perceptual stability in function than do vision and hearing, although metastability can be observed in all modalities. Those senses characterized by low relative stability in their representation of stimuli were termed metastable by Geldard. While he did not discuss pain in this context, the summation phenomenon described by Price et al. (60) indicates that pain has metastable characteristics. Numerous clinical phenomena also lend evidence to this conclusion.

Referred pain phenomena illustrate the metastability of pain. Noxious sensory impulses arising in visceral or other deep tissue structures may give rise to an experience of pain in superficial areas of the body, sometimes in locations quite removed from the diseased organ. Angina pectoris, for example, originates from the ischemia of cardiac tissue but it is commonly felt in the chest and in a thin strip along the volar surface of the left arm. In some patients it is manifested as throat or shoulder pain. The ache associated with gall bladder disease is commonly experienced at the shoulder tip. Stimulation of the central zone of the diaphragmatic pleura is typically referred to the shoulder and neck. Labor pain is often felt in the sacral and lumbar areas of the back. In addition to visceral structures, joints and teeth may also give rise to referred pain. Temporo-mandibular joint disorders may generate peculiar patterns of temporal headache, and dental disease may similarly give rise to pain localized in the face, eyes, or head. These few common clinical examples illustrate that substantial distortions in spatial location of sites of pathology do occur in the perceptual process of pain.

Frank hallucination can occur in association with migraine headache, and such experiences extend into visual perception as well as certain other modalities such as taste. Migraine victims often report seeing peculiar angular visual patterns during the prodroma preceding the headache. Bright colors often characterize a "castle fortification" visual pattern. Normal vision is disturbed and objects may appear to be missing parts so that a traffic "stop" sign may be missing its "o". These phenomena suggest that the headache itself may be in part a hallucinogenic experience. Indeed, the relationship of the pain to tissue stress or damage cannot be specified, nor is it known whether any tissue stress actually exists. Bakal (7), after reviewing the physiological evidence on migraine headache, concluded that the pain is generally associated with hyper-responsivity of the cranial vasculature and instability of the autonomic nervous system. However, these are correlated response patterns rather than causes.

The term "migraine" is sometimes used by physicians in a less than formal manner in diagnosis of abdominal or pelvic pain that defies explanation. Patients sometimes present with an intense, incapacitating pelvic pain that seems analogous to a migraine headache, and like the headache it seems to bear no relationship to disease. Such phenomena have never been studied in the context of perceptual psychology, but the data and clinical observations available suggest that such problems may be related to disorders of perceptual mechanisms.

PERCEPTION AND MEASUREMENT

The technology of measuring perceptual processes in man is that of psychophysics. Psychophysical methods have been employed to study virtually all sensory modalities, and pain researchers have used them extensively in laboratory studies of human subjects. Classical methods have been reviewed by Wolff in another chapter of this book and they will not be detailed here. In brief, the traditional approach to measuring pain has involved pain threshold estimation and related subjective judgment procedures. In recent years, however, some investigators have advocated the use of an alternative methodology, Sensory Decision Theory (SDT) for laboratory pain research. The purpose of the following material is to introduce, broadly overview, and describe SDT methodology for pain research. In addition, a brief review of selective literature using this approach will be presented.

Basic Similarities and Differences Between Classical and SDT Models

Broad Communalities: One common ground shared by classical psychophysics and SDT is that both camps construe perceptual experiences as unobservable phenomena of human consciousness that cannot be directly measured. Perceptual experiences can only be inferred from some form of behavioral or physiological response that implies the existence of subjective awareness, e.g., a verbal report, a withdrawal motor response, an increase in heart rate.

A second communality that both threshold researchers and SDT investigators share is the assumption that perceptual abilities can best be evaluated by studying detection and discrimination. Detection tasks involve the identification of a faint stimulus intensity presented against a background of no stimulation (sometimes considered a background of internal noise), i.e. in contrast to blank trials. By establishing the detectability of a stimulus for a subject, the investigator defines the sensitivity of the sensory system for that individual. In pain research, specification of the sensitivity of the subject to nociceptive input provides a measure of sensitivity to painful events.

Discrimination of two intensities of stimulation is also an initial measure of perception, since it reflects the subject's information processing capabilities. While detection measures indicate the level of stimulation at which sensory processing can occur, discrimination indices reveal how well the perceiver can process sensory input. Perception is best appraised by examination of both detection and discrimination performances.

Broad Differences: The fundamental difference between classical psychophysics and SDT may be described as a difference in research paradigms (i.e., implicit conceptual schemes on which the models are based). Paradigms tend to be implicit rather than formally articulated (49) and it may be useful to construe the paradigm differences here in terms commonly used in experimental psychology. By drawing a parallel between these two paradigms in the field of perception and a classical distinction evident in the history of human learning research, one could describe classical psychophysics as an S-R (stimulus-response) paradigm and SDT as an S-O-R (stimulus-observer-response) paradigm. The S-R conceptualization in psychophysics is based on the assumption that a stimulus (S) delivered to a receptive field will give rise to a response (R) that provides a reasonably accurate estimate of the sensation experienced, so that $R=f(S)$. This paradigm is still influential since the magnitude estimation procedures of Steven's Power Law scaling (66) are based on this assumption. It is assumed in the S-R framework that a subjective report is a valid and accurate indicator of the information processed by the subject. All work on pain threshold could be classified as S-R research.

In contrast, the S-O-R paradigm stresses the role of the observer, as a modulator in the data collection sequence. Before the stimulus gives rise to a response, the observer must process the input through the attentional filter and central organizational mechanisms before making a decision about what response he will give. That decision will be determined in part by the sensory input he receives, but, in addition, his perceptual habits, beliefs, expectations, potential costs and rewards, and memory of previous events will also control his decision. The O factor is broadly conceptualized, taken into account, and actually measured in SDT procedures, whereas it often contaminates measurement in S-R research.

The SDT paradigm accounts for the O factor by postulating that a decision process is an intrinsic part of the perceptual experience leading to a response. The nature of this process is, of course, determined partly by the restrictions and rules established in the social context of the experiment (e.g., subjects may be asked to judge the intensity of a stimulus or to give certainty ratings about the occurrence of a stimulus) as well as by the psychologic, social, or economic consequences of the decision. The SDT model can provide a measure to indicate whether a subject is conservative, fair, or liberal in labeling a stimulus intensity as painful.

Basic Principles of Sensory Decision Theory

SDT employs a probability theory model for perception that has proven useful for the study of several forms of human sensory function such as vision, audition, and olfaction. While the methodology of SDT differs from the more traditional measurement of sensory thresholds in several specific ways, the most significant difference is its emphasis on the importance of decision processes in perceptual report. It is assumed that an external event impinging on sensory organs generates an internal sensory signal that varies from trial to trial about some average value along a continuum of subjective intensity. This concept implies that the same event is experienced somewhat differently each time it is repeated, so that the perceiver must exercise some judgment in reporting detection of the event or in discriminating one intensity of a given event from another. It is assumed that he makes such judgments by employing one or more decision criteria. Internal sensory signals that exceed one of the criteria on the internal continuum are reported in one way, while those that fail to exceed it are reported in another.

The SDT framework defines the fundamental aspects of perception as sensory sensitivity, i.e. the ability of the perceiver to detect signals from the environment, and response bias or the way in which the perceiver locates his decision criteria along the internal continuum. This location may be conservative or liberal with regard to the number of errors in judgment that are made, and it reflects the motivational or attitudinal state of the perceiver.

A Synopsis of Sensory Decision Theory Methodology: In its classical form, SDT analysis was applied to data collected in a task where a perceiver judged the presence or absence of a weak signal in a background of noise; i.e., actual (noise plus signal) and blank (noise alone) trials were presented repeatedly in random order, and the perceiver guessed whether the signal had occurred after each presentation. The experimenter specified whether the perceiver's guesses were right or wrong; that is, a response was right if he correctly identified the signal when it was present, but wrong if he mistakenly called the noise trial a signal. Over many trials the rate of <u>correct</u> <u>positive</u> responses could be specified. This was termed hit rate (HR). Similarly, the rate of <u>erroneous</u> <u>positive</u> <u>guesses</u> over many trials was termed the false affirmative rate (FAR).

When HR and FAR have been examined over several conditions of an experiment, such as three types of instructions (e.g., "be conservative when guessing," "be moderate," or "be liberal and don't worry about mistakes"), it becomes evident that the rate of correct responses and the rate of errors are related. Green and Swets (36) have explained in detail how a plot of several sets of HR and FAR values yields a function that contains information about the subject's perceptual abilities as well as his response tendencies.

Statistically, it is possible to obtain two measures from the function that relates HR to FAR. The first, sensory sensitivity (generally symbolized as d'), indicates the ability of the subject to detect the difference between an actual stimulus and a blank trial or, alternatively, the intensity difference between two stimuli. The second reponse index is termed response bias. It reflects the willingness of the subject to make many false-affirmative responses in order to increase the number of hits, or, conversely, to decrease the number of hits in order to minimize false-affirmative errors. The response bias factor is statistically independent of d', and behaviorally it reflects the perceiver's attitude, expectancy, or strategy. Of course, bias changes may be functionally related to changes in d' since the experience of sensory analgesia may bias subjects to respond in certain ways in a study involving an analgesic agent. The basic SDT methodology has been extended to include the use of a rating scale for the subject's responses. The advantages of this procedure are 1) that the scale helps clarify the characteristic of the stimulus being judged for the subject (e.g., he can use it to judge the subjective intensity of a noxious stimulus), thus facilitating testing, and 2) all of the rating scale categories used by the subject, except for the lowest one, yield a pair of hit rate and false-affirmative rate values, so that the rating scale is an efficient way of establishing the function needed for estimation of d' and response bias. When rating scales are used, it sometimes seems inappropriate to designate certain responses as right and others as wrong, so the terms hit and false-affirmative often are, in the strictest sense, misnomers. Nonetheless, the calculations of d' and response bias are exactly the same as in classical experimental procedures. The plot which relates a set of hit rate values to false affirmative rate values over several conditions of an experiment is called a receiver operating characteristic (ROC). Figure 1 (40) presents the mean ROCs for a group of 10 elderly women and a group of 10 young women who were required to make rating judgments about each of two painful dental

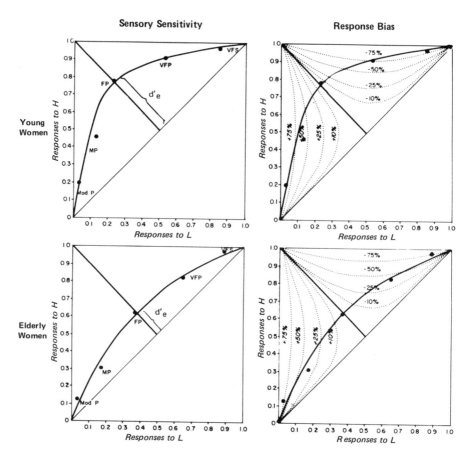

FIG. 1. Mean receiver operating characteristics (ROCs) representing the effect of age on d'$_e$ (left side) and per cent bias (right side) for young (top set) and elderly women (bottom set). These functions are a plot of the percentage of responses to the higher stimulus (ordinate), cumulated over the rating scale categories, and the percentage of responses to the lower stimulus (abscissa) cumulated in a similar manner.

stimuli. The greater the distance of the ROC is from the principal diagonal, the better the discrimination performance of the subjects. Here, young women performed significantly better than old women. Each of the plotted points is a rating scale category.

It is possible to estimate d' at each of the rating scale categories where the subject has provided both HR and FAR. The original formulation of Sensory Decision Theory holds that d' should be identical at each category, save for the random influences of measurement error. In reality, however, consistent tendencies for d' to be slightly higher at one end of the response scale than at the other are more often observed than not (36). A variety of statistical procedures are available which adjust quite adequately for this problem. These include a special way of calculating d', termed d'_e (36), averaging of d' across rating scale categories (22), and calculation of an overall d' with correction for systematic trends across scale categories (62). Substantial unsystematic variations in d' across rating scale categories for a subject indicate a poor quality of measurement.

Response bias can be scaled in several ways including likelihood ratio scores (36) which depend on the assumptions just discussed, Per Cent Bias measures which require very few assumptions (45) and Ingham's C Index (47) which conveniently scores response bias in the same units used to measure d'.

In applying SDT to pain, investigators have assumed that the fundamental building block of the pain experience is the ability of the individual to detect and process information about tissue injury or stress. It has further been assumed that analgesia is most pragmatically defined as an impairment of the ability of the perceiver to process nociceptive sensory information. SDT research thus focuses on the sensory-discriminative aspect of pain rather than on the total pain experience.

The report of pain given by a perceiver may be determined by his sensory ability, his motivational state, and his judgmental processes. The latter two variables are reflected in the location of the decision criterion, or the response bias, of the perceiver. Recently, Rollman (63) has criticized the application of SDT to pain research in the laboratory, and Chapman (14) has defended this practice. While SDT does not provide a perfect solution to the difficult problem of measuring pain, it is less likely to generate erroneous conclusions than other alternatives and it is the best way to approach laboratory pain problems.

Mathematical Models and Pain: While the pain experience is a complex phenomenon, it must be acknowledged that sensory input is the fundamental component of pain, and therefore a factor that needs to be measured.

Concomitant measurements of such variables as motivational drive, emotional arousal, and cognitive functioning can only be done very crudely, at best, with the tools available at present. Psychophysical models such as SDT offer sensory measurement with good precision but at the cost of oversimplification. Watson (68) has described the logic of the psychophysicist in the following terms:

"...the builders of mathematical models have approached psychophysics with an array of intentional oversimplifications, based on the idea that one way to make a terribly complex set of problems manageable is to define many of them out of existence, at least for the moment. What this may mean in practice is that a set of inputs to a system, which are multidimensional in character, and for which several of the dimensions have previously been shown to be individually systematically, related to behavior, are treated as though they are homogenous in their effects." (6B, p. 284)

Watson goes on to justify the use of mathematical models for perception.

"The advantages of such seemingly unrealistic restrictions are that the pared-down models can be completely described and comprehended by the model builder, and that as they are refined until they fit as well as possible (i.e., that they come as close to possible to describing the data from the relevant experimental procedure), they can tell us how much of the results <u>could</u> be accounted for by a simple system such as the one they postulate." (68, p. 285)

The investigator aspiring to measure human pain thus faces two choices. He may elect to assess pain in a global, relatively crude way, which gives him efficiency and convenience, but he must bear the frustration of lacking the precision so often necessary for critical progress. Alternatively, he may caricature pain by employing a psychophysical model that yields precise measures. Unfortunately, the model builder may operationalize pain in such a sterile manner that his results cannot be generalized to any practical issues.

As with other areas of science (49) mathematical modeling is characterized by a series of evolutionary and revolutionary changes. Progress in model development may be evaluated as improvement in approximation of naturally occurring events by reliable models. For pain, as for other modalities of perception, SDT provides a model that offers a limited approximation of the natural perceptual experience. However, for other types of perception SDT has proven to be a better model than its predecessor, the sensory threshold and evidence available to date suggests that it may well be the best model for pain research.

Application of SDT to Pain Research

SDT methods have been used for pain research in several laboratories. A thorough review of this area is not within the scope of this chapter, but the following material illustrates SDT application in the pain field.

Work by Others: Clark used SDT procedures to demonstrate that a placebo increased response bias against reporting pain, but that it had no effect on the detectability of painful stimuli (22). Clark and Mehl (25) compared perceptual performance in young adults and older (late middle age) individuals. They reported that young men had the same sensitivity to radiant heat stimuli as older men, but that older women showed a reduced sensitivity to pain. Complex differences in response bias among age and sex groups were also observed. Their results suggested that there are developmental changes in pain responsivity. Clark and Goodman (24) applied SDT to examine the effects of verbal suggestion on the perception of radiant heat pain, and they reported that suggestions did not affect sensitivity to painful stimulation although they did change the subject's pain reporting habits. Additional work by Clark and Dillon has provided information about basic procedural variables in SDT pain research (23).

Craig et al. (26, 27) used SDT in a study of the influence of social factors on pain perception. Applying painful cutaneous shocks to subjects, they studied the analgesic effects of a tolerant model, i.e., a confederate of the experimenter ostensibly undergoing the shock experiment in the presence of the subject. They found no response bias changes, but sensory sensitivity to pain was reduced in subjects who observed the model while experiencing pain themselves. Hall (38) carried out a series of studies using SDT procedures and addressed the issue of whether this methodology was suitable for pain research. He concluded that the research to date supported the claims made for the SDT approach and that criticisms had failed to refute these claims.

Work by Our Group: The following material delineates the application of SDT methods in our work over a period of several years. The narrative illustrates how such procedures can be employed in a systematic series of studies.

Our first study was concerned with determining whether changes in pain report induced by suggestion were sensory effects or attitudinal shifts in response bias. Feather, Chapman, and Fisher (30) studied the effects of a placebo, coupled with strong suggestion, on the perception of radiant heat pain in student nurses. A group of women was tested in an SDT task, once under control conditions and once following placebo ingestion. Sensory sensitivity to pain remained unchanged, but willingness to report pain decreased significantly with placebo treatment, thus illustrating that the placebo generated an attitudinal shift rather than a sensory change.

We were also intrigued by the reports of clinicians that diazepam had analgesic effects, since manufacturers of the drug claimed that it had no analgesic properties. Chapman and Feather (17) examined the effects of 10 mg diazepam on tolerance of tourniquet pain, as well as on state anxiety as evaluated by the State-Trait Anxiety Inventory. Using a double blind design, placebo and aspirin (600 mg) were compared with diazepam. The length of time subjects would bear the painful tourniquet was significantly increased by diazepam, and state anxiety was lower during pain tolerance testing when diazepam was administered. A second experiment in the same subjects using cutaneous radiant heat was analyzed using SDT. Diazepam had no effect on either sensory sensitivity to pain or response bias. It was concluded that the apparent analgesic properties of the drug, i.e., its ability to increase pain tolerance, were due to its effects on the motivational-emotional dimension of pain, and that it had no effect on the sensory-discriminative dimension.

In another study, Chapman and Feather (18) examined the effects of painful electric shock delivered in a classical conditioning paradigm on the perception of a visual stimulus. Subjects receiving conditioning showed a significant increase in sensory sensitivity to the visual stimulus although volunteers subjected to the same number of shocks delivered in a sham-conditioning situation and subjects tested on the same number of trials as controls, but with no shocks, showed no changes. This study suggested that painful experiences may affect perception in other sensory modalities via conditioning.

To further determine whether the SDT model was useful for evaluating drug-induced analgesia, we decided to test a well-known pharmacological agent. The effects of 33% nitrous oxide were studied by Chapman, Murphy, and Butler (20) in order to determine whether this clinically-proven analgesic drug could significantly reduce sensory sensitivity to pain. Comparing SDT measures of response to radiant heat pain under control and gas inhalation conditions, we observed a significant decrease in sensitivity to pain with treatment and a concomitant increase in response bias against reporting the stimuli as painful (i.e., an attitude shift).

After these radiant heat studies, we attempted to develop a better laboratory dolorimetric model. We can now produce a graded pain sensation by electrical stimulation of the human tooth pulp. Using tooth pulp dolorimetry, Chapman, Gehrig, and Wilson (19) replicated the observation of sensory analgesia with 33% nitrous oxide in a study that compared the inhalation analgesic with acupunctural stimulation. Interestingly, a significant reduction in sensory sensitivity to pain was also observed in the acupuncture subjects. Both groups showed significant changes in response bias (willingness to report the dental shocks as painful) as well.

To confirm the observation of acupunctural analgesia, Chapman, Wilson, and Gehrig (21) replicated the finding of reduced sensory sensitivity to painful dental shock after acupuncture stimulation at a classical Oriental medicine treatment site (Hoku) on the hands. In addition, we stimulated the same site in other subjects with a surface electrode and carried out acupuncture in other volunteers at a point on the hands that is unrecognized in Oriental medicine (i.e., placebo acupuncture). We observed that the surface electrode had the same effects as the penetrating needle (both modalities delivered strong, pulsing electrical stimulation at 2 Hz), but those stimulated at a non-acupuncture point showed no effects. Changes in response bias did not occur in the placebo group because they were not given any special instructions. Such changes were observed in the two treatment groups.

The only other laboratory doing extensive work on the effects of acupuncture and transcutaneous electrical stimulation on pain evoked from tooth pulp stimulation is that headed by Andersson in

Sweden (4, 5, 46). Their investigations have used threshold measures, and they have stimulated facial acupuncture points (i.e., sites in the same neurologic segment as the teeth) to demonstrate a strong acupuncture effect. Chapman, Chen, and Bonica (16) attempted a replication of their threshold findings using SDT procedures to determine whether the threshold increase was due primarily to reduced sensory sensitivity to dental stimulation or to attitudinal changes in the subjects such as those associated with a placebo effect. We observed a remarkable fit of our findings to the Swedish data. SDT measures indicated that a profound level of analgesia did indeed occur, such that sensory sensitivity changed significantly (and substantially) with treatment, while response bias did not. Interestingly, subjects demonstrated that they could accurately detect stimuli below the sensory threshold during acupuncture analgesia. This observation suggested that sensory threshold is not an adequate form of measurement for acupuncture analgesia.

We have also been interested in collecting basic normative data to support our laboratory pain model. Harkins and Chapman (39) compared old and young men with regard to their abilities to discriminate between painful signals. Using dental dolorimetry, post-retirement men performed the same task as a group of college students. The results indicated that the perceptual discrimination performance of older men (as assessed by the sensory sensitivity measure) was inferior to that of the younger ones. However, ability to detect painful stimulation (threshold) was the same for the two groups. This study suggested that older people have greater difficulty judging the differential strength of painful signals than younger people.

To further examine individual differences in ability to perceive noxious input, we replicated and extended our normative investigations to include young and elderly women (40). Threshold and nociceptive discrimination were evaluated in 20 healthy women ranging in age from 20–84. A significant age effect was observed for d' but not for detection thresholds. This observation replicated the earlier study by Harkins and Chapman. A failure to observe an effect of age on threshold for noxious dental stimulation is at variance with research by others employing radiant heat dolorimetry. This suggests that laboratory dental pain is a different phenomenon than cutaneous radiant heat pain, and it stresses the importance of cross modal studies of various laboratory induced pain experiences within the same subjects.

Chapman and Butler (15) used SDT methodology to evaluate the effect of doxepin, a tricyclic antidepressant, on the perception of pain. Since we have observed that most patients in our chronic pain clinic who are treated with tricyclic antidepressants show a positive response, and that most of the individuals show such a response within one week after treatment, we hypothesized that tricyclic agents may have analgesic properties. We divided 18 subjects into two groups of nine each. Half the subjects received doxepin for one month while the other half received a visually

identical placebo under double blind conditions. Subjects were
tested at baseline and again three different times for a one month
period. Measures consisted of d' and response bias from a SDT
task and a variety of psychometric measures. We observed that
the drug had no significant effect on ability to perceive painful
dental shocks in the laboratory, but there was a dramatic change
in response bias following ingestion of the drug or the placebo in
all subjects and this high level of response bias was maintained
until the end of the study. This finding suggests that the good
effects of the drug may be due in part to placebo effect and may
be linked with the instructions given at the time the drug is
prescribed for the patient. We noted that the drug may be beneficial for chronic pain patients because it relieves disturbed
sleeping patterns and has other beneficial side effects even
though it does not alleviate pain and it is effective too early
to be a true antidepressant therapy.

SUMMARY

A review of the literature on the peripheral mechanisms subserving perception of painful events suggests that there are two
kinds of nociceptors. The first contributes information about
harmful environmental stimuli while the other informs the brain
about the disturbed well-being of body tissues. When these
structures are viewed in relation to their central transmission
pathways, and behavioral data are integrated with these observations,
it appears that there are two kinds of pain: that which serves as
an injury warning system and that which functions as an injury
reminding system. The warning system indicates immediate tissue
damage and serves to provoke the organism into escape or avoidance responses. The reminding system, in contrast, provides an
ongoing source of information about tissues that are stressed or
injured. This can be used by the organism to guard injured areas
from further stress and to avoid behaviors that would be maladaptive
during injury.

Except in the laboratory of the physiologist, nociceptors are
virtually never stimulated singly. Natural injury always involves
the activation of several receptor cell populations, both nociceptive and non-nociceptive, in a broad receptive field. The sensory
messages that provide the basis of pain are thus more than simple
indicators of stimulus energy. Complex patterns of information
with potentially infinite variety routinely result from tissue
damage.

When a barrage of noxious sensory impulses has been generated
by tissue injury or stress, transmission of these impulses may be
altered by attentional filtering at higher central levels in the
neuraxis. Such filtering may reduce or amplify the perceived
intensity of the painful stimulation. In some instances where pain
is chronic, patients develop perceptual habits of attending closely
to somatic signals while partially ignoring events in the physical
and social environments.

The relationship between tissue damage, as detected by certain classes of receptors, and emotional-motivational arousal has long been considered reflexive. However, recent perceptual research strongly suggests that emotion is not an intrinsic characteristic of the pain experience, but rather a correlate that emerges when ongoing perceptual routines are disrupted by the occurrence of pain. The literature on psychologic control of acute pain states indicates that perceptual disruption can be minimized by prophylactic counseling and teaching of patients in critical situations where pain is likely to be experienced. When such controls are employed, pain behavior is reduced and patients show much lower levels of arousal during tissue injury or stress.

At higher levels of perceptual functioning, pain is experienced as a configuration or Gestalt of sensory events rather than as a simple sensation. That is, perception occurs in natural units that may be described as perceptual "wholes." Experiences of pain stand out against the background of other experiences, and this can be usefully construed as a figure-ground relationship.

The figure-ground organization of pain experiences tends toward stability when pain becomes familiar and is accepted as part of the normal perceptual routine. For chronic pain patients the tendency toward stability in experience is quite strong, and the pain tends to resist therapeutic interventions that would threaten the familiar, albeit unpleasant, perceptual experience. Research on the stability of perceptual wholes suggest that patterns of sensory experience are maintained even when certain elements are withdrawn from the patterns. This provides a hypothesis for explaining the perseveration of chronic pain states in patients subjected to nerve blocks or other therapies that remove or block the pathways noxious information transmission.

In considering perceptual organization it is necessary to remember that pain always occurs against a background of other experiences or in the context of other experiences. As in other senses, contextual changes can generate illusions in perception, and this tendency toward illusion can play a major role in pain. Furthermore, pain is characterized by high metastability; i.e., the phenomenon often bears a poor relationship to energy changes in environmental events. The relationship of tissue-damaging events to the intensity, duration, and localization of pain experiences is poor especially for pain of visceral origin. Distortions in perception and illusions are further engendered by personality and cultural factors, which have not been discussed because they are beyond the scope of this paper.

Current methodologies for quantifying perceptual abilities are termed psychophysical procedures. These methods focus on detection and discrimination abilities, relying on verbal report or subjective judgment. Psychophysical methods are examples of the intentional oversimplification of perceptual processes, since they reduce complex issues of perception to laboratory measures of detection and discrimination. Sensory Decision Theory has recently been applied in psychophysical pain research. This approach appears to yield more information and more precise measurement than traditional threshold estimation.

Pain has not been previously examined within the framework of perceptual psychology, but it seems clear that perceptual psychologists can make significant contributions to the pain field and that, conversely, pain may provide many fascinating phenomena that will help to further progress in the field of perceptual psychology.

REFERENCES

1. Acupuncture Anesthesia in the People's Republic of China. (A trip report of the American Acupuncture Anesthesia Study Group) National Academy of Sciences. Washington D.C., 1976.

2. Anderson, D.J. (1975): Brit. Med. Bull. 31:111-114, 1975.

3. Anderson D.J., Hannam, A.G. and Matthews, B. (1970): Phys. Rev. 50(2):171-195.

4. Andersson, S.A., Erickson, J., Holmgren, E. and Lindqvist, G. (1973): Brain Res. 63:393-396.

5. Andersson, S.A. and Holmgren, E. (1975): Amer. J. Chin. Med. 3(4):311-334.

6. Avant, L.L. and Helson, H. (1973): In: Handbook of General Psychology, edited by B.B. Wolman, 419-448, Prentice-Hall, Inc., New Jersey,

7. Bakal, D.A. (1975): Psych. Bull. 82(3):369-382.

8. Barber, T.X. (1963): Psychosom. Med. 25:303-333, 1963.

9. Benedetti, C., Chapman, C.R. and Bonica, J.J.: Pain and its modulation by endogenous and exogenous opioids: Implication for anesthesiology. (submitted).

10. Bonica, J.J. and Albe-Fessard, D. (1976): Advances in Pain Research and Therapy, Vol. 1, pp.v-vi, Raven Press, New York.

11. Bruegel, M. (1971): Nurs. Res. 20(1):26-31.

12. Chapman, C.R. (1976): Psychologic aspects of cardiac pain. Presented at the National Conference on Cardiac Pain. Sponsored by International Association for the Study of Pain. Henry Chauncey Center. Princeton, New Jersey.

13. Chapman, C.R. (1977): Arch. Surg. 112:767-772.

14. Chapman, C.R. (1977): Pain, 3:295-305.

15. Chapman, C.R. and Butler, S.H.: Pain, (in press).

16. Chapman, C.R., Chen, A.C., and Bonica, J.J. (1977): Pain, 3:213-227.

17. Chapman, C.R. and Feather, B.W. (1973): Psychosom. Med. 35(4):330-340.

18. Chapman, C.R. and Feather, B.W. (1972): J. Exp. Psychol. 93:338-342.

19. Chapman, C.R., Gehrig, J.D. and Wilson, M.E. (1975): Anesthesiology 42(5):532-537.

20. Chapman, C.R., Murphy, T.M. and Butler, S.H. (1973): Science, 179:1246-1248.

21. Chapman, C.R., Wilson, M.E. and Gehrig, J.D. (1976): Pain, 2(3):265-283.

22. Clark, W.C. (1969): J. Abnorm. Psychol. 74(3):363-371.
23. Clark, W.C. and Dillon, D.J. (1973): Perception and Psychophysics 13(3):491-493.
24. Clark, W.C. and Goodman, J.S. (1974): J. Abnorm. Psychol. 83(4):364-372.
25. Clark, W.C. and Mehl, L. (1971): J. Abnorm. Psychol. 78(2):202-212.
26. Craig, K.D. (1975): Pain, 1(4):375-378.
27. Craig, K.D. and Coren, S. (1975): J. Psychosom. Res. 19:105-112.
28. Dalrymple, D.G., Parbrook, G.D. and Steel, D.F. (1973): Brit. J. Anaesth. 45:589-598.
29. Dam, W. and Vive Larsen, J.J. (1974): In: Monographs in Anesthesiology: Relief of intractable pain, edited by M. Swerdlow, pp. 130-147, (Vol. 1), Exerpta Medica Foundation.
30. Feather, B.W., Chapman, C.R. and Fisher, S.B. (1972): Psychom. Med. 34:290-294.
31. Finneson, B.E. (1962): Diagnosis and Management of Pain Syndromes, Saunders, Philadelphia.
32. Fordyce, W.E. (1976): Behavioral Methods for Chronic Pain and Illness. The C.V. Mosby Company, Saint Louis.
33. Freeman, G.L. (1940): J. Exp. Psychol. 26:602-608.
34. Garner, W.R. (1970): Amer. Sci. 58:34-42.
35. Geldard, F.A. (1975): Sensory Saltation: Metastability in the Perceptual World, John Wiley & Sons, New York.
36. Green, D.M. and Swets, J.A. (1974): Signal Detection Theory and Psychophysics, Robert E. Kruger Publishing Company, New York.
37. Gregory, R.L. (1968): Sci. Am. 219(5):66-76.
38. Hall, W. (1977): Psychological processes in pain perception: the prospects of a signal detection theory analysis. Doctoral dissertation. University of New South Wales.
39. Harkins, S.W. and Chapman, C.R. (1976): Pain, 2(3):253-264.
40. Harkins, S.W. and Chapman, C.R. (1977): J. Gerontol. 32(4):428-435.
41. Helson, H. (1964): Adaptation-level Theory: An Experimental and Systematic Approach to Behavior. Harper & Row, New York.
42. Hilgard, E.R. (1971): Am. Sci. 59(5):567-577.
43. Hilgard, E.R. and Hilgard, J.R. (1975): Hypnosis in the Relief of Pain. William Kaufmann, Los Altos, California.
44. Hilgard, E.R., Ruch, J.C., Lange, A.F., Lenox, J.R., Morgan, A.H. and Sachs, R.B. (1974): Amer. J, Psychol. 87(1-2):17-31.
45. Hodos, W. (1970): Psychol. Bull. 74:351-354.
46. Holmgren, E. (1975): Effects of conditioning electrical stimulation on the perception of pain. Doctoral thesis. Dept. of Physiology. University of Göteborg; Göteborg, Sweden.
47. Ingham, J.G. (1970): Acta. Psychol. 34:39-50.
48. Knox, V.J., Morgan, A.H., and Hilgard, E.R. (1974): Arch. Gen. Psychiatry. 30:840-847.

49. Kuhn, T.S. (1962): The Structure of Scientific Revolutions. The University of Chicago Press, Chicago.
50. Lassner, J. (1967): Hypnosis and Psychosomatic Medicine. Proceedings from the International Congress for Hypnosis and Psychosomatic Med. Springer-Verlag, Berlin.
51. Licklider, J.C.R. and Miller, G.A. (1951): In: Handbook Handbook of Experimental Psychology, edited by S. S. Stevens, pp. 1040-1074, Wiley, New York.
52. Mackworth, N.H. (1950): Medical Research Council. Special Report No. 268, London: H.M. Stationery Office.
53. Mandler, G. (1975): Mind and Emotion. John Wiley & Sons, Inc., New York.
54. Melzack, R. (1971): Anesthesiology 35(4):409-419.
55. Melzack, R. and Wall, P.D. (1965): Science, 150(3699): 971-979.
56. Mumford, J.D. and Bowsher, D. (1976): Pain, 2(3):223-243.
57. Parbrook, G.D., Steel, D.F., Dalrymple, D.G. (1973): Brit. J. Anaesth., 45:21-32.
58. Pilowsky, I. (1967): Brit. J. Psychiat. 113:89-93.
59. Pilowsky, I. (1970): Acta. Psychiatr. Scand. 46:273-285.
60. Price, D.D., Hu, J.W., Dubner, R. and Gracely, R.H. (1977): Pain, 3(1):57-68.
61. Read, G.D. (1955): The Natural Childbirth Primer. Harper and Brothers, New York.
62. Richards, B.L. and Thornton, C.L. (1970): Education and Psychological Measurement. 30:885-889.
63. Rollman, G.B. (1977): Pain, 3:187-211.
64. Ruch, J.C. and Patton, H.D. editors (1965): Physiology and Biophysics. W.B. Saunders, Philadelphia.
65. Sternbach, R.A. (1974): Pain Patients-Traits and Treatment Academic Press, New York.
66. Stevens, S.S. (1975): Psychophysics, John Wiley & Sons, New York.
67. Vellay, P. (1960): Childbirth without Pain. E.P. Dutton & Company, Inc, New York.
68. Watson, C.S. (1973): In: Handbook of General Psychology, edited by B.B. Wolman, Englewood Cliffs, N.J.: Prentice-Hall.
69. Wertheimer, M. (1974): In: Handbook of Perception. Vol. 1 edited by E.C. Carterette and M.P. Friedman, pp. 75-91, Academic Press, New York.

The Psychology of Pain, edited by R. A. Sternbach.
Raven Press, New York © 1978.

Psychodynamic Aspects of the Pain Experience

I. Pilowsky

The University of Adelaide, Department of Psychiatry, Royal Adelaide Hospital, Adelaide, South Australia, 5000

Although pain was a prominent feature of the clinical pictures described in Freud and Breuer's "Studies on Hysteria" (14) relatively scant attention was paid by Freud to the subject thereafter. Considering how central a role pain plays in human existence it is somewhat surprising that the topic was neglected in this way. Engel (10) has suggested that this was due to the changing nature of Freud's clinical practice, as he became less a neurologist and more an analyst. Be that as it may, it would patently be foolish to hope to understand so complex a phenomenon as pain without taking into account its interaction with the total personality, and the psychodynamic approach is particularly suited to this task, since it views the individual as a psychobiological system in which innate and environmental forces interact, compete and must be reconciled in the interests of adaptive functioning. Furthermore, it postulates that an individual's personality is shaped from birth by repeated attempts to reconcile inner drives with environmental realities so that innate and acquired needs may be satisfied.

Since psychodynamic theory has its origins in psychoanalysis it is useful to review briefly the major domains of psychoanalytic theory. These "domains" are essentially paradigms which complement each other but differ in their utility for clinical or research objectives, depending on the population under consideration and the particular dimension of behavior which is the focus of interest. Taken together, these paradigms of human behavior and mental life constitute the *psychoanalytic metapsychology*, and include the topographic, structural, dynamic, genetic-developmental, adaptive and cultural schemata.

The *topographic* view emphasises the existence of both conscious and unconscious mental life and holds that behavior is controlled and shaped to a large extent by motives of which the individual is not consciously aware. The *structural* view describes a model of personality involving relatively stable psychological systems which constitute the internal representations of forces and objects that shape and modulate the organism's behavior. These systems are named the id, ego and superego and relate to instinctual forces, integrating functions and internalized value systems respectively.

The *dynamic* approach emphasizes the interplay between "psychic" energies derived from basic drives and other needs. It focuses particularly on the instinctual influences on behavior. This view is complemented by the *economic* approach which stresses the organism's attempts to achieve satisfactions with the least possible expenditure of psychic energy.

The *genetic* paradigm describes the orderly unfolding of personality through a series of biologically determined, developmental stages, and the influences of the individual's successful or unsuccessful passage through these critical oral, anal and phallic periods on the ultimate personality configuration.

The *adaptive view* emphasizes the demands of the environment and delineates the strategies and styles used in coping with them. Finally, the psychosocial or *cultural* approach stresses the part played by social and cultural factors in shaping human behavior.

Since pain is encountered throughout the life cycle, its role in personality development can hardly be doubted, although the size and prominence of its contribution must vary from one individual to another. It would seem useful, therefore, to consider the part played by pain experiences in human functioning in terms of all the view points constituting the psychoanalytic metapsychology. In addition, the part played by pain in certain clinical syndromes will also be discussed since psychodynamic processes are often more clearly demonstrated in relation to psychopathological states.

At this point, it is no longer possible to avoid some remarks concerning the *definition of pain*. Two particularly useful definitions are those of Sternbach (34) and Merskey (21). Together they make clear the complex nature of the experience, as well as the advantage of discussing it within a number of conceptual frameworks. Sternbach (34) defines pain as "an abstract concept which refers to (1) a personal, private sensation of hurt; (2) a harmful stimulus which signals current or impending tissue damage; (3) a pattern of responses which operate to protect the organism from harm". Taking a somewhat different position, Merskey (21) defines pain as "an unpleasant experience which we primarily associate with tissue damage, or describe in terms of tissue damage or both". Both these definitions stress the subjective nature of the pain experience and by implication shift the focus of the search for causal factors from the somatic to the psychosocial domain. This is an important realignment, but it is interesting to reflect that however much behavioral scientists may justify their interest in pain by highlighting the subjective component, the fact that pain (and its "organic" connotation) is a cardinal indication for the possible need to provide health care, leads inevitably to a wish on the part of most doctors to demonstrate that no matter how obvious the role of "psychological" variables in the aetiology of pain, "organic" inputs are nonetheless present.

Indeed, even when it appears clearly demonstrated that certain types of mental imagery can provoke or intensify pain (17,29) there remain inevitable doubts as to the precise nature of the relationship, and the possible mediating effects of processes (such as muscle activity) operating at the periphery rather than within the central nervous system. It is interesting to consider the arbitrary nature of the division between inputs from the "periphery" and those from the "centre". At what point, one may ask, does an input become peripheral? Must it arise from an organ or tissue which is not part of the nervous system? Must it be unable to reach conscious (or even unconscious) awareness? It can be seen that attempts at such distinctions must, to a large extent, remain arbitrary, but the need to draw them remains strong nonetheless. Certainly, the danger of over-looking "organic" factors is frequently stressed and rarely far from the minds of clinicians treating patients in pain, even when a fairly confident decision has been made that psychological determinants are preeminent.

PSYCHOANALYTIC BEGINNINGS

Freud (14) regarded pain as a common conversion symptom, and leaned to the view that pains encountered in "hysteria" were originally of a somatic origin. In discussing the leg pains of Fraulein Elisabeth Von R he states: "The circumstances indicate that this somatic pain was not *created* by the neurosis but merely used, increased and maintained by it.....I have found a similar state of things in almost all the instances of hysterical pains into which I have been able to obtain an insight. There had always been a genuine,

organically-founded pain present at the start".   (Note
the use of the word "genuine" to denote an "organic"
pain.)

Similarly when Freud (14) found that he was able to
relieve this patient's facial pain by hypnosis, he
states that he "began at that time to harbour doubts of
the genuineness of the neuralgia".

Freud (14) concluded that conversion pains were not
a consequence of a symbolization process but that the
patient "picked out from among all the pains that were
troubling her at the time, the one particular pain
which was symbolically appropriate".   Finally, he
acknowledged the difficulty, in many instances, of
deciding whether sensations arose from a process of
symbolization or whether indeed both the sensations and
the symbols (as expressed in the everyday language of
emotions) arose from the same source; an awareness of
the bodily changes which characteristically accompanied
responses to certain stressful situations.

This approach to pain avoids the problems which flow
from a search for simple causal relationships.   It
highlights, instead, the interactive role of pain
experiences in psychic functioning, and leads naturally
to a consideration of pain in the context of the
Freudian metapsychology.

The Dynamic View

The *dynamic view* emphasizes the part played by
psychic "energies" derived from the individual's
innate drives, of which those related to sexuality,
aggression and dependency, are considered preeminent.
Clearly, the pain experience may be associated with the
gratification or frustration of any of these drives.
The fact that inflicting or receiving pain can occur as
part of sexual excitement or indeed constitute the
individual's only sexually satisfying activity, is well
known.   Pain may, therefore, acquire a sexual
connotation which renders it pleasurable to a greater
or less degree.

Even more obvious is the relationship between pain
and aggressive feelings.   Pain is often the end result
of aggression - either inflicted upon others or
inflicted by them on oneself.   The relationship is, of
course, a complex one, since pain may lead to anger as
easily as anger to pain.   Suffice to say that pain may
serve to alter psychic dynamics by mobilizing anger as
well as by being involved in its discharge.

Finally, dependency strivings are often gratified in
the context of a pain experience.   In fact, of all
behaviors, those indicating the presence of pain, most
predictably evoke the altruistic impulse, but it is

important to bear in mind the ambivalent nature of
this response (26).

The pain experience has yet a further dynamic role
in so far as it is a "result of some local breaking
through of the barrier against stimuli (13).   As a
consequence "an immense 'countercharge' is set up, in
favour of which all other psychic systems are impover-
ished, so that a widespread paralysis or diminution of
other psychic activity follows".   Thus pain is
associated with a withdrawal of psychic energy
(cathexes) from a greater or lesser number of
activities and attachments in order to cope with the
intrusion.   Such a withdrawal may clearly bring other
benefits (secondary gains) not directly related to the
task of coping with pain.

The Structural View

We may turn now to the *structural view* of behavior
and consider the relationship between pain and the id,
ego and superego, as well as the body image, self-
image and internal object representations.

The body image consists of mental representations of
the physical body but may be quite different from it.
It is invested with various emotional connotations
relating to the gratification of basic drives and the
conflicts associated with them.

Analytic writers have stressed particularly the
closeness of the ego and the body image.   In Freud's
words "The ego is first and foremost a body ego" (13).
And in the same vein, Fenichel (11) points out that
the body image is formed during the earliest stages of
development, that it "constitutes the idea of I and is
of basic importance for the further formation of the
ego".   Engel (10) has also suggested the concept of a
"body pain image" referring to areas of the body
previously involved in pain, and of "pain memories"
which are the "ideational complexes, conscious and
unconscious associated with past pain experiences,
stimulation of which may later give rise to pain".

The close association between the ego, the body
image, the self image and internalised objects, is
taken further by Szasz (35) who points out that the
individual may react to his body (or more precisely his
body image) as he might react to another person.
Indeed, attitudes may be projected onto the body as
they might be projected on to others.   Thus pain may
be perceived as a hostile attack emanating from the
body in much the same way as hostility may be perceived
to emanate from another person.

Certain internalised objects - the mental representations of significant others and their values - form

the basis for the development of the ego ideal and the conscience, which together constitute the superego. These mental structures play an important role in the modulation and control of drives in the light of social and cultural norms transmitted to the individual through parental figures. The pain experience often plays a role in the formation of the superego - in particular that component referred to as the conscience. Parents may use actual or threatened pain to shape the behaviors of children. In this way, pain becomes associated with the contravention of standards, the incurring of punishment and the expiation of guilt. On the other hand, the parent who is often in pain may provide a model for identification, which results in the incorporation of pain and illness behavior as key components of the self image and the ego ideal.

In addition, the extensive use of pain infliction by parents may result in the formation of a cruel unyielding superego with an associated chronic sense of guilt and low self esteem, and the perception of pain as a means of expiation and tension reduction. In more general terms, it can be seen that pain can thus come to play a crucial role in an individual's intrapsychic and interpersonal dynamics. The latter outcome is of particular significance to the understanding of the transference and countertransference problems encountered by chronic pain patients in the clinical situation.

The Developmental Approach

This view of behavior stresses the importance of early critical psychosexual phases of development from the initial oral, to the later anal and genital, stages. In the face of later frustrations, the individual regresses to the fixation point which represents the developmental stage at which greatest difficulty was experienced. Psychoanalytic writers have traced the origins of specific psychiatric syndromes to predisposing vulnerabilities arising from problems at specific psychosexual stages of development. Thus hysterical illnesses have been limited to oedipal (genital stage) problems, obsessional neuroses to difficulties in the anal phase, and psychoses to the oral stage.

All the stage-specific sites of sexual excitation, i.e. the oral, anal and genital zones, may also be involved coincidentally in painful processes during childhood and such experiences may also constitute a barrier to the proper resolution of a phase. In addition, since the oral, anal and genital areas have special sexual significances, pain experienced in these locations will require to be understood in terms of these special attributes of the body image.

The Adaptational Approach

This view emphasizes the coping and defensive strategies employed by the individual in adjusting to environmental demands. Of particular relevance, is the defence of somatization, i.e. the turning away from unacceptable thoughts and situations towards a focus on physical problems. This is a process akin to conversion but in many ways it represents a more general coping strategy.

The pain experience does, of course, assist in coping with difficulties by warning of danger but it may also facilitate denial and repression, thus leading to a more defensive and less adaptive response.

In addition, pain may lead to the use of illness behavior (from which it is virtually inseparable) in both its adaptive (19) and pathological (25) forms. The latter possibility - described as *"abnormal illness behavior"* (25) refers to syndromes in which the individual's mode of perceiving, evaluating and responding to those aspects of himself which he assesses in terms of illness and health, is maladaptive; and, furthermore, it persists even though a doctor or other suitably qualified social agent provides a proper assessment of the person's health status and the course to be followed in relation to it. The various forms of abnormal illness behavior have been classified (27) on the basis of whether motivation is conscious or not, whether reality testing is intact or impaired, whether illness is affirmed or denied and whether the focus is physical or psychological.

In this context only those forms of abnormal illness behavior which are germane to the elucidation of the pain experience will be considered. They are the neurotic and psychotic forms of somatically focussed, illness-affirming syndromes. The neurotic forms include conversion reactions, hypochondriacal reactions and obsessional neuroses. The psychotic forms are represented by hypochondriacal delusions occurring in depressive or schizophrenic psychoses.

PAIN AND NEUROTIC ABNORMAL ILLNESS BEHAVIOR

Conversion Reaction

Pain is a common *conversion reaction*. The more restricted psychoanalytic explanation of this symptom

viewed it as transformation into physical symptoms of
repressed sexual drives, as a consequence of unresolved
oedipal conflicts.   In more recent times, the concept
of conversion has been considerably broadened until it
is sometimes difficult to perceive what precise meaning it may have.   In the case of pain it is often
particularly difficult to postulate the precise
symbolic significance of the symptom.   However, what
is striking in the case of a conversion reaction, is
the patient's illness behavior.   Characteristically
the attitude is one of dissatisfaction with the
position one is placed by the pain, but denial of any
preoccupation with the illness or any concern over
what the cause of the pain might be.   The famous
"belle indifference" is thus not often present, but
anxiety or depression - or more precisely "suffering"
is reported as a consequence of the pain.   Other
personal problems are strenuously denied or, if
acknowledged, attributed to the pain.   Indeed, if
indifference is present, it relates to the patient's
life situation rather than to the pain.

In these patients the pain may be seen to serve a
number of functions apart from the hypothesized
symbolic expression of repressed libidinous strivings.
It may function as an expression of hostile dependency
and allow the punishment of parental figures (such as
doctors) for not gratifying dependency and sexual
needs.   At the same time, the attention derived from
doctors, especially in the form of physical examination, allows covert gratification of sexual needs -
much as do the "doctor games" of childhood.   Indeed,
fantasizing such a possibility may provide a source of
sexual stimulation.   Of course, the pain experience as
such, may be experienced as sexually stimulating while,
at the same time, providing the punishment required
for expiation of the guilt which is inevitably aroused.

Hypochondriacal Reactions

These syndromes may be grouped into two main overlapping types - the phobic and somatic forms (24).
In the phobic form the pain forms the basis for a fear
of impending illness of some sort.   Since the
physical focus is usually a physiological accompani-
ment of anxiety, the focus is often on headache or
"cardiac pain".   In these instances the fear usually
involves a transformation of anxiety over instinctual
wishes into fears of illness by a process of displacement.   Typically, the anxiety has been provoked by the
mobilization of sexual or aggressive drives over which
the patient fears a loss of control with subsequent

retaliation or abandonment by significant others. Illness behavior in these patients takes the form of fearful self awareness and, at times, a paradoxical reluctance to report anxieties in case they will be found to be justified.   Rapport is usually good and it may be possible to reassure the patient, at least for a time.   Indeed, the irrational nature of the fear may be ruefully acknowledged.

In the case of somatic hypochondriasis the patient shows a focussing of interest on the pain with no marked anxiety or depression.   The patient concentrates a great deal of attention on the pain and its possible origin.   He is prepared to discuss it at length with doctors and can rarely be reassured.   In these syndromes the pain allows a withdrawal of interest from the external world and a preoccupation with illness and bodily functions.   To some extent the hypochondriacal reaction appears as a response to perceived rejection by others (often following a significant loss) and allows the discharge of hostile and sadistic feelings onto relatives and physician by persistent complaining.

PAIN AND PSYCHOTIC ABNORMAL ILLNESS BEHAVIORS

Psychotic Depression

Pain associated with hypochondriacal delusions may occur as part of a psychotic depression.   A study of such patients which sheds interesting light on the interaction between somatic symptoms and depression, is that of Giberti (16) who found hypochondriasis was commoner in male depressives, and was associated with mild organic dysfunction and chronic organic disease, older age groups, lower incidence of cyclothymic personality traits, lower socioeconomic status, less likelihood of delusions of guilt and unworthiness,few previous episodes of depression and greater duration of the current episode.   It would seem from this study that the depressed patient who is preoccupied with pain (or other physical symptoms) is less severely depressed and less likely to be guilty.   These findings would support the view that pain can serve to neutralize guilt and also (possibly by allowing the discharge of aggression through complaint behavior) cause an amelioration of depression.

The role of pain in *schizophrenia* is a complex one. Pain and hypochondriasis, often diffuse, may at times be an early symptom of the illness and may be part of a general narcissistic withdrawal.   Pain may also be the focus of a delusional system and be explained as a

consequence of some form of attack by enemies on the
patient's physical integrity.   Interestingly, Cowden
and Brown (3) proposed that hypochondriasis should
have an integrative effect in schizophrenia since it
was a more acceptable form of symptomatology from a
social point of view.   To demonstrate their point
they treated a 43 year old male with a longstanding
schizophrenic illness by focussing on his "back pain"
over a period of three months.   They report that as a
result, he was able to leave hospital free of delusions
and hallucinations and appeared to have made a better
adjustment than on previous discharges.   Delaney (6)
also provided clinical evidence to support the view
that pain (in this case atypical facial pain) could act
as a defense against psychosis.   He described three
women who developed psychotic symptoms 24-48 hours
before neurosurgical treatment for the pain.   All
responded to major tranquillizers with disappearance
of the psychosis and relief of pain.

Finally, we may consider patients who present with
chronic pain as their most prominent symptom and who
are frequently referred to pain clinics.   In these
patients diagnosis in conventional terms is difficult
and the differentiation between conversion and hypochondriacal reactions often unsatisfactory.   It has
been suggested elsewhere (28,32) that "abnormal
illness behavior" may be a useful description of this
clinical constellation.   This emphasizes the close
link between pain, illness behavior and the sick role,
and provides a useful framework for the consideration
of personal and environmental determinants of pain.

The intrapsychic functioning and interpersonal
relationships of these patients has been most penetrat-
ingly described by Engel (10).   He concludes that they
are prone to use pain as a "psychic regulator" and show
among other features, prominent guilt, a masochistic
character structure, a strong aggressive drive which is
not fulfilled and a sadomasochistic type of sexual
development.

THE VALIDITY OF PSYCHODYNAMIC FORMULATIONS

A considerable body of research concerned with
testing psychoanalytic theory, has accumulated over
the past fifty years.   Despite much criticism of the
testability (or "verifiability" or "falsifiability")
of these theories, a great deal of work has been undertaken to examine their validity (12).   Systematic
investigations into the validity of psychodynamic
theories of pain have, however, been relatively
uncommon.   In the main reports have been based on
clinical studies of very small numbers of patients and

have concentrated in particular on the relationship between drives such as aggression, and the complaint of pain.

The work of Eisenbud (9) although involving a single patient, demonstrates the way in which experimental techniques can be applied fruitfully to psychodynamic issues. He was able to show in the case of a male patient, that hypnotically induced conflicts relating to hostility and aggression, generated headaches. Similarly, Marcussen and Wolff (18) were able to induce headaches in patients prone to migraine by placing them in situations where they were intensely angry and frustrated but unale to take action.

These findings tally to some degree with those of Furmanski (15) who studied the personalities of 100 patients with migraine. He found that they showed marked narcissim and a "strongly developed aggressive instinct". Affectively cold parents or a strict childhood training, had frustrated these needs and produced "ambivalences and an ultramoral and rigid superego". Attacks of migraine began when "hostilities accumulated beyond the individual's capacity for tolerance of frustration".

It is of considerable interest to relate these reports to those of Dudley (8). In order to examine the effects of a noxious stimulus on respiration, headache was induced in 26 subjects by the use of a metal headband equipped with adjustable rubber-tipped screws. All subjects reacted with what is described as "action-orientation": anger, anxiety, resentment and a strong desire to end the experiment. However, three subjects, who showed minimal changes in respiratory function although they were visibly tense, restless and irritable, denied that they wanted to take action to terminate the stimulus (which they admitted was noxious to them). One patient claimed that he had experienced a great deal of pain and hospitalization as a child with many surgical operations for foot deformities and had, over the years, learned to cope with pain by emotional detachment.

These findings highlight the complex nature of the anger or hostility experience and the need to take more than the subjective state into account. They underline the fact that the context in which a pain is felt may be critical to the precise nature of that pain experience, and that individuals who wish to act out their anger, but feel they cannot, may suffer a more uncomfortable type of pain experience.

Pilowsky and Spence (31) have examined the relationship of pain to anger and illness behavior. Their study used the Illness Behavior Questionnaire (30) to compare 100 patients referred to a pain clinic for the management of intractable pain, with 40 general hospital out-patients who also reported pain as a prominent symptom. It was found that the pain clinic group reported a greater incidence of anger inhibition (but not frequency) than the control group. Within the pain clinic group it was found that patients with extreme combinations of anger experience and anger inhibition were more likely to show hypochondriasis and affective disturbance.

Yet another study supporting the view that the suppression of emotions predisposes to the development of pain is that of Parkes (22) who examined the correlates of phantom pain in a group of 46 amputees. Of the variables studied two relating to personality were significantly associated with the persistence of pain: rigidity and compulsive self-reliance. Parkes (22) describes these individuals as being quite unable to accept the need to be dependent on others. Their watchword is "never show your feelings to others". He suggests that a relationship in which the vulnerable amputee felt safe to express his feelings of "grief, anger and helplessness" might well reduce the need for repression and consequently prevent the persistence of phantom limbs.

PAIN IN CHILDHOOD

It is plain that most studies of the psychodynamics of pain have tended to focus on the structural and dynamic views. It may be supposed that a developmental approach could also be fruitful in demonstrating the importance of early childhood events to the shaping of the pain experience. At least one might hope that information gathered concerning family interactions could prove more reliable than that provided by adult patients.

Apley and Naish (2) surveyed one thousand school children and found that 10.8% suffered from recurrent abdominal pains. By comparing this group to controls they were able to show that organic disorders did not play a causal role. They found a peak incidence at the age when schooling began. Until that time there was no sex difference, but thereafter, pain was commoner in girls. They found that a high incidence of abdominal pain and other somatic complaints was present in the families of children with pain. In addition, these children tended to be anxious, timid, fussy and over-conscientious. These findings underline the importance of identification, separation, anxiety and superego factors in the genesis of pain. Also significant is the finding of a longterm followup study by Apley and MacKeith (1) which indicated that one-third of such children continued to have abdominal pain, one-third had developed other symptoms and one-third were well.

Poznanski (33) points out that it is difficult to establish the age at which neonates begin to feel pain, but notes that by the end of the first week or ten days most infants show a reaction to focal stimulation in the form of diffuse bodily movements or crying. Furthermore, individual differences in responses to sensations can be noted between four to twelve weeks of age. As early as four months, the infants' reactions "are modified patterns that have emerged both from his innate perceptual response and the care-taking environment". Poznanski (33) points out that recurrent psychogenic pain syndromes do not seem to arise before the age of four years. In her own series of 14 patients anxiety and other emotional factors played an obvious role, and in some children there was a tendency to respond to pain in a style characteristic of their family. Secondary gain in the form of the opportunity to withdraw from a difficult situation was often present.

Other clinical studies have noted the importance of loss and guilt (23) in the genesis of abdominal pain; and the frequent occurrence of domestic conflicts, school difficulties, parent-child disagreements and peer problems in children present with chest pain (7). In addition, the latter patients report of knowing relatives or acquaintances with chest pain related to heart disease suggested the presence of an identificatory process.

Overall, the literature suggests that the meaning ascribed to the word "pain", as is the case with all words, is acquired during childhood in the family context. That social influences continue to be important throughout life is indicated by the work of Craig, Best and Ward (4) who found that subjects paired with a tolerant model (who rated the intensity of electrical shocks lower than the subject) accepted greater shocks than did subjects paired with an intolerant. The authors concluded that in their study "meaning appears to have been defined by the social context in which the aversive stimulation was delivered".

In a similar study, employing a signal detection analysis, Craig and Coren (5) found that "if you tell a patient that the ongoing stimulation is painful it is not the internal sensory experience which is influenced but the willingness to report distress is reduced". These findings suggest that the effect of parental models on childhood pain may be extremely complex and may be worth studying in the light of these findings.

OVERVIEW

The word "pain" has intrapsychic, interpersonal and societal significances of a sort possessed by few other descriptors of personal experience. This must surely flow from its potential for disrupting every form of human and social activity, by virtue of its function as a signal of bodily danger and its high value as a releaser of altruistic impulses.

The meaning of this word for an individual clearly depends on the same factors which determine his entire personality and this review has attempted to elucidate some of these from a psychodynamic point of view. The pathways through which these various influences flow to produce an individual's pain experience and pain statements, can be variously conceptualised but for the moment are difficult to synthesize in a psycho-biological sense. Certainly, Melzack and Loeser's (20) suggested central "pattern generating mechanism" has many attractions as an explanation for the ways in which the influences of psychological, emotional and somatic variables combine to produce pain. It seems certain, however, that any attempt to fully understand pain will require us to tolerate life in a house of many paradigms.

REFERENCES

1. Apley, J., and MacKeith, R. (1968): The Child and His Symptoms. Blackwell, Oxford.
2. Apley, J., and Naish, N. (1958): Arch. Dis. Child, 33:165-170.
3. Cowden, R. C., and Brown, J. E. (1956): J. Abnorm. Soc. Psychol., 53:133-135.
4. Craig, K. D., Best, H., and Ward, L. M. (1975): J. Abnorm. Psychol., 84:366-373.
5. Craig, K. D., and Coren, S. (1975): J. Psychosom. Res., 19:105-112.
6. Delaney, J. F. (1976): Am. J. Psychiatry, 133: 1151-1154.
7. Driscoll, D. J., Glicklich, L. B., and Gallen, W. J. (1976): Pediatrics, 57:648-651.
8. Dudley, D. L., editor (1969): Psychophysiology of Respiration in Health and Disease. Appleton Century Crofts, New York.
9. Eisenbud, J. (1937): Psychiat. Quart., 11:592-619.
10. Engel, G. L. (1959): Am. J. Med., 28:899-918.

11. Fenichel, O. (1945): The Psychoanalytic Theory of Neuroses. W. W. Norton, New York.

12. Fisher, S., and Greenberg, R. P. (1977): The Scientific Credibility of Freud's Theories and Therapy. Basic Books, New York.

13. Freud, S. (1942): Beyond the Pleasure Principle. Hogarth Press, London.

14. Freud, S., and Breuer, J. (1974): Studies on Hysteria. Pelican, London.

15. Furmanski, A. R. (1952): Arch. Neurol. Psychiat., 67:23-31.

16. Giberti, F. (1965): Evolut. Psychiat., 30:97-110.

17. Hilgard, E. R., Morgan, A. H., Lange, A. F., Lenox, J. R., MacDonald, H., Marshall, G. D., and Sachs, L. B. (1974): Psychophysiology, 11: 692-702.

18. Marcussen, R. M., and Wolf, H. G. (1969): Psychosom. Med., 11:251-256.

19. Mechanic, D. (1968): Medical Sociology, Free Press, New York.

20. Melzack, R., and Loeser, J. D. (1978): Pain, 4: 195-210.

21. Merskey, H. (1964): An Investigation of Pain in Psychological Illness. D. M. Thesis, Oxford.

22. Parkes, C. M. (1973): J. Psychosom. Res., 17: 97-108.

23. Pedersen, W. M. (1975): Clin. Pediatr., 14:859-861.

24. Pilowsky, I. (1967): Br. J. Psychiatry, 113:89-93.

25. Pilowsky, I. (1969): Br. J. Med. Psychol., 42: 347-351.

26. Pilowsky, I. (1977): Br. J. Med. Psychol., 50: 305-311.

27. Pilowsky, I. (1978): Br. J. Med. Psychol., (in press).

28. Pilowsky, I., Chapman, C. R., and Bonica, J. J. (1977): Pain, 4:183-192.

29. Pilowsky, I., and Kaufman, A. (1965): Br. J. Psychiatry, 111:1185-1187.

30. Pilowsky, I., and Spence, N. D. (1975): J. Psychosom. Res., 19:279-287.

31. Pilowsky, I., and Spence, N. D. (1976): J. Psychosom. Res., 20:411-416.

32. Pilowsky, I., and Spence, N. D. (1976): Pain, 2:61-71.

33. Poznanski, E. O. (1976): Clin. Pediatr., 15: 1114-1119.

34. Sternbach, R. A. (1968): Pain: A Psychophysiological Analysis. Academic Press, New York.

35. Szasz, T. (1957): Pain and Pleasure, Tavistock Press, London.

The Psychology of Pain, edited by R. A. Sternbach.
Raven Press, New York © 1978.

Hypnosis and Pain

Ernest R. Hilgard

Department of Psychology, Stanford University, Stanford, California 94305

The usefulness of hypnosis in the relief of pain was demonstrated early in the 19th century, before chemical anesthetics had been introduced. Limb amputations and other major operations were done painlessly with hypnosis as the only anesthetic (14). The new method met immediate resistance, something that often happens when new procedures are proposed for medical practice. In 1842 Mr. Edward Ward, a surgeon in Nottinghamshire, amputated a thigh during a mesmeric trance, as hypnosis was then designated. The patient lay perfectly calm during the operation, and not a muscle was seen to twitch. The case was adversely received when it was reported before the Royal Medical and Chirurgical Society. Dr. Marshall Hall, eminent in the history of reflex action, suggested that the man was an impostor because if he had not been withholding response there should have been twitching in the other leg. Another physician member added that even if the painless operation were true the fact was unworthy of consideration, because pain was a wise provision of nature, and patients ought to suffer pain while they were being operated. They were all the better for it, and recovered better because of it (6). He succeeded, in fact, in having any mention of the paper deleted from the minutes. Eight years later Marshall Hall stated that the man had confessed that he had suffered during the operation. However, the man was still living and testified in a signed declaration that the operation had been absolutely painless. Among those who suffered strong opposition because they practiced hypnosis was Dr. John Elliotson, Professor of the Practice of Medicine at University College, London. He had earlier met opposition for introducing the stethosocope, because any competent physician could use his unaided ear to listen to a heart; he had no need for this new gadgetry. Elliotson lost his position because of his defense of hypnosis in surgery.

In those days hypnosis was called animal magnetism, and the objections were raised in part because of the magnetic theory, which was patently false. Despite the false theory the pain reduction was genuine, as was repeatedly demonstrated after hypnosis was explained as the result of psychological processes. Ether and chloroform were introduced while the controversies were still active. The convenience of the chemical agents settled the argument temporarily. Even today that convenience tends to hold back the use of hypnosis in instances in which it may be the method of choice.

Hypnosis became more acceptable after the upsurge of interest during World War II. While it was no longer taboo, its acceptance commonly was not enthusiastic among either medical doctors or psychologists. However, it was given official sanction as appropriate to teach in medical schools by both the British and the American medical associations, the former in 1955, the latter in 1958.

THE CLINICAL APPLICABILITY OF HYPNOSIS

Hypnosis should be considered a tool to be used wisely and with discrimination, only when circumstances are appropriate. It may be used as the sole anesthetic, or, more often, in conjunction with chemical anesthetics or analgesics. Just as the anesthesiologist has a variety of chemical agents to be used with discretion, so too hypnosis has its appropriate and inappropriate uses. Pain is so ubiquitous that a more extended account is required to deal in detail with the variety of its clinical applications (29). A few illustrations may serve to illustrate some of the conditions in which hypnosis has been successfully applied.

Cancer

Sacerdote (55) reported the case of a 60-year old man whose primary lesion was in the throat, with an extension into a large, painful indurated mass involving most of the right side of the neck, jaw, and cheek. After hypnotic induction, Sacerdote suggested to him that he could experience a pleasant tingling sensation -- like a weak electric current -- wherever the tumor extended. The patient was able successfully to substitute the pleasant tingling for the pain.

In cases of terminal cancer it is humane to employ hypnosis to relieve the pain without the use of narcotics, so that the patient is able to communicate comfortably with friends and relatives before the final coma begins.

Burns

Many complications arise in the course of recovery from severe burns. These include not only the severe and constant pain, but loss of appetite, painful procedures such as debridement of scar tissue, contractures resulting from failure to exercise because of pain, and associated psychological problems that may greatly slow recovery (10). In a number of instances hypnosis has proved successful in managing these problems.

The case of a 30-year-old man with thermal burns covering 45 percent of his body surface was cited by Crasilneck and Jenkins (11) as illustrating the appropriateness of hypnotic treatment. The patient had become increasingly fearful of the frequent anesthetics needed for dressing changes, the painful manipulation of the extremities, and debridements. Because of his fears and complaints, it was decided to substitute hypnoanesthesia. With the aid of hypnosis, bandages could be changed and areas extensively debrided without any perception of pain prior to, during, or following the procedures. With further surgery under hypnosis, a donor split-thickness skin graft was removed from the patient's leg and placed on the burned areas, which had again undergone extensive debridement in preparation for these grafts. There were no problems during this extensive treatment under hypnosis.

Obstetrics

Hypnosis has been used frequently to relieve the pain and discomfort during normal labor and delivery. In this it competes with the closely related methods, such as the Lamaze method of psychoprophylaxis that grew out of Russian experience with hypnosis. Satisfactory comparative studies are lacking, although the best of these by Davidson (13) showed hypnosis superior to the Dick-Read method of painless childbirth.

Hypnosis has also been used in connection with caesarean sections, either planned in advance or in emergencies. A patient who presented an obstetrical emergency illustrates the advantages of having available someone familiar with hypnotic procedures. A woman expecting a baby had been poorly handled on the ward of the hospital. She had been there for hours with an impacted breech before Cucinotta, as the ward consultant, became aware of her. At that time she had a high fever, a systolic blood pressure of over 200, and a heart rate of more than 150 beats per minute. She evidently needed a caesarean operation, but the anesthetist refused to give any general chemoanesthesia, and the operation under local anesthesia was not judged feasible. Hence Cucinotta, who was to do the surgery, determined to use hypnosis. Although he had not seen her before and she was completely naive to hypnosis, he hypnotized her during the ten to fifteen minutes in which he was scrubbing and preparing her abdomen. The record obtained by the anesthetist during the course of the operation showed that the vital signs steadily returned to normal despite the progress of the surgery. A normal infant was delivered, and the mother's recovery was uneventful. The record was later reviewed by a senior obstetrician who described it as remarkable.[1]

---

[1] The case has not been published, but has been authenticated by Dr. George L. Hoffman, Jr., Professor of Surgery, the University of Pennsylvania Medical School (29).

Dentistry

As with burns, dental procedures are accompanied by many symptoms other than pain, such as anxiety ("dental phobia"), and gagging. These ancillary symptoms can often be dealt with by hypnosis, even though the dental procedures themselves are carried out ultimately with the usual local anesthetics. Sometimes, however, there are unfavorable reactions to the chemical anesthetics, and pain reduction is then a central problem.

A 36-year old woman had previously reacted to procaine with edema of the face and body, urticaria, nausea, and vomiting. As a result, even minor dental procedures had been carried out under general anesthesia. Because of her unfortunate experiences, she had refused to return to her dentist; by now most of her teeth had developed cavities. She needed a series of sessions with her dentist, and it was judged impractical to place her under a general anesthetic each time. She then came to the attention of Crasilneck, McCranie, and Jenkins (12). A personality evaluation indicated that she was relatively free of emotional symptoms other than her extreme fear of dental procedures. After a discussion, hypnosis was induced; she proved to be an excellent subject and was soon capable of reaching a profound hypnotic state. Thereafter, on five separate occasions, dental procedures lasting approximately two hours each were successfully performed. On all five occasions the patient achieved analgesia through hypnotic suggestion alone. She was free of all pain and apprehensiveness. Eventually her fears of dentistry were greatly diminished and she could accept minor procedures without hypnosis.

In the preceding cases the sources of the pains to be alleviated were all of evident organic origin, regardless of the psychological components in the total responses to the traumatic aspects of the illness or to the procedures in treatment. In such instances the effectiveness of hypnosis clearly cannot be explained away by saying that the pain is "merely psychological." It does not follow that hypnosis will be either more (or less) successful with pains that have larger psychosomatic components. In some instances a pain of deep psychological meaning to the patient may be more difficult to remove by psychological means than one that is clearly associated with a tumor growth or accidental injury, but no universal generalization is possible.

Headaches

Headache is one of the symptoms in which there are evidently large psychological components, regardless of the organic involvements that may also occur. Persistent or repeated head pains classified as migraine headaches are estimated to affect about five percent of the adult population. They commonly respond to hypnotic treatment. Harding (20) has reported his successes and failures in hypnotic treatment of 90 patients, 26

males and 64 females, who came to him with intractable migraines.
The number of sessions with each patient ranged from four to
seven; the sessions averaged 30 minutes in length. An inquiry
six months to eight years after hypnotic treatment showed that
38 percent had obtained complete relief; 32 percent found moderate relief; and the remaining 30 percent either had no relief or
were lost to follow-up. The degree of success is sufficient to
encourage further trials with the method; Harding has in fact
continued, and his success rate with 200 patients is at least
as great as that reported for the first 90.

Phantom Limb Pains

The complex psychological features of phantom limb pain, often
following amputation, have been reviewed by Kolb (41), and later
by Melzack (48). Hypnosis has been applied most widely, with
encouraging results, by Cedercreutz and Uusitalo (7). Their
results in more than 100 cases have been so encouraging that
they believe that hypnosis should always be tried before any
other treatment when phantom pain appears. In 37 cases in which
the patient had lost either an arm or a leg, 20 lost all of
their symptoms immediately after hypnosis, and ten more felt
that their condition had improved. As with surgical treatments
for pain, symptoms may recur; in follow-ups ranging up to eight
years the researchers found that eight remained fully symptom-
free, 10 were still improved, but the others in this group showed
no residual benefit. Of course, when symptoms recur, it is
easier to reinstate the hypnosis than to perform another operation, and the danger of untoward side effects is less.

Many other symptoms have been treated hypnotically, such as
tic douloureux (trigeminal neuralgia), neck and lower back pains,
whiplash injuries, and various gynecological conditions.
Illustrations can be found in recent books dealing with clinical
hypnosis, such as those of Cheek and LeCron (8), Crasilneck
and Hall (10), Frankel (16), and Kroger (42).

PAIN REDUCTION IN THE LABORATORY

Research in a clinical setting is known to be extremely difficult. Motivational conditions vary widely, in part because some
painful illnesses are death-threatening while others are not,
some pains are of long and uncertain duration while others are
brief, owing to the conditions of their production. Under these
conditions appropriate controls with well-matched untreated
patients, or double-blind procedures, are difficult to arrange
and under some circumstances may be unethical.

The laboratory has many advantages, with the major disadvantage that the motivational condition of a suffering patient
cannot be duplicated, and the typical doctor-patient relationship cannot be capitalized upon. For example, placebo effects
appear to be more prevalent in real life setting than in the
artificial laboratory (37). At the same time the laboratory

setting permits parametric studies in which the influence of
known variables can be investigated according to their presence
in varying amounts. To study with some precision the influence
of hypnosis upon pain it is necessary to measure hypnotizability
(the degree of reponsiveness or susceptibility to hypnotic
procedures), and to measure pain responsiveness to standard
conditions of normally painful stress, with and without hypnosis.
Such a comparison of hypnotic susceptibility and reaction to
pain sounds straight-forward, but there are many choices to be
made, and these often affect the interpretation of the experimental findings. For example, standardized scales for measuring
hypnotizability can be used with or without a prior induction
of hypnosis, because hypnotic-like suggestions without a prior
induction, called "waking hypnosis," may yield results similar
to those obtained after a hypnotic induction. This issue is
of more interest to theoreticians than to those who are concerned with the practical utility of hypnotic procedures.
Furthermore, debates still go on as to the extent that hypnotic
susceptibility can be improved with practice. If all people are
fundamentally alike in hypnotizability, but have not learned
the skill, measurement of their entering hypnotizability might
not be relevant. However, careful studies tend to show that,
despite the small gains that are made in hypnotic susceptibility
with practice, the initial responsivity is a fair indicator of
the ultimate hypnotic performance. What this means, specifically,
is that there is a positive correlation between initial and final
measurements of hypnotizability when practice has intervened,
as summarized by Perry(52).

There are a number of methods for producing and measuring pain
in the laboratory, and the available methods are not all
equivalent (27). In addition to the choice of painful stressor,
it is necessary to select among available subjective and
objective indicators of pain. Subjective measures include
magnitude estimation of pain on a numerical scale, or the signal-
detection methods (9). Quasi-objective measures make use of
time to first pain (threshold pain) and time to some end-point
(tolerance time). The measure is objective (time) but the
decisions that enter into the initial and final criteria are
subjective. Physiological indicators may be used to substitute
for or to accompany subjective reports. Subjective distinctions
may also be rated in some manner to reflect anxiety, depression,
sensory pain, discomfort, or the quality of the pain experience
as proposed by Melzack and Torgerson (49). With all these
choices to be made, it is not surprising that those who choose
differently may find that their investigations yield somewhat
inconsistent results.

How the Studies Have been Conducted

Primary attention is given here to the studies from the
Stanford Laboratory of Hypnosis Research. The usual scale for

measuring hypnotic responsiveness has been the Stanford Hypnotic Susceptibility Scale, Form A (62). This scale has been supplemented on occasion by its alternate form (SHSS:B) or by other scales such as SHSS:C (63), or by the Stanford Profile Scales of Hypnotic Susceptibility: Forms I and II (SPS:I, SPS:II) (64). All of these scales give the subject a fixed number of opportunities to respond in the manner characteristic of the highly hypnotizable. When 12 such opportunities are given, as in SHSS:A or SHSS:C, scores vary between 0 and 12. Those who score 0 yield none of the responses characteristic of the hypnotizable, while those who score 12 yield the characteristic responses to all opportunities. As in other measures of individual differences, most people earn in-between scores. The scales have been shown to be satisfactorily consistent and valid as measures of hypnotizability (21, 28).

The stressors used to produce pain in the laboratory have been chiefly two: cold pressor pain, in which a hand and forearm are placed in circulating ice water for a standard period of time not exceeding 60 seconds (sec)and ischemic pain, in which pain is produced by the occlusion of circulation in an arm through a tourniquet above the elbow, followed by a standard amount of exercise of the occluded hand (59). After the exercise stops, the pain mounts gradually in the motionless arm over a period of minutes. It may require as much as 20 minutes for the pain to reach the same magnitude as that reached in 60 sec in the ice water. The qualities of the two pains are somewhat different; the ischemic pain corresponds more nearly to that of postsurgical pain.

The report of pain called for in studies from this laboratory has been a magnitude estimate on the basis of a numerical scale in which 0 represents no pain and 10 a pain sufficiently high to be so disagreeable that the subject would wish to terminate it. The scale is open at the top, however, so that magnitude estimates above 10 are given as the pain continues to rise toward the end of the period of stimulation. The advantages of a scale unbounded at the top are readily demonstrated (36). The magnitude estimates are requested from the subject at standard intervals from the onset of stimulation. In some of our studies reports of sensory pain have been supplemented by corresponding reports of the subjective distress that the sensory pain causes as it continues. In some instances the differentiation of these two reports is of crucial importance (18).

Many physiological indicators of pain have been employed by investigators. In our experiments we have studied chiefly cardiovascular responses as recorded by way of plethysmographic transducers and sphgmomanometer cuffs attached to the fingers of the non-stimulated hand. The derived measures have been heart rate and systolic blood pressure. These measures have in no instance proved as reliable or valid as the verbal responses in reflecting felt pain, although they have provided useful information in other respects.

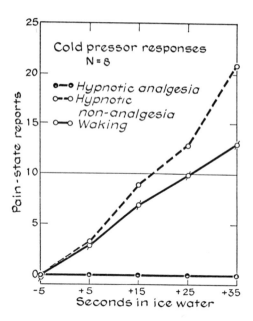

FIG. 1.   Cold Pressor Pain in Waking, Hypnosis without
Analgesia Suggestions, and Hypnosis with Analgesia Suggestions.
The eight subjects report no pain whatever in hypnotic analgesia.
The mean differences between waking and hypnotic non-analgesia
are not significant.   From Hilgard (24).

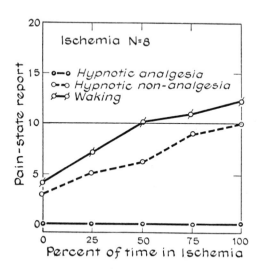

FIG. 2.   Ischemic Pain in Waking, Hypnosis without Analgesia
Suggestions, and Hypnosis with Analgesia Suggestions.   The same
subjects who reported no cold pressor pain (Figure 1), also
report none in hypnotic analgesia when the stress is produced
by the tourniquet-exercise method.   Mean differences between
waking and hypnotic non-analgesia are not significant.
From Hilgard (24).

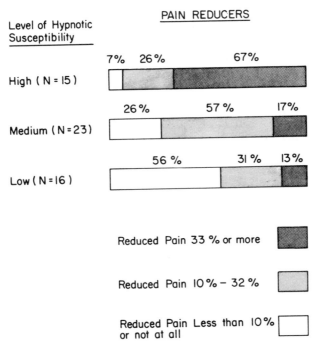

FIG. 3. Hypnotic Analgesia in Cold Pressor Test as Related to Level of Hypnotic Susceptibility. The amount by which pain is reduced is probabilistically related to previously measured hypnotizability. From Hilgard and Morgan (33).

Pain Reduction as Correlated with Hypnotic Susceptibility

For some highly susceptible hypnotic subjects the laboratory-produced pains can be completely eliminated by hypnotic suggestion. Results for cold pressor pain are given in Figure 1 and for ischemic pain in Figure 2. The general finding, however, is that there is a probabilistic relationship between pain reduction through hypnosis and previously measured hypnotizability (Figure 3). That is, the more highly hypnotizable subjects can reduce pain more successfully than the lows, although an occasional low is able to reduce pain by suggestion.

PHYSIOLOGICAL CORRELATES OF FELT PAIN
AS A SOURCE OF CONFUSION

In most but not all of the reports on the hypnotic reduction of pain the physiological indicators of pain have been found to persist even when it is clear that the person following hypnotic suggestion feels no pain or greatly reduced pain (4, 15, 22, 34, 57, 61). This result led Sutcliffe (61), for example, to characterize as a "delusion" the hypnotic pain reduction that was reported to him by his subjects. Such a characterization attributes primacy to the physiological indicators of stress as representing pain, rather than to the pain as experienced by the person. This sounds as though hypnotic pain reduction might be at best a placebo effect, but McGlashan, Evans, and Orne (46) have shown that this is not the case.

The occasional reports in contradiction to the generality that the physiological indications remain even though the subjective responses are no longer present can be illustrated by an early study by West, Neill, and Hardy (65). They concluded from their study of the effect of hypnosis in the reduction of the pain of radiant heat: "The experimental results leave no doubt that hypnotic suggestion of analgesia diminishes the galvanic response to noxious stimuli." However, a reexamination of their data in some detail by Shor (58) pointed out that the reduction of the GSR was uncorrelated with the amount of pain reduction, and even the subject whose pain perception was unchanged by hypnosis had a significant reduction in the GSR as a consequence of the hypnotic procedure. Whatever the GSR was measuring, such as relaxation or reduced anxiety, it was a poor indicator of pain.

Anxiety Reduction Does Not Account for Hypnotic Pain Reduction

Shor (57, 58) found that by careful instructions he could reduce anxiety when rather severe electric shocks were administered. The physiological indicators of pain were reduced to trivial levels by the anxiety-reducing instructions independent of hypnosis or of hypnotic susceptibility. He stated as a consequence: "In other words, hypnotic analgesia did not lessen physiological reactions to pain." In this his results agreed with those of the majority of studies. However, he went on to state a hypothetical conclusion: "Hypnotic analgesia is one means of eliminating the incidental anxiety component of the total pain experience." This conclusion may very well be correct, but it was not demonstrated in his experiments because hypnosis failed to alter the physiological indicators beyond what the nonhypnotic procedures had done. The conclusion has been widely interpreted to mean that anxiety reduction is the primary mode of operation of hypnotic analgesia. Actually the results of the experiment directly contradict this interpretation, since hypnotic analgesia reduced the experience of pain despite its failure to further reduce anxiety, and those who reduced their anxiety but were not hypnotizable did not reduce their felt pain. The amount of pain reduction, according to Shor's original dissertation (57) correlated with hypnotic susceptibility at about the same level as found in our laboratory.

Anticipatory Responses Modify the Interpretation of Physiological Responses to Stressful Stimulation

Another source of confusion in interpreting the relationship between hypnotic analgesia and physiological correlates of pain arose in our own laboratory. A study by Lenox (44) appeared to show that hypnotic analgesia in ischemia reduced, or eliminated, the rise in either blood pressure or heart rate associated with normal ischemic pain. I referred to this finding and accepted it as a warning that it was essential to sample more than one kind of pain before arriving at generalizations because this result with ischemic pain contradicted our findings with cold pressor pain (23). On the basis of subsequent experimentation, however, we have concluded that Lenox's results may have been misleading because of inadequate attention to anticipatory responses. We have since found that, despite expecting successful analgesia because of prior hypnotic success, a subject's heart rate and systolic blood pressure commonly rise prior to the stress (31, 33). Levels reached before the onset of stress may be so high that there is little further rise during the period of stress. The course of anticipatory rise in heart rate, prior to placing the hand and forearm in circulating ice water (cold pressor test), is presented in Figure 4. The subjects served as their own controls. The lower curve shows that, in the non-analgesic condition, when the pain was to be experienced at its normally painful level, there was no rise in heart rate. The upper curve shows that subjects who anticipated analgesia after the hand and forearm would be placed in the ice water, showed an increase in heart rate prior to the stress, averaging about five BPM. The explanation is doubtless complex, perhaps involving effects of attention on heart rate as explored by Lacey (43) in other connections. In any case, changes in heart rate within a pain experiment will reflect changes other than felt pain.

The fuller story of the significance of anticipatory responses as modifying the interpretation of physiological responses to stress is shown in a partial replication of Lenox's experiment. Eight highly hypnotizable subjects were studied both in waking and in hypnotic analgesia, this time in the ischemic test, as reported by Hilgard and Morgan (33). The results replicated Lenox's findings in part, because, if measured from a relaxation baseline, the total rise in blood pressure, in our experiment as in his, was greater in waking than in hypnotic analgesia (Figure 5). When the whole picture is examined, however, there is very little difference between the blood pressure responses in waking and in hypnotic analgesia during the stress period itself. It should be noted that corrections can be made when indicators are studied over short intervals of time as in these studies. In studies that use indicators of stress such as chemical or hormonal products in

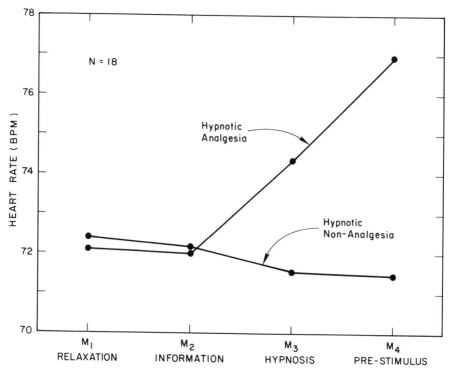

FIG. 4.   Heart Rate as a Function of Anticipated Cold
Pressor Stress under Conditions of Hypnotic Analgesia and
Non-Analgesia.   The final pre-stimulus period occurs at the
time that it is announced that the hand and forearm are soon
to be lowered into the ice water.   From Hilgard, E. R.,
Macdonald, H., Marshall, G., and Morgan, A. H.   Anticipation of
pain and pain control under hypnosis: Heart rate and blood
pressure responses in the cold pressor test.   J. Abnorm.
Psychol., 38: 561-568.   Copyright 1974 by the American
Psychological Association.   Reprinted by permission.

the blood or urine, the difficulties of distinguishing between
anticipatory changes and those associated with the actual stress
must be more difficult to overcome.

The "Hidden Observer" Findings:
Covert Cognitive Responses to Pain in the
Absence of Overt Cognitive Responses

The generalizable finding that there is a discrepancy between
physiological indicators of stress and felt pain lead to a
paradox in the hypnotic findings that such indicators of stress
as we have persist even when the subject is subjectively free of

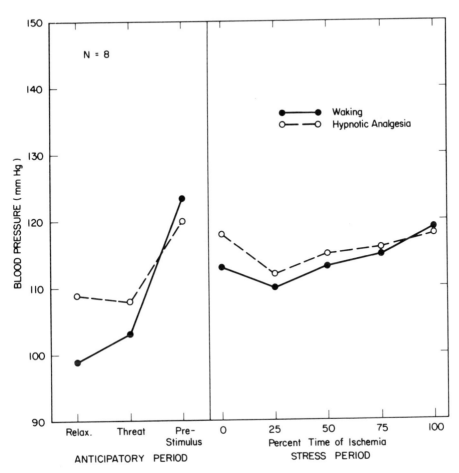

FIG. 5. Blood Pressure as a Function of Anticipated Stress in Tourniquet-Exercise Ischemia. Time in ischemia is expressed as percent because of the varied rates at which pain rises in waking. Time in waking and ischemia alike for each subject, but different from subject to subject. From Hilgard and Morgan (33).

pain in hypnotic analgesia. This paradox has been partially resolved by further studies in which it has been shown that some part of the person's cognitive system may be registering and processing pain while that person is hypnotically analgesic, so that the pain is not being cognitively processed at a conscious level. The concealed or covert cognitive apparatus has been described as a "hidden observer" who knows things that the overt cognitive apparatus in hypnotic analgesia is not aware of (Hilgard, 25, 26).

The method for exploring the hidden experience is a simple supplement to the ordinary hypnotic procedures. The hypnotized person, after the test of analgesia has been completed, can be told that the hypnotic consciousness knows only a limited part of the total information being processed, some of which is processed subconsciously. This is plausible because the hypnotized part commonly fails to attend to voices other than the hypnotist's, or comes out of hypnosis with amnesias for memories that are obviously stored in some manner because they can be recovered when the amnesia is reversed. To get access to such a part, if there is one, the hypnotist explains that a hand will be placed on the subject's shoulder, after which a conversation may take place between the hypnotist-experimenter and the hidden or covert part. When the hypnotist-experimenter later removes his or her hand, everything will be as before, until any residual amnesias are reversed according to a prearranged signal. With a hand on the subject's shoulder, the hypnotist-experimenter may ask the subject to indicate by raising an index finger if any hidden part has been uncovered. Not all of those who are both highly hypnotizable and analgesic will respond, but when a response is made, a sensible conversation can take place.[2] This covert part of the subject is able to recall the highest pain report given in waking and in hypnosis, and can add a supplementary report on what the pain was like to the concealed part while the subject was analgesic. Commonly the covert pain is reported as near to but below the normal waking pain, and above the hypnotically reported overt pain. If questioned about the distress felt at the concealed level, the distress is often reported as less than was felt at the same level of sensory pain when not hypnotized or when not hypnotically analgesic.

An alternative but equivalent method for exploring the "hidden observer" is provided by automatic writing. The subject may be instructed prior to the analgesia experiment to report the felt pain verbally according to the familiar magnitude scale. At the same time, felt pain will be reported

---

[2]Those familiar with the design of experiments in hypnosis will recognize the desirability of controlling for "demand characteristics," when a strong suggestion is given to a highly hypnotizable subject under hypnosis. A familiar control is to use instructed simulators, subjects insusceptible to hypnosis who attempt to behave as they would expect highly hypnotizable subjects to react. The design was proposed by Orne (50, 51). Such controls have been used in the pain experiments, first by Shor (57), and later by our laboratory, both for the simple analgesia (32) and for the "hidden observer" in pain (30), with satisfactory demonstration of the reality of the reported phenomena.

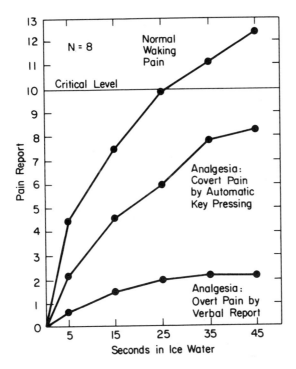

FIG. 6. Normal Waking Pain, Overtly Reported Pain in
Hypnotic Analgesia, and Covert Pain Revealed by Automatic Key
Pressing ("Hidden Observer" Method). Data from Hilgard, Morgan,
and Macdonald (35); reproduced from Hilgard and Hilgard (29).

automatically by the nonstimulated hand concealed in a box
equipped with keys appropriate to reporting numerical pain
magnitude estimates. The subject will then be giving two reports
simultaneously, one <u>overt</u> by word of the mouth, the other <u>covert</u>
via key-pressing by a hand of which he is not conscious.

An illustration of reports by automatic writing in the cold
pressor experiments is given in Figure 6. All of the subjects
whose results are averaged yielded "hidden observer" reports (32).
The covert report is seen to rise as the painful stress increases,
well above the report given overtly (verbally) in hypnotically
suggested analgesia. The covert report lies below the normal
pain report.

A corresponding set of reports in ischemic pain is given in
Figure 7. Here, however, the relatively simultaneous reports
were not by automatic writing but were given every two minutes
with the experimenter's hand on the subject's shoulder briefly
to elicit the covert report (39).

These findings, that some part of the person is processing
the information about the pain in parallel to the conscious
absence of pain, provides at least a partial resolution of the

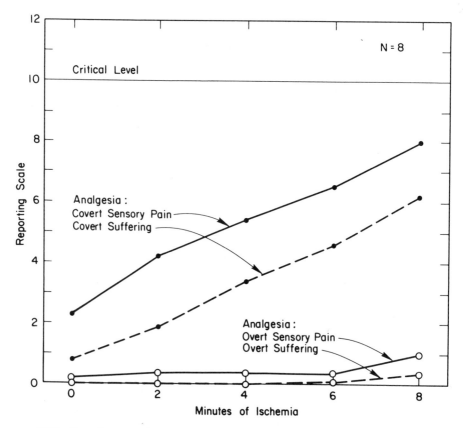

FIG. 7. Pain and Suffering (Distress) as Overtly Reported
in Hypnotic Analgesia, and Covert Pain and Suffering as
Revealed by Intermittent Questioning by "Hidden Observer"
Method. Data from Knox, Morgan, and Hilgard (39); reproduced
from Hilgard and Hilgard (29).

paradox of the persistence of some physiological signs of stress
even when the subject feels no pain.

It should be pointed out that the physiological signs used
are not indicative of major threats to the body within hypnotic
analgesia, because the physiological changes are of an order
that can be produced without painful stress by anticipatory
responses, as was shown in Figure 5. That is, where it is
successful, hypnotic analgesia is a safe anesthetic, and there
is no danger of physiological shock as a consequence of the
presence of some covert detection of the sensory pain. Covert
experiences may even be present under general chemical
anesthesia (45).

There are many lingering uncertainties about the psychophysiology and psychopharmacology of pain, not confined to
hypnotic phenomena. That hypnotic analgesia occurs primarily

at higher cognitive levels is attested also by the failure
of naloxone to reduce hypnotic analgesia, as reported by
Goldstein and Hilgard (18). If release of a naturally occurring
morphine equivalent (endorphin) were responsible for the pain
reduction, naloxone would be expected to reverse it. It has
been reported that naloxone reverses the effect of acupuncture
analgesia (47). Despite the controls that were used, however,
there must be some lingering doubts about this finding because
of the positive correlations that have been reported between
successful pain reduction by hypnosis and by acupuncture
(38, 60), and other reports of the failures of acupuncture as an
analgesic agent (17, 40).

IRRELEVANCE OF THEORETICAL CONTROVERSIES OVER HYPNOSIS

The nature of hypnosis has been the subject of controversy
ever since Mesmer in the 1700's explained its action by
animal magnetism. A century later Charcot wrongly thought
it to reflect a nervous disorder limited to hysterics; Bernheim
correctly led to a general acceptance of the role of suggestion
in producing the phenomena. However, identifying hypnosis
with suggestion did not explain why some were more suggestible
than others, and did not itself set limits on what hypnosis
could do. As long as there are uncertainties over factual
relationships there will be those who commit themselves to
the acceptance of relationships not scientifically established,
and such premature commitments inevitably lead to controversies.
Many of the disputes are not over empirical matters at all,
but reflect conceptual preferences, including the best language
to use in describing and interpreting well-established findings.
For the practical purposes of using hypnotic procedures to
relieve pain, many of these "insider" arguments are irrelevant,
yet the "outsider," just familiarizing himself with hypnosis,
may be misled by them.

As one example, T. X. Barber, in his reviews of hypnosis in
relation to pain (e.g., 3, 5), has given the impression that
most surgery is not very painful, and only in such instances is
hypnosis likely to be useful. For example: "This chapter has
attempted to place this dramatic phenomenon in perspective by
emphasizing that most tissues and organs of the body, with the
notable exception of the skin, are rather insensitive to the
surgeon's scalpel" (5, p. 97). The exception is however, noteworthy, for skin pains are well controlled by hypnosis, and it
is one-sided to downgrade the effectiveness of hypnosis by
ignoring its successful use in dermabrasion and debridements
following burns. Furthermore, Barber's tendency to use "hypnosis"
in quotation marks is a way of indicating that at the time of
writing he felt there was something artificial about it.
Sarbin and Coe (56), who recognize the importance of role
enactment in hypnosis, have become strongly committed to
that position. They cite the undocumented case of a patient who

felt no pain when his wrist was burned while it was hypnotically
anesthetic. "The patient had to choose between disclosing
that he felt the burn, thereby embarrassing and perhaps
displeasing the therapist on whom he had become dependent, or
not disclosing the private fact that he felt the burn and thus
avoiding the risk of weakening the relationship" (56, page 136).
The implication that the person reports no pain only because he
wishes to keep a secret from the hypnotherapist is a misleading
exaggeration of social role theory.

Some other issues between clinicians and experimenters are of
more importance in practice than the conceptual problems just
referred to. Many clinicians do not accept the experimental
findings that individual differences in hypnotizability are
quite stable and persistent. They believe, instead, that
everyone is hypnotizable if his or her resistances are overcome, or if they become properly "trained" to experience deep
hypnosis. However, whenever measurements have been made, in
clinical practice as well as in the laboratory, the success in
pain reduction through hypnotic procedures has been found
correlated with the responsiveness to hypnosis (Hilgard and
Hilgard, 29).[3]

One possible reason for the widespread belief among practicing
hypnotists that measured hypnotizability is unimportant is that
for many psychotherapeutic purposes depth of hypnosis is less
critical than the therapeutic skill of the practitioner. In
fact, what the Russians have called the Bekhterev-Bernheim
method requires only that the patient be cooperative enough
to keep his eyes closed while therapeutic suggestions are
given (53). In the case of pain, we have been able to show
that insusceptible subjects can reduce their pains by about 20
percent of normal through waking suggestion. This much reduction
is probably mediated by lessened anxiety and fear (32).
That much easing of pain, achievable by the low hypnotizable,
may be enough to make the pain tolerable. However, the truly
hypnotizables can reduce their pains far more, so that
hypnotizability is still important as a determiner of what can
be achieved.

An additional issue has to do with the role of hypnotic
induction, the "non-trance" theorists arguing that, because
there is no "trance," an induction ceremony is unnecessary.
At an empirical level, "waking hypnosis," that is, hypnotic

---

[3] One exception is the report by Joseph Barber (2) that
success in relieving dental distress in actual dental practice
was uncorrelated with measured hypnotic susceptibility. This
finding disagrees with an earlier one by Gottfredson (19),
and the nature of the disagreement remains to be explained.
Our own efforts to use Barber's hypnotic procedures with ice
water pain have not substantiated the advantages of his approach
in overcoming the differential effects of hypnotic
susceptibility.

suggestions without a prior induction, lead to consequences that correlate with those following an induction, the more highly hypnotizable responding to a greater extent than the less hypnotizable. At the same time, the general level of hypnotic performance is increased when a trance-induction precedes the later test suggestions (54). Sometimes methods roughly equivalent to an induction are used in control groups for comparison with a standard induction. These alternatives include prolonged relaxation, the exercise of imagination, or so-called "task motivation" instructions. Substitute procedures may be equivalent to inductions, even though they are not identical, for there are many alternative acceptable procedures for entering hypnosis. Most practicing hypnotists recognize that induction procedures can be widely varied with only slight differences in the consequences; an "active-alert" induction yields results very like the usual "passive-relaxed" induction (1).

The efficacy of hypnotic or hypnotic-like procedures in the reduction of pain is well established. At the same time, there is room for differences of interpretation of the mechanisms according to which pain control operates.

References

1. Banyai, E. I., and Hilgard, E. R. (1976): *J. Abnorm. Psychol.*, 85: 218-224.
2. Barber, J. (1977): *Am. J. Clin. Hypn.*, 19: 138-147.
3. Barber, T. X. (1963): *Psychosom. Med.*, 25: 303-333.
4. Barber, T. X., and Hahn, K. W., Jr. (1962): *J. Abnorm. Soc. Psychol.*, 65: 411-418.
5. Barber, T. X., Spanos, N.P., and Chaves, J. F. (1974): *Hypnosis, Imagination, and Human Potentialities.* Pergamon Press, New York.
6. Bramwell, J. M. (1956): *Hypnotism: Its History, Practice and Theory.* Julian Press, New York. (Original date, 1903).
7. Cedercreutz, C., and Uusitalo, E. (1967): In: *Hypnosis and Psychosomatic Medicine*, edited by J. Lassner, pp. 65-66. Springer-Verlag, New York.
8. Cheek, D. B., and LeCron, L.M. (1968): *Clinical Hypnotherapy.* Grune and Stratton, New York.
9. Clark, W. C. (1976): In: *Pain: New Perspectives in Therapy and Research*, edited by M. Weisenberg and B. Tursky, pp. 195-222. Plenum Press, New York.
10. Crasilneck, H. B., and Hall, J. A. (1975): *Clinical Hypnosis: Principles and Applications.* Grune and Stratton, New York.
11. Crasilneck, H.B., and Jenkins, M. T. (1958): *J. Clin. Exp. Hypn.*, 6: 153-161.
12. Crasilneck, H.B., McCranie, E. J., and Jenkins, M.T. (1956): *J. Am. Med. Assoc.*, 162: 1606-1608.
13. Davidson, J.A. (1962): *Br. Med. J.*, 2, No. 5310: 951-953.

14. Esdaile, J. (1957): Hypnosis in Medicine and Surgery. Julian Press, New York. (Original date, 1846).

15. Evans, M.B., and Paul, G. L. (1970): J. Consult. Clin. Psychol., 35: 362-371.

16. Frankel, F. H. (1976): Hypnosis: Trance as a Coping Mechanism. Plenum Press, New York.

17. Galeano, C., and Leung, C. Y. (1978): Pain, 4: 265-271.

18. Goldstein, A., and Hilgard, E. R. (1975): Proc. Natl. Acad. Sci., 72: 2041-2043.

19. Gottfredson, D. K. (1973): Hypnosis as an Anesthetic in Dentistry. Unpublished Doctoral Dissertation, Brigham Young University.

20. Harding, H. C. (1967): In: Hypnosis and Psychosomatic Medicine, edited by J. Lassner, pp. 131-134. Springer-Verlag, New York.

21. Hilgard, E. R. (1965): Hypnotic Susceptibility. Harcourt Brace Jovanovich, New York.

22. Hilgard, E. R. (1967): Proc. Natl. Acad. Sci., 115: 470-476.

23. Hilgard, E. R. (1969): Am. Psychol., 24: 103-113.

24. Hilgard, E. R. (1972): In: Hypnose and Psycho-somatische Medizin, edited by D. Langen, pp. 152-157. Hippokrates Verlag, Stuttgart.

25. Hilgard, E. R. (1973): Psychol. Rev., 80: 396-411.

26. Hilgard, E. R. (1977): Divided Consciousness: Multiple Controls in Human Thought and Action. Wiley, New York.

27. Hilgard, E. R. (1978): In: Handbook of Sensory Physiology, vol. 8, edited by R. M. Held, H. W. Leibowitz, H-L. Teuber. Springer-Verlag, New York (in press).

28. Hilgard, E. R. (1978): Am. J. Clin. Hypn., 25 (in press).

29. Hilgard, E. R., and Hilgard, J. R. (1975): Hypnosis in the Relief of Pain. William Kaufmann, Los Altos, Calif.

30. Hilgard, E. R., Hilgard, J.R., Macdonald, H., Morgan, A. H., and Johnson, L.S. (1978): J. Abnorm. Psychol. (in press).

31. Hilgard, E. R., Macdonald, H., Marshall, G. D., and Morgan, A.H. (1974): J. Abnorm. Psychol., 38: 561-568.

32. Hilgard, E. R., Macdonald, H., Morgan, A. H., and Johnson, L. S. (1978): J. Abnorm. Psychol., 87: 239-246.

33. Hilgard, E. R., and Morgan, A. H. (1975): Acta Neurobiol. Exp., 35: 741-759.

34. Hilgard, E. R., Morgan, A. H., Lange, A. F., Lenox, J. R., Macdonald, H., Marshall, G. D., and Sachs, L. B. (1974) Psychophysiology, 11: 692-702.

35. Hilgard, E. R., Morgan, A. H., and Macdonald, H. (1975): J. Abnorm. Psychol., 84: 280-289.
36. Hilgard, E. R., Ruch, J.C., Lange, A. F., Lenox, J. R. Morgan, A. H., and Sachs, L. B. (1974): Am. J. Psychol., 87: 17-31.
37. Jospe, M.L. (1974) The Placebo Effect. Unpublished Doctoral Dissertation, University of Minnesota.
38. Katz, R. L., Kao, C. Y., Spiegel, H., and Katz, G. J. (1974): In: Advances in Neurology, Vol. 4: International Symposium on Pain, edited by J. J. Bonica, pp. 819-825. Raven Press, New York.
39. Knox, V. J., Morgan, A.H., and Hilgard, E. R. (1974): Arch. Gen. Psychiatry, 30: 840-847.
40. Knox, V. J., and Shum, K. (1977): J. Abnorm. Psychol., 86: 639-643.
41. Kolb, L. C. (1954): The Painful Phantom. Thomas, Springfield, Illinois.
42. Kroger, W. S. (1977): Clinical and Experimental Hypnosis (Second Edition). Lippincott, Philadelphia.
43. Lacey, J.I. (1967): In: Psychological Stress, edited by M. H. Appley and R. Trumbull, pp. 14-37. Appleton-Century-Crofts, New York.
44. Lenox, J. R. (1970): J. Abnorm. Psychol., 75: 199-206.
45. Levinson, B. W. (1967): In: Hypnosis and Psychosomatic Medicine, edited by J. Lassner, pp. 200-207. Springer-Verlag, New York.
46. McGlashan, T. H., Evans, F. J., and Orne, M.T. (1969): Psychosom. Med., 31: 227-246.
47. Mayer, D. J., and Price, D. D. (1977): Brain Res., 121:368.
48. Melzack, R. (1971): Anesthesiology, 34: 409-419.
49. Melzack, R., and Torgerson, W. S. (1971): Anesthesiology, 34: 50-59.
50. Orne, M.T. (1962): Am. Psychol., 17: 776-783.
51. Orne, M.T. (1971): Int. J. Clin. Exp. Hypn., 19: 183-210.
52. Perry, C. (1977): Int. J. Clin. Exp. Hypn., 25: 125-146.
53. Platonov, K. I. (1959): The Word as a Physiological and Therapeutic Factor. (2nd. Edition) Foreign Languages Publishing House, Moscow.
54. Ruch, J.C., Morgan, A. H., and Hilgard, E. R. (1973): J. Abnorm. Psychol., 82: 543-546.
55. Sacerdote, P. (1970): Int. J. Clin. Exp. Hypn., 18: 160-180.
56. Sarbin. T. R., and Coe, W. C. (1972): Hypnosis: A Social Psychological Analysis of Influence Communication. Holt, Rinehart and Winston, New York.
57. Shor, R. E. (1959): Explorations in Hypnosis: A Theoretical and Experimental Study. Unpublished Doctoral Dissertation, Brandeis University.
58. Shor, R. E. (1967): In: Handbook of Clinical and Experimental Hypnosis, edited by J. E. Gordon, pp. 511-549. Macmillan, New York.

59. Smith, G. M., Egbert, L. D., Markowitz, R. A., Mosteller, F., and Beecher, H. K. (1966): J. Pharmacol. Exp. Ther., 154: 324-332.

60. Stern, J.A., Brown, M., Ulett, G. A., and Sletten, I.(1977): In: Conceptual and Investigative Approaches to Hypnosis and Hypnotic Phenomena, edited by W. E. Edmonston, Jr., pp. 175-193.   Ann. N.Y. Acad. Sci.,   vol. 293, New York.

61. Sutcliffe, J.P. (1961): J. Abnorm. Soc. Psychol., 62: 189-200.

62. Weitzenhoffer, A.M., and Hilgard, E. R. (1959): Stanford Hypnotic Susceptibility Scale: Forms A and B. Consulting Psychologists Press, Palo Alto, California.

63. Weitzenhoffer, A.M., and Hilgard, E. R. (1962): Stanford Hypnotic Susceptibility Scale: Form C. Consulting Psychologists Press, Palo Alto, California.

64. Weitzenhoffer, A. M., and Hilgard, E. R. (1967) Revised Stanford Profile Scales of Hypnotic Suscepti- bility, Forms I and II. Consulting Psychologists Press, Palo Alto, California.

65. West, L. J., Neill, K.C., and Hardy, J.D. (1952): Arch. Neurol. Psychiatry, 68: 549-560.

The Psychology of Pain, edited by R. A. Sternbach.
Raven Press, New York © 1978.

Clinical Aspects of Pain

Richard A. Sternbach

Scripps Clinic Medical Group, Inc., La Jolla, California 92037

Although much of the research described in the preceding chapters has led to new developments in the assessment and treatment of pain, not all of it has.
This incomplete translation of research findings to
clinical applications may be due in part to the fact
that most research has been on acute pain, and the
clinical problems are usually chronic in nature. And
it may be due in part to the lack of awareness on the
part of clinicians of the implications of these research findings. However, some recognition must be
given the fact that the human patient with chronic
pain due to illness or injury is unlike the subject in
the laboratory.

As Finer has observed, the consequences of chronic
pain usually ". . . contribute to an egocentric, hypochondriacal, agitated depression" (19, p. 578). This
succinct summary of the problems caused by pain can
serve two purposes: it can serve as a test of the
usefulness of the concepts of pain which come from the
laboratory; and it can serve as a challenge for new
research to alleviate chronic pain.

What follows, then, is a description of the clinical problems in several different "languages": psychodynamic, behavioral, transactional, etc., and a similar description of the current approaches to the assessment and treatment of patients with pain.

Clinical Mechanisms

The early psychiatric literature was usually vague
in specifying whether their descriptions of mental
processes applied to organic or psychogenic pain, and
to acute or chronic states. The early psychological
literature was concerned with thresholds and the question of whether pain was a sensation or a feeling
state, and had little clinical relevance.

Pain Prone Patients and Psychogenic Pain.   Engel (17) has reported a series of patients who repeatedly suffer painful disability, with or without detectable lesions. These patients typically have excessive guilt feelings, conscious or unconscious, and the experience of pain serves as punishment which serves to relieve these guilt feelings. The patients are intolerant of success in their lives. They repeatedly get themselves into situations or relationships in which they are hurt or defeated, and that is when their health is best. Conversely, when their life situation improves, they suffer again from pain.

Engel observed that these patients usually were reared in a family situation in which pain and aggression were prominent. The patients may have experienced frequent abuse, or else parents were attentive only when the children were sick or hurt. A pattern of suffering was established in childhood, and frequently reinforced in adolescence when the expression of unacceptable sexual or aggressive impulses was punished. Tinling and Klein (70), students of Engel reported on a series of men with chronic psychogenic pain, whose anger was only partly sublimated by solitary hunting and driving fast cars.

Szasz (65) proposed a general psychoanalytic theory of pain. Pain results from the perception of a threat to the integrity of the body. The threat may be real or imagined - what is necessary for pain is the perception of it. The instances of injury without pain illustrate the threat to integrity without the perception. The instances of pain without injury illustrate the perception in the absence of the threat. Whether or not the pain is classified as "real" or "imaginary" depends on whether an observed finds objective evidence of the threat. Usually that decision is made by a physician looking for signs of physical injury; however, the threat may be psychological, rather than physical.

Merskey and Spear (36) presented several lines of evidence to suggest that a complaint of pain was about equally likely to be a symptom of a psychological as a physical disorder. However, it is important to point out that a diagnosis of psychogenic pain cannot be made by exclusion of physical causes. There must be adequate findings, from psychiatric interviews and/or psychological tests, to make such a judgment. It is also quite important to recognize that such dynamic mechanisms can result in illnesses or injuries so that the pain has both a somatic and a psychologic generator, operating in parallel. The causative labels "psychogenic" and "somatogenic" need not be, and frequently are not, mutually exclusive.

Pain Effects, Acute and Chronic. From a review of
the experimental and the clinical literature (54,56),
it appears that there is a significant difference between acute and chronic pain. Acute pain, meaning
pain of recent onset or of short duration, is typically associated with changes in autonomic activity
roughly proportional to the intensity of the stimulus.
There are increases in cardiac rate and stroke volume,
systolic and diastolic pressures, pupillary diameter
and striated muscle tension. There are decreases in
gut motility, salivary flow, and superficial capillary
flow. There are associated changes in bronchiole
diameter, and release of glycogen, and epinephrine and
norepinephrine.

The overall pattern is one of emergency response,
the fight or flight reaction. It is also the pattern
of responses seen in anxiety attacks. Patients with
acute pain usually experience anxiety, either about
the severity of the pain itself, or about the meaning
of the pain. When anti-anxiety medications are given,
or other anti-anxiety maneuvers performed, such as explanations, reassurance, etc., patients report less
pain. Similarly in laboratory studies, manipulations
which reduce anxiety also diminish pain responses.

Chronic pain, meaning pain of at least several
months' duration, presents a rather different picture.
If the pain is constant rather than intermittent,
there appears to be an habituation of the autonomic
responses. A pattern of "vegetative" signs emerges:
patients report sleep disturbance, appetite changes,
decreased libido, irritability, withdrawal of interests, weakening of relationships, and increased somatic preoccupation.

This pattern is also that seen in depressive reactions. Psychological testing usually shows chronic
pain patients to be depressed, although they may not
experience a depressed mood; the depression may be
masked by the absorption in the somatic symptoms (55).
It has been reported that treatment of depression frequently results in a significant reduction of pain
(11,35,68), but there is also evidence that reduction
or abolition of pain reverses the neurotic depression
caused by the pain (8,63).

These clinical studies are obviously empirical.
The association of chronic pain and depression has not
been adequately investigated because there is no good
animal model of chronic pain which has been studied
(58), and because it has not been possible to produce
laboratory manipulations of depression comparable to
those which have been performed on anxiety. As a consequence, we are still unclear as to the underlying
pathophysiology, although there is suggestive evidence

that disturbances in brain serotonin activity may be involved (3,5,29,61).

Pain Expression.   It was formerly assumed that there was a 1:1 relationship between the perception of pain and the expression of it.   Therefore, those who complained of pain in situations where others did not must either be neurotic or have "low pain thresholds". It turns out, however, that neurotic patients may be quite inhibited in pain expression (7,9,10,43), and pain thresholds vary little among patients. The problem, rather, seems to be one of communication style.

There seem to be two major determinants of pain expression.   One is cultural background, or ethnic membership.   Zborowski (79) showed that two groups which inhibit pain expression, Old Americans and Irish-Americans, do so for different reasons.   The former "take it in stride", the latter are afraid to appear "like babies".   Similarly, two groups which encourage pain expression, Italian-Americans and Jewish-Americans, also do so for different reasons.   The former rally support and expect and are satisfied with relief, the latter believe in the value of catharsis, and wish attention directed to the underlying cause. These differences in attitudes can influence pain tolerance (not pain threshold), and also physiological responses to repeated pain stimuli (64,72).

The other major determinant of pain expression seems to be the extent to which a person may be introverted or extraverted.   The expression of pain appears to be associated with extraversion, and the inhibition of such expression with introversion (18,28).   These findings appear to apply to the clinical situation as well.   In a series of studies of patients with advanced cancer, Bond and his colleagues (7,8, 9,10,43) have examined the relationships among perceived pain, requests for analgesics, neuroticism, and introversion/extraversion.   They found that the degree of pain experienced is positively correlated with the degree of neuroticism, but the complaint of pain (and the receipt of analgesics) is associated with the degree of extraversion.   Of those with the greatest amount of pain (by rating), the amount of pain expression seemed to be a function of extraversion.   Thus neurotic introverts might suffer silently, with little relationship between pain severity and pain complaint, but those with high extraversion scores had little difficulty communicating.

It therefore seems that the readiness to communicate pain, and the style of doing so, reflect both cultural and psychological factors.   These are not the factors formerly assumed to be involved, but represent the effects of both social learning and relatively stable personality characteristics.

Operant and Respondent Pain. Fordyce (20,21) has pointed out the advantage of substituting a learning model of pain for a disease model. The disease model infers an underlying cause which must be sought and treated. This is useful when the problem is acute pain and the pain is a symptom. It may not be a useful concept, and may be irrelevant, when the problem is chronic pain whose cause is understood but not correctable. In such cases, a learning model may be more helpful, because in such a model the pain itself, and not some underlying process, is the subject of attention.

Respondent pain behaviors are those elicited by antecedent noxious stimuli, and thus are usually reflex in nature: vocalization, sudden withdrawal, and increased pupillary diameter, for example. Such respondent are conditioned in the Pavlovian manner; any stimulus regularly paired with the noxious stimulus will itself acquire the ability to elicit similar responses - the doctor's office, or a parent's angry voice, for example.

In contrast, operants are emitted behaviors which are governed by the reinforcers which follow them: moaning behavior, rewarded by attention from the family; being bedridden, reinforced by respite from unpleasant duties, etc. These operant pain behaviors are conditioned in the Skinnerian manner; any pain behavior followed by a favorable consequence (positive reinforcer) is more likely to recur - it will show an increase in frequency. Any behavior followed by an aversive consequence (negative reinforcer, punishment) will be less likely to recur, and will show a decrease in frequency if there are no positive consequences. It should be noted that a decrease in pain is almost always a positive reinforcer, and whatever behavior diminishes pain is likely to be repeated.

In practice, one usually encounters chronic pain patients who show a mixture of respondent and operant behaviors. There is usually both reflexive behavior to antecedent pathogenic stimulation, and operant behavior maintained by contingent environmental consequences. The analysis of any patient's pain may not be advanced by questions as to "psychogenic" versus "somatogenic", but it may be furthered a great deal by attention to reflex-like respondents and contingent-controlled operants. The application of these principles will be discussed in the section on therapies below.

The Economics of Pain. In this section and the one immediately following, we direct our attention to topics usually neglected in discussions of pain mechnisms. By "economics of pain" is meant, not the cost of treatment, or the social effect of pain, but rather the economic factors which contribute to pain.

It has been shown (36) that in both medical and psychiatric patients with pain, as compared to controls without pain, those with complaints of pain are more likely to come from a lower socioeconomic class, i.e., from the working or laboring class. Furthermore, such patients are more likely than controls to have had painful experiences in the past, and to have had more relatives who had pain experiences. These findings suggest that being poor, and engaging in physical labor, predispose to pain - a common observation.

In addition, it is a frequent observation that those who are poor are less well educated. Those who are less educated are not usually familiar with psychological concepts, nor psychologically minded. Poor people are thus more likely not to be able to express emotional stress or conflict in psychological terms, but in social "acting-out" or in somatic complaints including pain. For such persons, the complaint of pain may be the final common expression for physical stress, emotional strain, and financial deprivation.

The problem is compounded by the economic reinforcement system for pain and disability. Some health plans support physical treatment, but not psychological. Some systems provide disability payments for those whose pain and/or disability prevent them from working. This is particularly important for laboring persons, whose ability to function on the job is more dependent upon body integrity than those of other classes. The reward system of disability payments is more important to laborers, too, because disability income will more nearly approximate their earned income than it will for other classes, and because the labor itself is more demanding and less satisfying. Thus there is some benefit to obtaining disability income, and somewhat less incentive to risking getting well. For laborers who are poorly educated, middle-aged, and tired, pain may be the only alternative.

The Politics of Pain. In his patienthood, the person with pain is involved in a struggle for power which is primarily a vertical relationship. The middle class patient can usually negotiate a treatment contract with the physician on a horizontal basis, as a social peer, for the physician is usually also of the middle class. The working class patient, however, is likely to perceive himself as having to deal with an authority figure - and resents it.

The patient's resentment arises from several sources. He is a petitioner for aid, and the petitioner always is angry at those from whom he must seek help, whether banker or doctor. More importantly, the pain patient - the disabled working class pain patient - seeks aid for his livelihood, his career. He knows how much he is handicapped, and how much he needs to be restored to wholeness. He sees sitting across from him a wealthier person who is not in pain, and whose career would not be much jeopardized even if he did have pain.

The patient would like to be able to negotiate a treatment contract as he would with his plumber or mechanic - people in his own class: do the job right, and get paid; do it wrong, and the job goes to someone else. But the patient cannot - he must be polite. The doctor has the power not merely to withold treatment ("It's all in your head"), but to report to insurance companies and governmental agencies that the patient is well enough to return to work.

The patient knows very well that his relationship to the doctor is not a confidential one. The doctor's report goes to every agency that pays the bills or makes employment decisions. These agencies are not going to pay the doctor or hospital without the reports. Thus, the doctor is in the role of a double agent, ostensibly working for the patient, but really working for his sources of income.

The patient is also engaged in a power struggle with the agencies which pay his bills and determine his income. These bureaucracies, insulated from the patient as a human being by mounds of papers, are staffed by clerks and administrators whose allegiance is not to the patient, but to their superiors who rate them and determine their promotions. The laboring class patient is quite at a disadvantage in dealing with such persons, because of his deficiences in language skills and his financial impotence.

Such patients are thus easy prey for lawyers, who represent to the patients that the patients are victims of society, that the pain and illness behavior are symptoms of their oppression, and that the lawyers can help redress their grievances. Since the patient by himself has little chance with the doctor, and no chance with the bureaucracies, he has little to lose - especially if the lawyer's fee is on a contingent basis.

As the lawyer is usually from the same social and economic class as the doctor, he does not feel defen-

sive in his dealings with him.   And as the   lawyer's
language skills are usually excellent, he has few difficulties in negotiating with governmental agencies or
insurance companies.   Thus the lawyer frequently   suc-
ceeds in obtaining disability   income - or similar litigation benefits - and thrives.

In order to increase the amount of settlement,   and
therefore attorneys' fees, there is an increasing tendency   to ask   for rewards   for   "pain and suffering".
This concept, originally   invented by lawyers (for similar reasons)   for use in damage suits,   is more frequently now being applied to   routine disability cases
as well.   It has the effect of   increasing the financial rewards to the applicant and lawyer, and the bur-
den on all taxpayers, and by so widening the base   of
support, makes more democractic the increase in attorneys' incomes.

Another point,   not to be minimized, is the obvious
superiority   of attorneys to medical researchers,   for
the   lawyers have managed to measure   pain and suffering, whereas the researchers have not.

Finally,   we should note that   pain is not merely a
commodity at the local and national levels, but inter-
nationally   as well.   There have been   widespread reports of how the United States,   through the CIA,   has
instructed several   military dictatorships in advanced
techniques of torture.   In this way, pain exported to
less well developed countries in exchange for   loyalty
to United   States policies,   becomes an   instrument of
international diplomacy.   Those of   us working in the
area of   pain can be proud that   our subject is deemed
so valuable,   and thankful   for the   generosity of the
United States in sharing it with others.

Diagnostics

The distinction between   research and clinical work
is more apparent than real.   In each case the investigator must ask the right questions, and   must make observations   in a way that avoids bias from unsuspected
sources.   Results or   findings must be   objective and
replicable.   Conclusions (diagnoses)   should stand up
to testing (response to treatment).   The situation is
the same with pain patients in particular.

In diagnosing   patients with pain there are   really
two separate but interrelated tasks.   One is to assess
the pain itself,   almost as though the patient did not
exist,   or were merely the carrier   of a tissue speci-
men.   This is what is   usually done in hospital emergency rooms,   and is clearly the first and most important step in diagnosing acute pain.   The working diag-

nosis of the referring physician should never be accepted without further questioning, for it is sometimes wrong. The second task is to assess the patient as a person, as one with pain and a unique exposure history.

With respect to both problems there are many different opinions as to the best approaches. There are several ways to "measure" pain, but there is not yet a purely objective physiological measure which can be used as well with animals, the way a thermometer measures body temperature. Lacking such a technique (which may soon be developed), several approaches may be combined to give an approximation. Similarly, with personality assessment, there is no unanimity of opinion as to the best approach.

In what follows we will cite some published reports and studies wherever possible, but many areas remain uninvestigated. Clinical experience is drawn upon to fill in the gaps.

Measurement and the Ethics of Pain. There are several possible ways of quantifying pain severity: magnitude production, cross-modality matching, or the matching of pain stimuli intensities, among other psychophysical methods. None is entirely satisfactory, because all rely on subjective report, with the many biases due to factors influencing pain expression (see above).

On a priori grounds it would seem that pain matching techniques would be most accurate and reliable, particularly when the qualities of the stimuli are similar. This has given rise to the clinical adaptation of experimental methods such as the tourniquet pain test (62). This in turn raises ethical questions.

The most obvious problem is that of inflicting pain on another, especially one who is already obviously in pain and suffering. What right has anyone to inflict pain on another? The act must be justified by an important need, and it must be approved by the patient giving fully informed consent.

What justification can there be, or what important need? It is the need of the therapist to know how much pain the patient is experiencing so that treatments will be appropriate, not too little for severe pain nor too drastic for mild pain. Is it always necessary to use a matching pain technique for this purpose? No - for most patients (approximately 2/3) other estimates appear adequate.

What if one wishes to compare another, non-painful technique with a pain-matching method? The justification can be made that it will help measure the severity of the patient's pain, and thus treatment will be appropriate. In such a case, it is usually possible to convince the patient that is is for his own benefit, ultimately, and he will consent. In actuality, the beneficiary is more likely to be the investigator, who wishes to validate one method or another, so he can have a useful dependent variable to use in clinical trials of some pain relieving procedure, and thus ultimately obtain more publications, promotions and grants.

It is very difficult to separate what is genuinely of benefit to the patient from what is a rationalization by the investigator. In general, investigators tend not to be critical in their thinking about the procedures by which they earn their living, and clinicians specifically tend to justify, rationalize, and even act cavalier about their income-producing activities.

With such an attitude it is a simple matter to get "fully informed consent" to carry out almost any procedure. The pain patient is a supplicant very much dependent upon the good opinion of the investigator. The very fact that the clinician is an investigator engaged in clinical research suggests that he probably has a good reputation, and the patient undoubtedly feels that he is in a court of last resort, and the investigator is the patient's last hope for relief. In such a circumstance, the patient will feel that he cannot risk rejection, he cannot offend, he must please. He is therefore likely to agree to almost any reasonable request, and accompany it with that commonly heard and most pathetic of statements, "Maybe this will help somebody else some day".

In general, if a principle were to be stated, it would be that the clinical investigator measuring a patient's pain should do no harm to the patient's dignity or welfare. If pain is to be inflicted, it should be because there is no satisfactory alternative, it will directly benefit the patient (not "science" or "others"), and the patient is under no obvious or subtle compulsion and has the opportunity of terminating both the induced pain and his participation in the procedure without compromising his care.

Severity of pain. Of the several attributes of pain, its severity is most important. As already indicated, the extent of efforts to provide pain relief will depend upon how severe the patient's pain is. Desperate straits call for desperate measures, but only desperate straits do so. Many patients demand pain relief, insisting their pain is unbearable and even excruciating, but sit calmly as they describe it, and can even be led into a joking conversation.

Careful quantification of their pain usually indicates it to be slight or moderate in severity, and their persuasiveness was part of their expressive style (see above). And I have seen patients whose pain level was trivial, but who were made worse by cordotomies and by implantation of electrodes in the brain and spinal cord.

On the other hand, there are also stoical patients, as well as neurotic inhibited ones, who do not verbalize their pain levels appropriately, and therefore suffer needlessly. They are not given adequate analgesics or other pain relieving attention. They tend to understate their pain, and thus are passed over in favor of those who are more expressive or demanding.

One way of quantifying pain is the traditional one of using the verbal descriptors: none, slight, moderate, severe, and unbearable; these comprise a nominal five-point scale. However, they are susceptible to expressive bias as the patient's spontaneous verbalizations. It has been shown that words are not adequate as measures of severity (1,2), and a factor analysis of such verbal descriptors shows a tendency to use affective rather than sensory terms (6,15).

In an attempt to avoid affective loadings and to obtain more "pure" sensory measures of clinical pain intensity, graphic representations of pain have been developed using visual analogue and graphic rating scales (48). These have been shown superior to simple verbal terms (1).

Similarly, attempts have been made to introduce other pain stimuli of known intensity, for the patient to match against his clinical pain level. This has been done with a calibrated pressure algometer (78), and with an adaptation of the submaximum effort tourniquet technique (62). The latter procedure expressed the matched level of clinical pain as a percentage of the patient's own maximum pain tolerance, rather than comparing it to a standardization group; this pain score was then compared with a previously obtained numerical rating of severity using a 0 to 100 scale. The method was shown to have good reliability (62). The numerical rating (magnitude production) of pain level was shown by canonical correlation to be associated with limitations due to pain, while the tourniquet pain score was associated with depression (69). The technique however was not sensitive to changes in pain level produced by analgesics of different strengths (50).

Other attempts at cross-modality matching have been made, but these always result in a number on a scale of physical intensity, which gives no information

about the severity of the patient's pain because it is
compared with others' scores, rather than the patient's own maximum tolerance. All things considered,
it is probably most useful now to have patients rate
their pain level on a numerical or visual analogue
scale, with careful attention to instructions about
scaling the intensity (rather than other qualities of
pain), and to definitions of endpoints on the scale.

Locus of pain. It is a curious fact, not well explained that handedness may be related to pain
perception and the localization of pain. In a study
on the relationships among different deep muscle and
cutaneous thresholds, Wolff and Jarvik (76) used radiant heat, ice water, hypertonic saline, and hypotonic saline injections. They noted consistent differences in lower thresholds for the left side as compared with the right. Later, Wolff, et al. (77) used
electric shock and again found the non-dominant side
to be consistently more sensitive to pain, using both
pain threshold and pain tolerance measures.

This finding is supported by reports from the
clinical literature. The reports of Edmonds (16),
Halliday (23) and Spear (all cited in 36), and supported by Agnew and Merskey (2), all show pain complaints to be more frequent on the non-dominant side.
It should also be noted that psychoanalytic lore has
long held the left or non-dominant side to represent
the weak, passive aspect of the self. It is unclear
what to make of all this. It is not simply a matter
of awkwardness resulting in more frequent injuries to
the extremities on the left, because headaches, when
unilateral, occur on the left more often as well.

Apart from this phenomenon, the precise localization of a pain complaint is important in the diagnosis
of the underlying pathology. Not all pain follows a
dermatomal distribution, and those that do not may yet
be "somatogenic" rather than "psychogenic". Pains associated with sustained muscle contractions may follow
a myotomal pattern, or may involve a limb in what may
seem like an "hysterical" distribution to an uncriti-
cal investigator. Vascular pains have a different
distribution still, and like muscle pains, may have a
characteristic pattern of qualities, precipitants, and
mechanisms of alleviation and exacerbation. Pains may
be perceived as superficial or deep, localized,
spreading, or radiating. All such characteristics
help to define the probable underlying pathophysiology.

Quality of pain. The adjectives used to describe
the nature of the pain sensation may also be of diagnostic value. These represent those attributes of

pain apart from its intensity, locus, or temporal characteristics. Such terms as sharp, dull, aching, throbbing, burning, tightening, etc. are of some importance. For example, pains associated with nerve damage or irritation are frequently described as jabbing, shooting, or lightning-like; these are seen in some spinal cord injuries and neuralgias. Causalgia is usually described as burning; and patients with causalgia often apply cold. The skin in causalgia and neuralgia is often hyperesthetic - very sensitive to light touch - but not tender to deep pressure.

Vascular pains may be throbbing with vasodilation, or tight and cramping with vasoconstriction. Muscle pains are usually aching, and worsened by remaining too long in one position, but changes in position, and certain activities, are associated with sharp pains. Visceral pains are usually deep, with local tenderness to pressure, and have an aching quality with, occasionally, intermittent radiating sharp pain.

Less well educated patients do not always have a range of adjectives at their disposal. They may say, "I don't know how you describe it - it's just a hard pain, that's all." In such cases, when it is clear that the patient is not merely being vague, it is helpful to offer a list of the commonest terms for the patient to choose from, or a series of pairs, such as: sharp or dull? burning or icy? swollen or tight?, etc.

Temporal aspects of pain. It is helpful to establish whether the pain may be constant, though waxing and waning in severity, or intermittent. If intermittent, what is the period - minutes, hours, days, or is it irregular? Are the pains precipitated or exacerbated by position, activity, emotion, events, weather, or other obvious causes? What has been the duration and what was the original cause, of the pain?

Pains which are intermittent and have a very short period, described as shooting, jabbing, etc. are often related to nerve injuries. Other pains are more steady, although vascular pains are sometimes throbbing, and some muscle pains involve spasms; these may also be periodic.

Headaches which are constant are usually muscle contraction in type, although a few may involve a space-occupying lesion. Vascular headaches tend to be more periodic, occurring every few days or weeks. Visceral pains, as previously noted, frequently have both a steady and an intermittent component. Pains which do not accompany activity, but follow it by several hours, are usually muscular in origin.

Is the pain greatest on awakening, then decreasing during the day, or least on arising and increasing

through the day?   Even more importantly, does it dis-
turb sleep?   Does it keep the patient from falling
asleep, or awaken him during the night, or both? How
does the patient medicate himself to treat the fluctuations in pain and sleep?

Affective and semantic aspects of pain.   It takes
just a few minutes to find out where the pain is, how
severe it is, how long the patient has had it, what it
feels like, how it varies, etc.   Initial questions of
this sort require the patient to separate himself from
his pain, to view his pain objectively, as something
outside himself.   This may be a useful prelude to
treatment, but the evaluation process must also consider the patient's emotional responses to the pain.
This is true whether the pain is clearly a symptom of
physical illness or of psychological illness.   The
reason for this is that affective responses can diminish or potentiate pain severity, or otherwise alter
other qualities of the pain.   Put in other terms, operant pain may continue or magnify respondent pain.

Patients may describe their pain as nauseating,
frightening, depressing, or otherwise emotionally up-
setting. The problem here, however, is that those who
are easily given to emotional expressiveness may over-
state their distress, whereas some who are inhibited
may nevertheless have a clinically significant affective disturbance.   The proper assessment of emotional
(or mental) problems requires the usual psychodiagnos-
tic techniques, but a simple statement of the emotional reaction the pain produces may also contribute to
and understanding of the pain itself.

Melzack and Torgerson (34) empirically developed a
list of pain descriptors which formed three major categories: sensory (throbbing, burning, cramping,
etc.); affective (sickening, terrifying, blinding);
and evaluative (annoying, miserable, unbearable). The
list was found to be able to be scaled on an intensity
class for each category (and subcategory), and such
rankings held up among subjects of different cultural,
socioeconomic and educational backgrounds.

The study led to the development of the McGill Pain
Questionnaire (32), which permits quantification of
these descriptors, as well as a measure of pain intensity. Melzack reports that the measure called the
Present Pain Intensity (PPI), a 5-point scale: mild,
discomforting, distressing, horrible, excruciating;
correlated more highly with the evaluative category
than with the others, and was more labile than the
other indices and more susceptible to influence by
variables other than the sensory dimensions of pain
(32).

This is in agreement with the finding by Timmermans and Sternbach (69) that the numerical estimate of pain severity was correlated with the impact of pain on daily functioning, and the tourniquet pain score was associated with the level of depression. Also in agreement is the report by Bailey and Davidson (6), who did a factor analysis of the descriptor terms with respect to the intensity ratings assigned them. The first factor obtained was an "intensity" factor, but the "intensity" appeared to relate to affective-evaluative terms rather than sensory ones.

Agnew and Merskey (2) used the descriptors in the McGill Pain Questionnaire on patients with chronic pain due to organic or psychiatric illness, and found that the former group used sensory-thermal words more than the latter group did. Female patients with pain attributed to anxiety used sensory-temporal words more frequently than those with other psychiatric diagnoses.

Crockett et al. (15) also performed factor analyses of the McGill Pain Questionnaire descriptive terms, using both a patient population and students undergoing experimental pain. Their results largely supported Melzack and Torgerson's (34) classification, but also suggested an even greater number of dimensions. Of five factors obtained, the first two loaded primarily on words from the affective category, the third from the sensory-evaluative categories, the fourth and fifth from the sensory.

These studies have in common the findings that the words patients use in describing their pain are as important as a measure of severity, and that the affective terms may be the most important of all.

Psychodiagnostics. With affective correlates of pain apparently so important, it is obvious that there should be a useful way of measuring this in patients with pain. We have already seen that acute pain is associated with anxiety, and chronic pain with depression. Both are frequently associated with hypochondriasis as well. It is important to be able to determine the extent to which anxiety, depression and hypochondriasis are present, so that appropriate treatment can be initiated.

Diagnostic interviews can be very misleading. The patient with pain usually is quite focused on the symptom, and ascribes all associated difficulties to it. He may not acknowledge the anxiety or depression at all, or, if he does, he insists it is due to the pain and will clear when the pain is gone. The patient may be quite correct in this (8,63), but it may not be possible to eliminate the pain. It is therefore helpful to the patient to attempt to control the pain as much as possible, and simultaneously treat those affects which tend to make pain more severe.

Objective tests are best, because they can be quantified so as to indicate the extent of abnormality. (They also make easier the research on various clinical pain populations). Unfortunately, only the MMPI has a clinically useful profile with sizeable medical and psychiatric patient norms, and with each passing year it is becoming more outdated. Yet there are several characteristic profiles which one obtains from a pain population with the MMPI (56).

We have several times noted that hypochondriasis accompanies pain. The hypochondriasis scale of the MMPI is really only a symptom checklist. Pilowsky (42) has shown that a factor analysis of attitudes to illness results in three primary factors: somatic preoccupation; disease phobia; and conviction of illness with non-response to reassurance. He and Spence have devised a scale which measures these, and it is useful (44,45). Usually, when a patient's depression is masked by his pain, it is a somatic preoccupation form of hypochondriasis, but it is quite helpful to know if the other factors may also be involved.

From a more behavioral point of view, the clinician is interested in learning which are the operant rather than respondent pain behaviors the patient displays, and what are the reinforcers which maintain them. Either a questionnaire or interview may provide such information. It is helpful to know what analgesics the patient uses, and how often; how much time the patient spends sitting or reclining each day; what changes have occurred in the occupational and family situation since the pain began; what the frequency of office and clinic visits has been, etc. It is also useful to get similar information from a family member, independently. These data provide baseline standards against which to measure the effects of behavioral intervention; they also provide clues to the reinforcers serving to maintain operant pain behavior.

Pain Games and the Practice of Pain. Szasz (66) first described the art of painmanship, in a classic paper which deserves to be read widely. He described the problem of psychogenic pain and how patient and doctor alike conspire to define it as a medical problem rather than a psychological one. The role identities of painful person, on the one hand, and the doctor on the other, are defined and perpetuated by the nature of the interactions in which they engage. In behavioral terms, we would say that each reinforces the other and thus maintains his own and the other's inappropriate behavior.

We have specified some of the commonest of the pain games, using a transactional analysis approach (56, 57). These apply not to the psychogenic pain patient, but to the patient with pain due to organic factors. Although only 10% of those with such pain may engage in such games (operants) to a significant degree, it is well to be aware of the games and alert to the players, for they may play havoc with an unsuspecting pain clinic.

It seems almost unbelievable that a person with pain due to an organic lesion would repeatedly sabotage attempts to relieve or minimize his pain, and yet not be psychotic. Such a patient is rare, but does indeed exist. He (she) engages in the practice of pain for reasons which may be variously described: relieving guilt due to unacceptable anger, or satisfying dependency needs; playing "stump the experts" to prove that the doctors cannot take proper care of one (as the parents could not); to maintain a disability because of need for an economic base; to insure an adequate supply of analgesics; to maintain a tyrannical role in the home, etc.

It should be obvious that these are clinical descriptions, and there is little in the way of objective data to support them. We are not aware of any test data or clinical research to advance such descriptions beyond this level. Yet awareness of this aspect of pain behavior makes the clinician's job much easier. Usually a good hint of a patient's practice of pain lies in the repetitive pattern documented in the medical records.

Therapies

Somatic Therapies. The attempts to abolish pain have been many and varied, and none is always effective. Traditionally, the surgical division of nerve pathways has been tried, but a careful analysis of follow-up data suggests that there are very few conditions, and very few techniques, with high long-term success rates (74). For most instances of chronic pain not associated with terminal disease, pain quite frequently begins to return after a variable period of 6-18 months. This applies to neurectomies, rhizotomies, cordotomies: where the pathology causing the pain persists, the pain will probably return. (In cases of malignant pain, death may well occur before the return of the pain). Brain ablation approaches tend to alter pain expressiveness more than pain levels, and are now quite rarely performed. New techniques of brain and spinal cord electrical stimulation seemed initially promising, but habituation seems to develop with continuous use.

Like surgical approaches, systemic chemical analgesia has a long history and serious limitations. Physical dependence, increasing tolerance, and in some instances psychological dependence, all complicate the regular use of narcotics. Local regional anesthesia (nerve blocks) have diagnostic value, and may temporarily interrupt "recurrent pain circuits". "Permanent" blocks with phenol or alcohol are usually not permanent, having the same limitations as surgical techniques. Neuroleptic or psychotropic drugs are helpful in treating the emotional concomitants of pain, anxiolytic agents for acute pain and antidepressants for chronic pain (35,68). They do not seem to do much for the pain itself, however, although there is some suggestion that agents promoting brain serotonin activity may directly increase pain tolerance (61).

Electrical stimulation of the implanted variety may have limitations, but peripheral transcutaneous stimulation, like acupuncture, does not seem to result in habituation, but for varying percentages of patients provides prolonged diminution of pain (60). It may even produce increasing sensitivity to the stimulation (33). The effect is clearly not a placebo response (14) but has a direct peripheral effect (26,67,71).

Many pain syndromes involve musculoligamentous conditions which may respond to physiotherapy. Heat, massage, ultrasound, and most importantly isotonic and isometric strengthening exercises, favorably affect chronic and recurrent strain and fibromyalgia. These procedures, properly used, also play an important part in behavior therapies.

Psychological Therapies. The somatic therapies, when they work, may abolish pain, but the psychological therapies seem to do so seldom. More frequently they reduce pain, but the effects may be longer lasting. Even the more dramatic results with hypnosis may be only partially effective. Hilgard (24) has noted that "hypnosis need not be thought of as competing with chemical analgesics, but rather as supplementing them when their use may be ill-advised, or when relief through smaller doses is desirable . . . in many instances hypnosis may be the sole anesthetic, but its success in completely suppressing severe pain requires highly hypnotizable patients, who are in the minority" (24, p. 213).

Unfortunately, although the recent experimental research on hypnosis itself is excellent (51), and experimental research involving hypnosis and pain is also (24,25), the clinical research on the use of hypnosis for pain is sparse and poor. Most of the reports are merely anecdotal case histories. There are few studies employing objective data or controls. Nevertheless the sheer weight of numbers reported in clinical studies, as well as the experimental studies, suggests that hypnosis may indeed be an effective treatment for pain (25).

One controlled study comparing hypnosis with prophylactic chemotherapy for migraine showed the former more effective (4). An interesting comparison was made of the effects of suggestions for (a) waking relaxation, (b) hypnotic relaxation, (c) waking analgesia, and (d) hypnotic analgesia, on pain thresholds and pain tolerance for electric shocks. Hypnotic analgesia was most effective (53). Such reports as these, though uncommon, tend to support the concept that hypnosis may indeed be of value as a part of a pain treatment program.

Biofeedback techniques have been much used in recent years, and have an extensive experimental background (37). Controlled studies of effectiveness in clinical pain conditions are few, however. More has been reported for headache than for other conditions. Budzynski et al. (12) found EMG feedback effective for muscle contraction headaches, as have others (75), but similar results have been reported for EEG alpha training (30,40) and for relaxation training alone without biofeedback (73). For vascular headaches, biofeedback training for peripheral vascular vasodilatation (a relaxation response) has been reported effective (46,47), and for some it is maintained at follow-up (52). Others have also reported success with the technique (1,31,38), but again, similar results have been obtained with behavioral techniques not using feedback (39,73). Which is most effective, and best maintained at long-term follow-up, is not yet clear. Applications to other pain states are still relatively rarely reported.

Behavior treatment for chronic pain has become relatively common in pain clinics since the impressive reports by Fordyce et al. (21,22). The essential elements of this approach to operant pain behaviors consist of extinguishing them by ignoring them, and shaping healthy, pain-incompatible behaviors with social and other positive reinforcers (20). Others have also shown that behavior modification techniques are effective for a variety of pain states, and that this approach does not merely teach stoicism, because subjective ratings of pain also are improved (13,27,49,50). Seres and Newman have introduced some novel objective measures of physical functioning, and have shown that improvements in these measures are sustained in follow-up studies (49,50). However, the reports of all these groups are of outcome studies of programs using a variety of treatments (group therapy, physical therapy, operant conditioning, etc.), so that their results reflect overall program effects rather than those of behavioral treatments along.

Needs for Clinical Studies. It should be noted here that clinical research on psychological therapies for pain are very sparse and unsophisticated as compared with research on the somatic therapies, but considering the recency of behavior therapies (for example) in pain treatment this is not too surprising. However, in a time when almost every published new drug study involves a double-blind crossover design with active and dummy placebo controls, it is not unreasonable to expect that psychological therapies should also develop such a sophisticated literature. It is quite possible to assign patients to A-B-A treatments involving, for example, hypnosis versus drugs, or to assign patients to a random groups or counterbalanced design involving biofeedback versus group therapy or drug versus operant conditioning paradigm.

It is one of the strengths of psychologists' training that experimental designs for clinical research are part of the program, and critical thinking about evaluation and outcome can co-exist with a readiness to explore new treatment approaches. Most pain treatment centers can easily accommodate such clinical research, and in my experience the physicians with medical responsibility for the patients involved, and the patients themselves, are eager to participate in any such reasonable study the psychologist may propose.

REFERENCES

1. Adler, C. S., and Adler, S. M. (1976): Headache, 16:189-191.
2. Agnew, D. C., and Merskey, H. (1976): Pain, 2: 73-81.
3. Akil, H., and Liebeskind, J. C. (1975): Brain Res., 94:279-296.
4. Anderson, J. A. D., Basker, M. A., and Dalton, R. (1975): Int. J. Clin. Exp. Hypn., 23:48-58.

5. Asberg, M., Thoren, P., Traskman, L., Bertilsson, L., and Ringberger, V. (1976): *Science*, 191: 478-480.
6. Bailey, C. A., and Davidson, P. O. (1976): *Pain*, 2:319-324.
7. Bond, M. R. (1971): *Brit. J. Psychiat.*, 119:671-678.
8. Bond, M. R. (1973): *J. Psychosom. Res.*, 17:257-263.
9. Bond, M. R., and Pearson, I. B. (1969): *J. Psychosom. Res.*, 13:13-19.
10. Bond, M. R., and Pilowsky, I. (1966): *J. Psychosom. Res.*, 10:203-208.
11. Bradley, J. J. (1963): *Brit. J. Psychiat.*, 109: 741-745.
12. Budzynski, T. H., Stoyva, J. M., Adler, C. S., and Mullaney, D. J. (1973): *Psychosom. Med.*, 35:484-496.
13. Cairns, D., Thomas, L., Mooney, V., and Pace, J. B. (1976): *Pain*, 2:301-308.
14. Chapman, C. R., Chen, A. C., and Bonica, J. J. (1977): *Pain*, 3:213-227.
15. Crockett, D. J., Prkachin, K. M., and Craig, K. D. (1977): *Pain*, 4:175-182.
16. Edmonds, E. P. (1947): *Ann. Rheum. Dis.*, 6:36-49.
17. Engel, G. L. (1959): *Am. J. Med.*, 26:899-918.
18. Eysenck, S. B. G. (1961): *J. Mental Science*, 107:417-430.
19. Finer, B. (1974): In: *Advances in Neurology, Vol. 4, International Symposium on Pain*, edited by J. J. Bonica, pp. 573-579. Raven Press, New York.
20. Fordyce, W. E. (1976): *Behavioral Methods for Chronic Pain and Illness*. Mosby, St. Louis.
21. Fordyce, W. E., Fowler, R. S., Jr., Lehmann, J. F., and De Lateur, B. J. (1968): *J. Chronic Dis.*, 21:179-190.
22. Fordyce, W. E., Fowler, R. S., Jr., Lehmann, J. F., De Lateur, B. J., Sand, P. L., and Trieschmann, R. B. (1973): *Arch. Physical Med. Rehab.*, 54:399-408.
23. Halliday, J. L. (1937): *Brit. Med. J.*, 1:213-217, 264-269.
24. Hilgard, E. R. (1975): *Pain*, 1:213-231.
25. Hilgard, E. R., and Hilgard, J. R. (1975): *Hypnosis in the Relief of Pain*. William Kaufmann, Los Altos, California.
26. Ignelzi, R. J., and Nyquist, J. K. (1976): *J. Neurosurg.*, 45:159-165.
27. Ignelzi, R. J., Sternbach, R. A., and Timmermans, G. (1977): *Pain*, 3:277-280.

28. Lynn, R., and Eysenck, H. J. (1961): Percept. Motor Skills, 12:161-162.
29. Maas, J. W. (1975): Arch. Gen. Psychiat., 32: 1357-1361.
30. McKenzie, R. E., Ehrisman, W. J., Montgomery, P. S., and Barnes, R. H. (1974): Headache, 13: 164-172.
31. Medina, J. L., Diamond, S., and Franklin, M. A. (1976): Headache, 16:115-118.
32. Melzack, R. (1975): Pain, 1:277-299.
33. Melzack, R. (1975): Pain, 1:357-373.
34. Melzack, R., and Torgerson, W. S. (1971): Anesthesiology, 34:50-59.
35. Merskey, H., and Hester, R. N. (1972): Postgrad. Med. J., 48:594-598.
36. Merskey, H., and Spear, F. G. (1967): Pain: Psychological and Psychiatric Aspects. Bailliere, Tindall and Cassell, London.
37. Miller, N. E. (1969): Science, 163:434-445.
38. Mitch, P. S., McGrady, A., and Iannone, A. (1976): Headache, 15:267-270.
39. Mitchell, K. R., and Mitchell, D. M. (1971): J. Psychosom. Res., 15:137-157.
40. Montgomery, P. S., and Ehrisman, W. J. (1976): Headache, 16:64-65.
41. Ohnhaus, E. E., and Adler, R. (1975): Pain, 1: 379-384.
42. Pilowsky, I. (1967): Brit. J. Psychiat., 113:89-93.
43. Pilowsky, I., and Bond. M. R. (1969): Psychosom. Med., 31:400-404.
44. Pilowsky, I., and Spence, N. D. (1975): J. Psychosom. Res., 19:279-287.
45. Pilowsky, I., and Spence, N. D. (1976): Pain, 2: 61-71.
46. Sargent, J. D., Green, E. E., and Walters, E. D. (1972): Headache, 12:120-124.
47. Sargent, J. D., Walters, E. D., and Green, E. E. (1973): Seminars in Psychiatry, 5:415-428.
48. Scott, J., and Huskisson, E. C. (1976): Pain, 2: 175-184.
49. Seres, J. L., and Newman, R. I. (1976): J. Neurosurg., 45:32-36.
50. Seres, J. L., Newman, R. I., Yospe, L. P., and Garlington, B. E. (1977): In: Pain Management: Symposium on the Neurosurgical Treatment of Pain, edited by L. J. Fletcher, pp. 33-53. Williams and Wilkins, Baltimore.
51. Sheehan, P. W. and Perry, C. W. (1976): Methodologies of Hypnosis. Erlbaum, Hillsdale, New Jersey (distributor, Halsted (Wiley), New York).

52. Solbach, P., and Sargent, J. D. (1977): Paper presented at 19th annual meeting of the American Association for the Study of Headache, San Francisco.

53. Stacher, G., Schuster, P., Bauer, P., Lahoda, R., and Schulze, D. (1975): *J. Psychosom. Res.*, 19:259-265.

54. Sternbach, R. A. (1968): *Pain: A Psychophysiological Analysis*. Academic Press, New York.

55. Sternbach, R. A. (1974): In: *Somatic Manifestations of Depressive Disorders*, edited by A. Kiev, pp. 107-119. Excerpta Medica, Princeton, New Jersey.

56. Sternbach, R. A. (1974): *Pain Patients: Traits and Treatment*. Academic Press, New York.

57. Sternbach, R. A. (1974): In: *Advances in Neurology, Vol. 4: International Symposium on Pain*, edited by J. J. Bonica, pp. 423-430. Raven Press, New York.

58. Sternbach, R. A. (1976): *Pain*, 2:2-4.

59. Sternbach, R. A., Deems, L. M., Timmermans, G., and Huey, L. Y. (1977): *Pain*, 3:105-110.

60. Sternbach, R. A., Ignelzi, R. J., Deems, L. M., and Timmermans, G. (1976): *Pain*, 2:35-41.

61. Sternbach, R. A., Janowsky, D. S., Huey, L. Y., and Segal, D. S. (1976): In: *Advances in Pain Research and Therapy, Vol. 1*, edited by J. J. Bonica and D. Albe-Fessard, pp. 601-606. Raven Press, New York.

62. Sternbach, R. A., Murphy, R. W., Timmermans, G., Greenhoot, J. H., and Akeson, W. H. (1974): In: *Advances in Neurology, Vol. 4: International Symposium on Pain*, edited by J. J. Bonica, pp. 281-288. Raven Press, New York.

63. Sternbach, R. A., and Timmermans, G. (1975): *Pain*, 1:177-181.

64. Sternbach, R. A., and Tursky, B. (1965): *Psychophysiology*, 1:241-246.

65. Szasz, T. S. (1957): *Pain and Pleasure*. Basic Books, New York.

66. Szasz, T. S. (1968): In: *Pain*, edited by A. Soulairac, J. Cahn, and J. Charpentier, pp. 93-113. Academic Press, New York.

67. Taub, A., and Campbell, J. N. (1974): In: *Advances in Neurology, Vol. 4, International Symposium on Pain*, edited by J. J. Bonica, pp. 727-732. Raven Press, New York.

68. Taub, A., and Collins, W. F., Jr. (1974): In: *Advances in Neurology, Vol. 4, International Symposium on Pain*, edited by J. J. Bonica, pp. 309-316. Raven Press, New York.

69. Timmermans, G., and Sternbach, R. A. (1976): In: Advances in Pain Research and Therapy, Vol. 1, edited by J. J. Bonica and D. Albe-Fessard, pp. 307–310. Raven Press, New York.

70. Tinling, D. C., and Klein, R. F. (1966): Psychosom. Med., 28:738–748.

71. Torebjork, H. E., and Hallin, R. G. (1974): In: Advances in Neurology, Vol. 4, International Symposium on Pain, edited by J. J. Bonica, pp. 733–736. Raven Press, New York.

72. Tursky, B., and Sternbach, R. A. (1967): Psychophysiology, 4:67–74.

73. Warner, G., and Lance, J. W. (1975): Med. J. Australia, 1:298–301.

74. White, J. C., and Sweet, W. H. (1969): Pain and the Neurosurgeon: A Forty-Year Experience. Charles C. Thomas, Springfield, Ill.

75. Wickramasekera, I. (1973): Headache, 13:74–76.

76. Wolff, B. B., and Jarvik, M. E. (1964): Am. J. Psychol., 77:589–599.

77. Wolff, B. B., Krasnegor, N. A., and Farr, R. S. (1965): Percept. Motor Skills, 21:675–683.

78. Woodforde, J. M., and Merskey, H. (1971): J. Psychosom. Res., 16:173–178.

79. Zborowski, M. (1969): People in Pain. Jossey-Bass, San Francisco.

SUBJECT INDEX

Subject Index